Diseases of the Abdomen and Pelvis

Diagnostic Imaging and Interventional Techniques

T0238916

J. Hodler • G.K. von Schulthess • Ch.L. Zollikofer (Eds)

DISEASES OF THE ABDOMEN AND PELVIS

DIAGNOSTIC IMAGING AND INTERVENTIONAL TECHNIQUES

**38th International Diagnostic Course
in Davos (IDKD)**
Davos, April 1-7, 2006

including the
Pediatric Satellite Course 'Kangaroo'
Davos, April 1-2, 2006

presented by the Foundation for the
Advancement of Education in Medical Radiology, Zurich

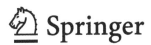 Springer

J. HODLER
Department of Radiology
University Hospital Balgrist
Zurich, Switzerland

G. K. VON SCHULTHESS
Universitätsspital
Nuklearmedizin
Zurich, Switzerland

CH. L. ZOLLIKOFER
Kantonsspital
Institut für Radiologie
Winterthur, Switzerland

Library of Congress Control Number: 2006922660

ISBN-10 88-470-0470-5 Springer Milan Berlin Heidelberg New York
ISBN-13 978-88-470-0470-2 Springer Milan Berlin Heidelberg New York

Springer is a part of Springer Science+Business Media

springer.com

© Springer-Verlag Italia 2006

Cover design: Simona Colombo, Milan, Italy
Typesetting: C & G, Cremona, Italy

Preface

The International Diagnostic Course in Davos (IDKD) offers a unique learning experience for imaging specialists in training as well as for experienced radiologists and clinicians wishing to be updated on the current state of the art and the latest developments in the fields of imaging and image-guided interventions.

This annual course is focused on organ systems and diseases rather than on modalities. This year's program deals with diseases of the abdomen and pelvis. During the course, the topics are discussed in group seminars and in plenary sessions with lectures by world-renowned experts and teachers. While the seminars present state-of-the-art summaries, the lectures are oriented towards future developments.

Accordingly, this Syllabus represents a condensed version of the contents presented under the 20 topics dealing with imaging and interventional therapies in abdominal and pelvic diseases. The topics encompass all the relevant imaging modalities including conventional X-rays, computed tomography, nuclear medicine, ultrasound and magnetic resonance angiography, as well as image-guided interventional techniques.

The Syllabus is designed to be an 'aide-mémoire' for the course participants so that they can fully concentrate on the lecture and participate in the discussions without the need of taking notes.

Additional information can be found on the IDKD website: www.idkd.ch

J. Hodler
G.K. von Schulthess
Ch.L. Zollikofer

Table of Contents

Seminars

Pediatric Satellite Course "Kangaroo"

List of Contributors

SEMINARS

Emergency Radiology of the Abdomen: The Acute Abdomen

B. Marincek[1], J.P. Heiken[2]

[1] Institute of Diagnostic Radiology, University Hospital Zurich, Zurich, Switzerland
[2] Mallinckrodt Institute of Radiology, Washington University School of Medicine, St. Louis, MO, USA

Introduction

The term 'acute abdomen' defines a clinical syndrome characterized by a history of hitherto undiagnosed abdominal pain lasting less than one week. A large number of disorders, ranging from benign, self-limited diseases to conditions that require immediate surgery, can cause acute abdominal pain. Eight conditions account for over 90% of patients who are referred to hospital and are seen on surgical wards with acute abdominal pain: acute appendicitis, acute cholecystitis, small bowel obstruction, urinary colic, perforated peptic ulcer, acute pancreatitis, acute diverticular disease, and non-specific, non-surgical abdominal pain ('dyspepsia', 'constipation').

Imaging Techniques

Clinical assessment of acute abdomen is often difficult because of the often non-specific findings of physical examination and laboratory investigations. In many centers plain radiographs of the abdomen, despite significant diagnostic limitations, serve as the initial radiological approach. Two views are usually taken, one supine and one erect. If the patient is unable to stand, a left lateral decubitus view is performed. For a systematic film analysis it is helpful to follow the mnemonic 'gas, mass, stones and bones' for the detection of (1) signs of mechanical bowel obstruction or paralytic ileus; (2) gas outside the bowel lumen in the peritoneal cavity (pneumoperitoneum), retroperitoneum, bowel wall, portal veins, or biliary tract; (3) mass or fluid collections, displacement of organs or bowel loops; (4) abnormal calcifications and/or calculi; (5) skeletal pathology.

The need for plain abdominal radiographs has declined due to the impact of cross-sectional imaging. The traditional indications for plain abdominal radiography – pneumoperitoneum, bowel obstruction, and the search for ureteral calculi – are better evaluated by unenhanced helical computed tomography (CT). A number of authors have shown that CT is clearly superior to plain radiography for diagnosing pneumoperitoneum, detecting a bowel obstruction, and for identifying ureteral calculi. The major obstacles to replacing plain abdominal radiography with unenhanced CT are its higher cost, more limited availability, and higher radiation dose.

Although ultrasonography (US) has gained widespread acceptance for evaluating the gallbladder in affected patients and the pelvis in children and women of reproductive age, CT is considered to be one of the most valued tools for triaging patients with acute abdominal pain. This is because it can provide a global perspective of the gastrointestinal (GI) tract, mesenteries, peritoneum, and retroperitoneum, inhibited by the presence of bowel gas and fat. Over recent years, most emergency centers have been equipped with newer helical CT scanners that permit imaging procedures to be performed in less time, with greater accuracy, and with less patient discomfort. The introduction of multidetector CT (MD-CT) technology, with advances in contrast dynamics and high-resolution volumetric data acqusition, has further enhanced the utility of CT in abdominal imaging. Image interpretation with helical CT and particularly with MD-CT is primarily performed at a workstation by manually paging or continuously scrolling up and down through the stack of reconstructed images. Additionally, multiplanar reformation (MPR) using coronal, sagittal, and curved planes, has evolved as a routine supplement to the axial images.

Three-dimensional volume rendered and maximum intensity projection (MIP) images are also easily produced from MDCT data sets. Inquiry about the site of abdominal pain facilitates the choice of imaging technique. For practical reasons, it is helpful to discuss the imaging strategies for acute pain localized in an abdominal quadrant separately from acute abdomen with diffuse pain and acute abdomen with flank or epigastric pain.

Acute Pain in an Abdominal Quadrant

Acute abdomen with pain localized in an abdominal quadrant can be classified as pain in the right upper, left upper, right lower, and left lower abdominal quadrant.

Right Upper Quadrant

Acute cholecystitis is by far the most common disease in the right upper quadrant. Other important diseases that resemble acute cholecystitis are pyogenic or amebic liver abscess, spontaneous rupture of a hepatic neoplasm (usually hepatocellular adenoma or carcinoma), hepatitis, and myocardial infarction.

US is the preferred imaging method for evaluating patients with acute right upper abdominal pain. It is a reliable technique for establishing the diagnosis of acute calculous cholecystitis. The primary criterion is the detection of gallstones. Secondary signs include the sonographic Murphy sign, gallbladder wall thickening by 3 mm or more, and pericholecystic fluid. Typically, a calculus obstructs the cystic duct in acute calculous cholecystitis. The trapped concentrated bile irritates the gallbladder wall, causing increased secretion, which in turn leads to distension and edema of the wall. Rising intraluminal pressure compresses the vessels, resulting in thrombosis, ischemia, and subsequent necrosis and perforation of the wall. Gallbladder perforation and complicating pericholecystic abscesses typically occur adjacent to the gallbladder fundus because of the sparse blood supply. CT may be useful for confirmation of the sonographic diagnosis. Emphysematous cholecystitis is a rare complication of acute cholecystitis and is associated with diabetes mellitus. US or CT demonstratation of gas in the wall and/or lumen of the gallbladder imply underlying gangrenous changes (Fig. 1). Acalculous acute cholecystitis accounts for approximately only 5% of cases of acute cholecystitis. It is especially common in intensive care unit patients. Prolonged bile stasis results in increased viscosity of the bile that ultimately leads to functional cystic duct obstruction.

US and CT are both accurate techniques for diagnosing liver abscesses. US usually reveals a round or oval hypoechoic mass with low-level internal echoes. Although the lesion may mimic a solid hepatic mass, the presence of through transmission is a clue to its cystic nature. Normally, pyogenic liver abscesses are the result of seeding from appendicitis or diverticulitis, or direct extension from cholecystitis or cholangitis. Amebic abscesses result from primary colonic involvement with seeding through the portal vein. In most cases, pyogenic and amebic abscesses are indistinguishable by US appearance. The CT appearances of pyogenic and amebic abscesses also show substantial overlap. Amebic abscesses are low attenuation cystic masses. An enhancing wall and a peripheral zone of edema surrounding the abscess are common but not universally present. Extrahepatic extension of the amebic abscess with involvement of chest wall, pleura, or adjacent viscera is a frequent finding. Whereas amebic abscesses are usually solitary and unilocular, pyogenic abscesses may be multiple or multiloculated and may demonstrate an irregular contour.

Spontaneous rupture of a hepatocellular carcinoma and subsequent hemoperitoneum represent a frequent complication found in countries with a high incidence of

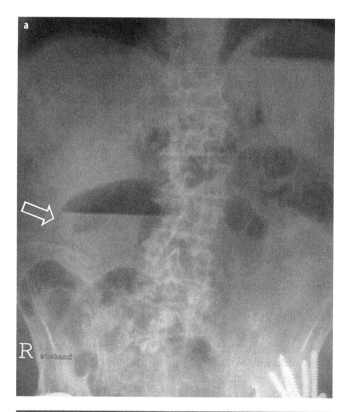

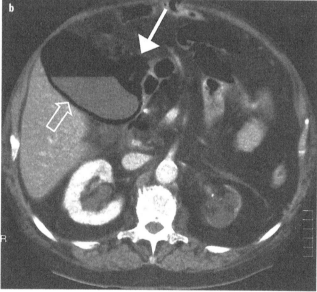

Fig. 1. A 74-year-old man with known diabetes mellitus presents with acute abdominal pain in the right upper quadrant. **a** Plain abdominal radiograph shows a fluid-gas level in the distended gallbladder and gas in the gallbladder wall (*open arrow*). **b** MDCT depicts the dilated gallbladder with intramural gas (*open arrow*), indicative of emphysematous cholecystitis. In addition, extraluminal/extramural gas is present due to walled-off gallbladder perforation (*arrow*). Hydronephrosis and parenchymal atrophy of the left kidney

this tumor, but uncommon in Western countries. Subcapsular localization and tumor necrosis have been implicated in pathogenesis. US, and especially CT, are the most useful techniques for diagnosing a ruptured hepatocellular carcinoma, which appears as a peripheral or subcapsular mass. Spontaneous hemorrhage within a hepatocellular adenoma occurs most commonly in women taking oral contraceptives. Capsular rupture with subsequent hemoperitoneum is an uncommon complication. On CT, high-density intraperitoneal fluid confirms the diagnosis of hemoperitoneum, and extravasation of contrast material is indicative of active bleeding.

Left Upper Quadrant

Acute abdomen with left upper quadrant pain is not frequent. Splenic infarction, splenic abscess, gastritis, and gastric or duodenal ulcer are the most important causes. US is usually used for screening, and CT enables accurate further evaluation. The diagnosis of gastric pathology is established by endoscopy, with imaging playing a minor role.

Common causes of splenic infarction include bacterial endocarditis, portal hypertension, and underlying splenomegaly. Pancreatitis that extends into the splenic hilum can also result in infarction. Splenic infarction may be focal or global. Typical focal splenic infarcts appear as peripheral wedge-shaped defects, hypoechoic at US and hypodense at CT, respectively. Most splenic abscesses are associated with hematogenous dissemination of infection, such as bacterial endocarditis or tuberculosis. Intravenous drug abusers are predominantly affected. Both US and CT are sensitive, but specificity is low. On US, most abscesses appear as hypo- or anechoic, poorly defined lesions; on CT, they typically appear as rounded, low-density lesions with rim enhancement.

Right Lower Quadrant

Acute appendicitis is not only the most frequent cause of acute right lower quadrant pain, but also the most commonly encountered cause of acute abdomen. Other diseases manifesting acute right lower quadrant pain include acute terminal ileitis (Crohn's disease), acute typhlitis, right sided colonic diverticulitis and, in women, pelvic inflammatory disease, complications of ovarian cyst (hemorrhage, torsion and leak), endometriosis, or ectopic pregnancy.

Most patients with typical clinical findings of acute appendicitis undergo immediate surgery without preoperative imaging. Since diagnosis is uncertain in up to one third of patients because of atypical symptoms, many centers today request appendiceal imaging for clinically equivocal patients. Although plain radiography continues to play a role in evaluating patients with acute right lower quadrant pain, its role is quite limited. Less than 50% of patients with appendicitis show an abnormality on plain radiographs. The most specific finding is the presence of an appendicolith, which is usually calcified, solitary, and rounded.

US has become an important imaging option in the evaluation of suspected acute appendicitis, particularly in children, pregnant women, and women of reproductive age. The prime sonographic criterion is the demonstration of a swollen, non-compressible appendix greater than 7 mm in

diameter with a target configuration (Fig. 2). Generally, the normal appendix cannot be defined with US, thus, clear visualization of the appendix is suggestive of inflammation.

Advantages of US include lack of ionizing radiation, relatively low cost, and widespread availability. On the other hand, US requires considerable skill and is difficult to perform in obese patients, patients with severe pain, and patients likely to have a complicating periappendiceal abscess. When the sonographic findings are unclear, CT can provide a rapid and definitive diagnosis.

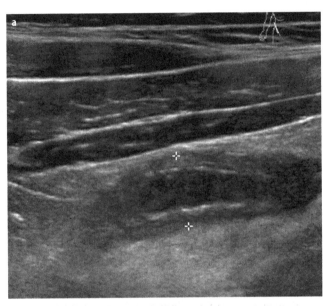

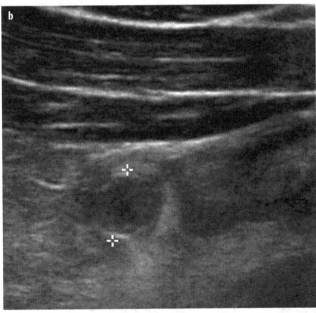

Fig. 2. A 25-year-old man presented with acute abdominal pain in the right lower abdominal quadrant. Physical examination and laboratory tests revealing elevated white blood cell counts, raised the suspicion of acute appendicitis. Longitudinal (**a**) and perpendicular (**b**) graded compression US shows an enlarged appendix (*cursors*, diameter > 10 mm) with edematous thickening of the appendical wall, confirming the diagnosis of acute appendicitis

CT has emerged in many centers as the primary imaging modality for patients with suspected acute appendicitis due to its exceptional accuracy. In the case of mild disease, the findings include a dilated, fluid-filled appendix with a calcified appendicolith or inflammatory changes of the mesenteric fat (Fig. 3). An inflammatory mass or an abscess may develop with disease progression and perforation.

Diverticulitis rarely manifests itself as a right-sided condition. Right-sided colonic diverticula are often congenital, solitary and true diverticula, unlike sigmoid diverticula. The normal appendix should be visible in right-sided diverticulitis. If the appendix cannot be identified, right-sided omental infarction or epiploic appendagitis must be considered in the differential diagnosis.

Left Lower Quadrant

Diverticulitis is the most common cause of acute abdominal pain in the left lower quadrant. Diverticulitis occurs in up to 25% of patients with known diverticulosis and typically involves the sigmoid colon. CT has replaced barium enema examinations because it is very sensitive and approaches 100% specificity and accuracy in the diagnosis or exclusion of diverticulitis. CT is also very useful in establishing the presence of pericolic complications and differentiating sigmoid diverticulitis from carcinoma – a major differential diagnostic consideration.

Superimposed on diverticulosis, the CT diagnosis of acute diverticulitis is based on the identification of segmental colonic wall thickening and pericolic inflammatory changes, such as fat stranding, inflammatory mass, gas bubbles, abscess, or free fluid (Fig. 4). Occasionally, patients with diverticulitis may manifest pneumaturia because of a complicating enterovesical fistula.

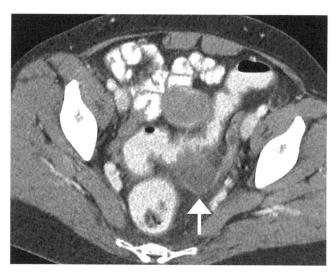

Fig. 4. 55-year-old man with known diverticular disease and acute abdominal pain in the left lower quadrant. MDCT shows a narrowed segment of the sigmoid colon with wall thickening, pericolic inflammatory changes, and an adjacent fluid-collection with marked peripheral enhancement (*arrow*), indicating an abscess after walled-off perforation in acute diverticulitis

Acute Abdomen with Diffuse Pain

Any disorder that irritates a large portion of the GI tract and/or the peritoneum will cause diffuse abdominal pain. The most common disorder is gastroenterocolitis. Other important disorders are bowel obstruction, ischemic bowel disease, and GI tract perforation.

Bowel Obstruction

Bowel obstruction is a frequent cause of abdominal pain and accounts for approximately 20% of surgical admissions for acute abdominal conditions. The small bowel is involved in 60-80% of cases. Frequent causes of small bowel obstruction are adhesions resulting from prior surgery, hernias, and neoplasms. In the large bowel, mechanical obstruction is commonly due to diverticular disease or colorectal carcinoma. 5-10% of cases of large bowel obstruction are caused by volvulus, which is most commonly in the sigmoid, followed by the cecum.

The diagnosis of bowel obstruction is established on clinical grounds and usually confirmed with plain abdominal radiographs. Because of the diagnostic limitations of plain films, CT is increasingly used to establish the diagnosis, identify the site, level, and cause of obstruction and determine the presence or absence of associated bowel ischemia. CT can be useful for differentiating between simple and closed loop obstruction. Closed loop obstruction is a form of mechanical bowel obstruction in which two points along the course of the bowel are obstructed at a single site. It is usually secondary to an adhesive band or a hernia. A closed loop tends to involve the mesentery and is prone to produce a volvulus, thus representing the most

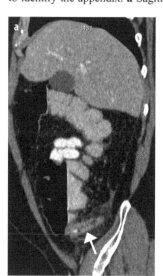

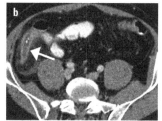

Fig. 3. 45-year-old man with elevated white blood cells and acute pain in the right lower abdominal quadrant. US examination was unable to identify the appendix. **a** Sagittal MDCT depicts marked enlargement of the retrocecal appendix (*arrow* in **a** and **b**), with wall thickening, mural enhancement, and adjacent fat stranding. **b** Transverse MDCT shows two appendicoliths within the appendical lumen. The US-diagnosis of acute appendicitis is difficult to establish in a retrocecal appendix

common cause of strangulation. However, only volvulus of the large bowel is associated with classic features on plain abdominal radiographs. The sigmoid volvulus produces a distended loop, with the twisted mesenteric root pointing to the origin of the volvulus, i.e., to the sigmoid.

CT is particularly reliable in higher grades of bowel obstruction. It has proved useful for characterizing bowel obstruction from various causes, including adhesions, hernia, neoplasm, extrinsic compression, inflammatory bowel disease, radiation enteropathy, intussusception, gallstone ileus, or volvulus. The essential CT finding of bowel obstruction is the delineation of a transition zone between the dilated and decompressed bowel. Careful inspection of the transition zone and luminal contents usually reveals the underlying cause of obstruction. However, the presumed point of transition from dilated to non-dilated bowel can be difficult to determine in the axial plane. MDCT facilitates this task by providing the radiologist with a volumetric data set that can be viewed in the axial, sagittal, or coronal plane or any combination of the three. These MPR views centered on the anticipated transition point help to determine the site, level, and cause of obstruction.

Mechanical obstruction has to be differentiated from paralytic ileus. Numerous causes exist for both diffuse and localized paralytic ileus. Paralytic ileus is a common problem after abdominal surgery. It may be secondary to ischemic conditions, inflammatory or infectious disease, abnormal electrolyte, metabolite, drug or hormonal levels, or innervation defects. A massively dilated colon with a thickened wall ('thumbprinting') caused by wall edema and inflammation is seen with toxic megacolon in pseudomembranous colitis. Toxic megacolon is the radiological manifestation of a paralytic ileus.

Ischemic Bowel Disease

Arterial or venous occlusion or thrombosis and hypoperfusion are predominant causes of bowel ischemia. Usually, a combination of these factors is observed. The predominance of one factor determines the outcome and the findings on CT. Diminished bowel wall enhancement is the only direct sign of vascular impairment of the bowel and has been reported in predominantly arterial disease, such as infarction, as well as in predominantly venous diseases, such as strangulation. Other CT findings are direct visualization of the thrombus in the superior mesenteric artery or vein. Bowel distention and bowel wall edema are nonspecific findings and can be seen with inflammatory or infectious causes. Bowel distention reflects the interruption of peristaltic activity in ischemic segments.

In closed loop bowel obstruction the closed loop can become strangulated, i.e., ischemic, although the progression of a closed loop obstruction to a strangulated one is not inevitable. The reported prevalence of strangulating obstruction ranges from 5-40%. Strangulation is a predominantly venous disease. The most frequent abnormality seen on CT is bowel wall thickening. The thickened bowel wall is sometimes associated with the target sign, alternating layers of high and low attenuation within the thickened bowel wall, which results from submucosal edema and hemorrhage. The bowel segment proximal to an obstruction can become ischemic due to severe bowel distention. CT findings that suggest subsequent infarction include non-enhancement of the bowel wall, gas in the bowel wall, mesenteric or portal veins, edema/hemorrhage in the mesentery adjacent to thickened and/or dilated bowel loops, and ascites (Fig. 5).

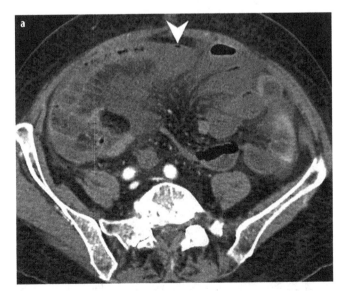 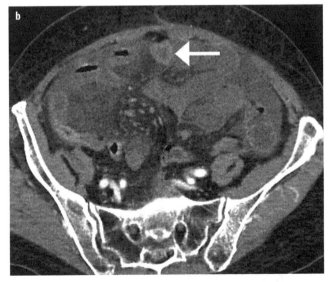

Fig. 5. 76-year-old man with acute diffuse abdominal pain and with a history of abdominal surgery performed five weeks previously. **a** Transverse MDCT demonstrates mesenteric edema and infarction of the distal ileum (*arrowhead*) with intramural gas. **b** Transverse MDCT at a level below depicts thickening of the bowel wall with irregular mucosal enhancement (*arrow*) indicative of bowel ischemia. Intraoperatively, a strangulating small bowel volvulus secondary to adhesion of the distal ileum was identified

GI Tract Perforation

Pneumoperitoneum usually starts with localized pain and culminates in diffuse pain after peritonitis has developed. It may result from a variety of causes. Gastroduodenal perforation associated with peptic ulcer or necrotic neoplasm has become less frequent in the last few decades due to earlier diagnosis and improved therapy. At the same time, the incidence of gastroduodenal perforations resulting from endoscopic instrumentation has increased. Perforation of the small bowel is relatively uncommon. Spontaneous rupture of the large bowel is more frequent and can occur in a markedly dilated colon proximal to an obstructing lesion (tumor, volvulus) or when the bowel wall is friable (ischemic or ulcerative colitis, necrotic neoplasm). Over the last decades, fiberoptic endoscopy has been increasingly performed for evaluation and biopsy of colorectal lesions, as well as for polypectomy; these procedures cause perforation in 0.5-3% of patients.

Pneumoperitoneum can be recognized by the presence of subdiaphragmatic gas on an erect chest radiograph or an erect or left lateral decubitus radiograph of the abdomen. An abundant pneumoperitoneum is indicative of a perforation complicating large bowel obstruction, and moderate quantities of free gas are seen in the perforation of the stomach. Only small quantities of gas escape with perforation of the small bowel, because the small bowel does not usually contain gas. Detection of subtle pneumoperitoneum is often difficult. CT is far more sensitive than conventional radiography for the detection of a small pneumoperitoneum, and it has thus become the modality of choice in cases that are unclear on a conventional radiograph. To enhance the sensitivity of CT for extraluminal gas, the images are also viewed at 'lung window' settings. On CT, small amounts of gas around the stomach and the liver are seen mainly after gastroduodenal or small bowel perforation.

Retroperitoneal perforations (duodenal loop beyond the bulbar segment, appendix, posterior aspect of ascending and descending colon, rectum below the peritoneal reflection) tend to be contained locally and remain clinically silent for several hours or days. Retroperitoneal gas has a mottled appearance and may extend along the psoas muscles. In contrast to intraperitoneal gas, retroperitoneal gas does not move freely when the patient's position is changed from supine to upright for plain abdominal radiographs.

Acute Abdomen with Flank or Epigastric Pain

Acute flank or epigastric pain is commonly a manifestation of retroperitoneal pathology, especially urinary colic, acute pancreatitis, or leaking abdominal aortic aneurysm.

Urinary Colic

For several decades, intravenous urography has been the primary imaging technique used in patients with flank pain thought to be caused by urinary colic. Abdominal radiograph and US are considered useful for those patients with contraindications to irradiation or contrast media. However, because of the low sensitivity of abdominal radiographs and US for urinary tract calculi, the role of unenhanced CT has grown rapidly. On CT, virtually all ureteral stones are radiopaque, regardless of their chemical composition. Uric acid stones have attenuation values of 300-500 Hounsfield units (HU), and calcium-based stones have attenuation values > 1,000 HU. In addition to the direct demonstration of a ureteral stone, secondary signs of ureterolithiasis may be seen, including hydroureter, hydronephrosis, perinephric stranding, and renal enlargement (Fig. 6). Perinephric stranding and edema result from reabsorbed urine infiltrating the perinephric space along the bridging septa of Kunin. The more extensive the perinephric edema as shown on unenhanced CT, the higher the degree of urinary tract obstruction. Focal periureteral stranding resulting from local inflammatory reaction or irritation and induced by the passage of a stone helps localize subtle calculi. MDCT is

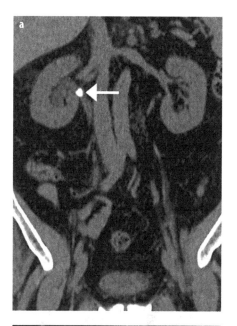

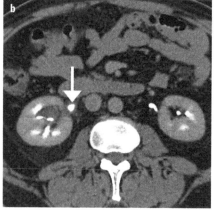

Fig. 6. 46-year-old man with right-sided flank pain. Coronal MDCT reconstruction (**a**) and transverse MDCT after intravenous contrast administration (**b**) demonstrate an obstructing stone at the uretero-pelvic junction (*arrow*) with dilatation of the renal pelvis and of the calices

favored over single-detector CT because it provides coronal MPRs, which often portray the urinary tract more effectively than axial images.

When no stone is detected, a search for an alternative diagnosis should be performed. Non-calculus urinary tract abnormalities causing symptoms of colic include acute pyelonephritis, renal cell carcinoma, acute renal vein thrombosis and renal infarction. Extraurinary diseases, such as appendicitis, diverticultis, small bowel obstruction, pancreatitis, and retroperitoneal hemorrhage may also simulate acute urinary colic. Occasionally, repeating the CT examination with intravenous, oral, or rectally administered contrast material may be required.

Acute Pancreatitis

Acute pancreatitis is an important disease causing epigastric pain. US is helpful for the demonstration of gallstones as a cause of acute pancreatitis and for the follow-up of known fluid collections. CT has become the imaging modality of choice to stage the extent of disease and to detect complications because CT findings correlate well with the clinical severity of acute pancreatitis. Pancreatic enlargement due to interstitial parenchymal edema may progress to pancreatic exudate collecting in the anterior pararenal space, the transverse mesocolon, the mesenteric root, and the lesser sac. The pancreatic parenchyma may undergo necrosis or hemorrhage. Severe pancreatitis is often complicated by thrombosis of the splenic and portal vein.

Acute pancreatic and peripancreatic fluid collections may evolve into pseudocysts. Pseudocysts exhibit defined capsules. A pseudocyst can erode peripancreatic vessels, resulting in bleeding or formation of a pseudoaneurysm. Larger aneurysms can be diagnosed by CT or sonographically with Doppler; angiography may be necessary to diagnose small pseudoaneurysms (< 1 cm).

Leaking Aneurysm of Abdominal Aorta or Iliac Artery

One of the most life-threatening alternative diagnoses in acute flank pain is a leaking aneurysm of the abdominal aorta or iliac artery. When a patient with suspected rupture of an abdominal aortic aneurysm is hemodynamically unstable, US is the initial imaging technique used. The examination can be performed rapidly using portable equipment in the emergency room. However, the diagnosis of para-aortic hemorrhage by US is poor.

In hemodynamically stable patients non-contrast-enhanced CT is the initial imaging test of choice. Non-contrast CT can almost always demonstrate a para-aortic hematoma if present and may show additional findings helpful in establishing the diagnosis, such as a high-attenuating crescent sign. If the non-contrast CT findings are equivocal or if endoluminal stent graft repair of the aorta is planned, contrast-enhanced CT should be performed.

Conclusions

The practice of radiology in imaging patients with acute abdomen has changed dramatically in the last few years. The time-honored plain abdominal radiographs have been largely replaced with US and CT. In particular, helical CT and more recently, MDCT permit the examination to be performed in less time, with greater diagnostic accuracy, and with less patient discomfort. The topographic classification of pain (i.e., localized pain in one of the four abdominal quadrants, diffuse abdominal pain and flank or epigastric pain) facilitates finding the answer to specific questions. Therefore, close co-operation with the referring physician prior to imaging remains essential for rapid and accurate diagnosis.

Suggested Reading

Bhalla S, Menias CO, Heiken JP (2003) CT of acute abdominal aortic disorders. Radiol Clin N Am 41:1153-1169

Freeman AH (2001) CT and bowel disease. Br J Radiol 74:4-14

Gore RM, Miller FH, Pereles FS et al (2000) Helical CT in the evaluation of the acute abdomen. AJR Am J Roentgenol 174:901-913

Macari M, Megibow A (2001) Imaging of suspected acute small bowel obstruction. Seminars in Roentgenology XXXVI:108-117

Mindelzun RE, Jeffrey RB (1997) Unenhanced helical CT for evaluating acute abdominal pain: a little more cost, a lot more information. Radiology 205:43-47

Novelline RA, Rhea JT, Rao PM, Stuk JL (1999) Helical CT in emergency radiology. Radiology 213:321-339

Smith RC, Varanelli M (2000) Diagnosis and management of acute ureterolithiasis. AJR Am J Roentgenol 175:3-6

Taourel P, Kessler N, Lesnik A et al (2003) Helical CT of large bowel obstruction. Abdom Imaging 28:267-275

Urban BA, Fishman EK (2000) Tailored helical CT evaluation of acute abdomen. Radiographics 20:725-749

Wiesner W, Khurana B, Ji H, Ros PR (2003) CT of acute bowel ischemia. Radiology 226:635-650

Trauma of the Abdomen and Pelvis I

P.J. Kenney

University of Alabama Medical Center, Birmingham, AL, USA

Introduction

Trauma has become a significant health problem, in part due to high velocity transportation and the use of penetrating weapons, especially firearms. Not only the young, but also the elderly and pregnant women are affected. Improvements for those affected include more rapid rescue, better organization of trauma centers, and advances in treatment. There are three recent trends: the increased tendency for non-operative care, the resulting increased need for accurate non-invasive imaging diagnosis, and a desire for cost-effective use of imaging. One aspect of the trend towards non-operative care is the desire to avoid non-therapeutic surgery; this is possible if imaging can identify those patients who require surgery. Another aspect is the realization that non-operative care can result in better long-term outcome, such as salvaging splenic and renal function. Lastly, imaging evaluation with a high negative predictive value may allow for discharge of trauma victims directly from the Emergency Department, avoiding hospital admission for observation.

CT versus Ultrasound

Controversy exists about the appropriate use of CT versus ultrasound (US). Each has advantages and disadvantages [1-3]. In general, CT has been shown to have the best statistical accuracy for detecting, characterizing and excluding injuries. If the volume of trauma justifies it, CT can be located in the trauma suite such that even unstable patients can be examined quickly and without compromise. This has been done in our institution and there is heavy reliance on CT for rapid accurate diagnosis, avoiding diagnostic peritoneal lavage and non-therapeutic laparotomies. CT is more reliable at excluding injury in those who may be discharged home, avoiding observation in hospital.

However CT may be overused – in one study only three of 100 patients had an alteration in clinical management after follow-up CT [4]. Sonography can detect significant injuries that can be treated; conversely, low risk patients with normal sonograms may be observed and possibly avoid CT [2, 3]. One of the strengths of US is its ability to detect peritoneal fluid, a significant but non-specific finding indicative of abdominal injury. However, abnormal US often requires further evaluation by CT. In a large study, US had 86% sensitivity and 98% specificity, with 43 false negative and 23 indeterminate studies, including six splenic, one liver, one renal, one pancreatic and one bowel injury [3]. Although the incidence of significant injury in the absence of free intraperitoneal fluid is low, it does occur. A multi-institutional study found a 28% incidence of splenic and hepatic injury in patients with no or minimal free fluid on CT [5]. In patients with seat belt marks, where bowel and mesenteric injury are common, US has been reported to miss up to 78% of significant injuries [6].

The advent of multidetector CT (MDCT) for trauma has allowed some improvements, although routine trauma CT of the abdomen has changed little. Use of MDCT allows for more rapid acquisition of high quality images of multiple body parts, such as examination of the head, neck, chest, abdomen and pelvis. It allows for better reformatting of images, with either thinner slice reconstructions, or other planes. In addition, if clinical circumstances warrant, a CT angiogram can be performed immediately followed by routine trauma imaging.

In traumatized pregnant women, US should be the first examination. It can evaluate the pregnancy, documenting fetal viability. US is nearly as accurate in detecting abnormal fluid in pregnant, as in non-pregnant patients [7]. If US shows fluid or other injury, CT is justified to obtain the best evaluation (Fig. 1). The best outcome for the fetus is assured by the best care of the mother. The radiation risk is reasonable if there is life-threatening injury, necessitating prompt diagnosis and treatment [8].

Urinary Tract

Installation of CT in the Trauma unit, and nearly universal use of CT, has altered our assessment of urinary tract trauma. While significant hematuria has been shown to be the best indicator of urinary tract injury, presently the decision to perform CT has little to do with presence or

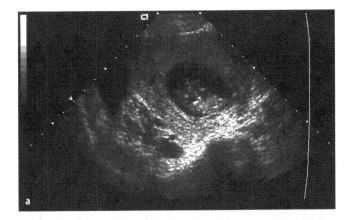

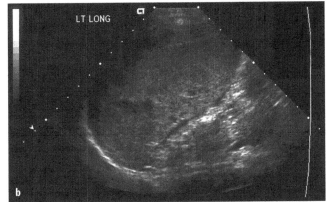

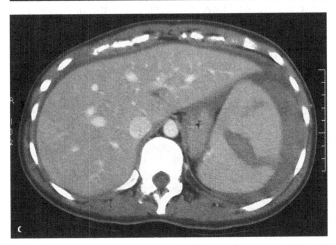

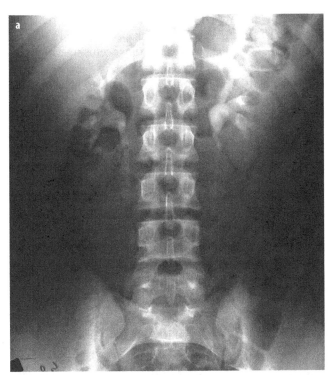

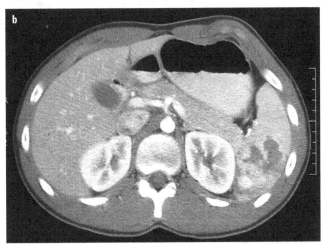

Fig. 2. Hematuria and left upper quadrant pain after football injury. **a** IVU shows no abnormality. **b** Subsequent CT for persistent pain showed free fluid in pelvis and extensive splenic laceration with extensive 'blush'. Surgery confirmed grade 4 splenic injury

Fig. 1. Pregnant female who suffered high speed motor vehicle collision. **a** US demonstrates intrauterine fetus (heart motion documented) and free pelvic fluid. **b** US shows perisplenic fluid with hypoechoic defect. **c** CT confirms splenic laceration; note higher density of perisplenic hematoma compared to rim of fluid about liver (sentinel clot sign)

absence of hematuria. CT is a primary investigation, after standard radiographs, for those patients with significant mechanism of injury or any signs or symptoms of significant injury. While intravenous urography (IVU) can detect renal injuries, it is less sensitive than CT, not accurate for grading the renal injury and cannot assess other organ systems (Fig. 2). US has a limited ability to evaluate renal injury [9]. Although screening US has val-

ue in trauma in general, it has severe limitations in detecting genitourinary (GU) injury. Free intraperitoneal fluid may not result from renal injury; although it may from bladder rupture, US cannot diagnose bladder injury. In a study of 4,320 trauma patients who had undergone US, 33 of 99 patients with urologic injury had false negative US. The sensitivity was only 56% for those with isolated urologic injury [10]. US is also not capable of grading renal injuries.

CT has excellent negative predictive value for renal injury. Presence and type of renal injury can be accurately indicated [11]. Renal contusion demonstrates ill-defined regions of diminished enhancement. Segmental renal infarction is identified as a wedge shaped, well-defined area of non-enhancement, and renal artery occlusion can be accurately diagnosed by its complete lack of enhancement or excretion by the kidney, usually with little to no associated hematoma. Angiography is thus not needed, and conservative therapy is now most often used. Most renal injuries are lacerations, with simple laceration limited to the cortex, and deep laceration extending into the collecting system, which may show extravasation. Scans delayed between 2 and 10 minutes aid in demonstrating or excluding extravasation (Fig. 3), although in most cases small amounts of extravasation will resolve with conservative therapy. Subcapsular hematoma is delimited by the renal cortex and may deform the renal surface; perinephric hematoma extends from the renal surface to fill Gerota's space, but does not deform renal contours, although it may displace the kidney. CT is excellent at demonstrating the extent of

hematoma, and evaluating enlargement on follow-up scans [11]. Renal fracture indicates a single complete fracture plane, often extending through the collecting system; multiple planes of disruption are seen with shattered kidney. CT can also diagnose ureteropelvic junction (UPJ) avulsion or ureteral injury, demonstrating lack of opacification of the ureter, retroperitoneal water attenuation collections adjacent to pelvis or ureter, and possibly extravasation of contrast on delay scans [11].

Although the American Association for Surgery of Trauma (AAST) Organ Injury Severity Scale for the kidney includes lesions with a different appearance in each category (1: contusion, small subcapsular hematoma, 2: < 1 cm laceration without extravasation, 3: > 1 cm laceration without extravasation, 4: deep laceration with extravasation or main renal artery or vein injury, 5: shattered kidney or UPJ avulsion), it has been shown to correlate with need for surgery and outcome [12].

Urethral injuries are predominantly seen in males. Anterior urethral ruptures are most commonly seen due to straddle injury. Posterior urethral ruptures most often are due to compressive force and resultant pubic bone fractures, although both anterior and posterior urethral injury can result from penetrating injury. Retrograde urethrography is the only accurate diagnostic imaging procedure. If a urethral injury is strongly suspected, a urethrogram should be performed before passage of a catheter (Fig. 4). However, in patients with moderate risk, a urethral catheter may be gently passed and the patient may go on to CT. A pericatheter urethrogram may then be performed after other injuries are stabilized. Urethral in-

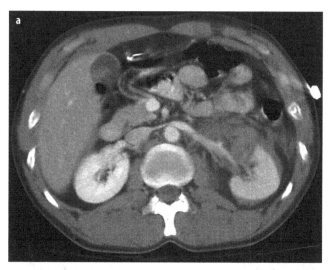

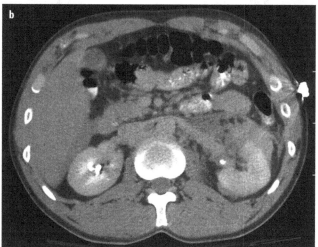

Fig. 3. Hematuria after fall from power line. **a** Initial CT shows left renal laceration with perinephric hematoma. **b** Delay image shows no leak from collecting system

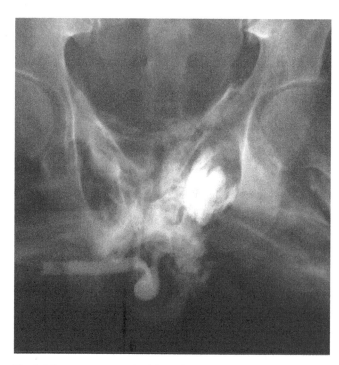

Fig. 4. Blunt trauma resulted in pubic rami fractures. Retrograde urethrogram reveals type 3 posterior urethral rupture

juries may be classified as Type 1: posterior urethra stretched but intact, Type 2: tear of membranous urethra above urogenital diaphragm, Type 3: tear of posterior urethra above and below urogenital diaphragm, Type 4: bladder neck injury and Type 5: anterior urethral injury [13].

Although urethrography remains the standard, CT findings have been described in urethral injury, which may be useful if CT is performed as the initial study. Obscuration of normal periurethral landmarks, in particular distortion or obscuration of urogenital diaphragm fat planes and hematoma of the ischiocavernosus muscle, are commonly seen in those with urethral injury [14]. Alternatively, completely normal perineal anatomy may exclude significant injury, but further investigation is needed.

Bladder injuries, which consist of contusions and ruptures, are most commonly extraperitoneal, less commonly intraperitoneal, or are combined in about 5% of cases. They have classically been detected with standard radiographic cystography (Fig. 5). While CT with only intravenous contrast may fail to identify extravasation from a ruptured bladder, several studies have shown very high accuracy for CT cystography, which is now our standard (Fig. 6). In those with suspected bladder rupture (primarily those with gross hematuria, over 25 red blood cells per high power field [rbc/hpf] with pelvic fractures, or unexplained pelvic fluid), we perform standard CT with the bladder catheter clamped. If there is no extravasation, the bladder is drained then refilled with 300-500 cc of dilute contrast and the pelvis is rescanned. Bladder ruptures are virtually always associated with fluid or hematoma in the pelvis, but such blood or fluid

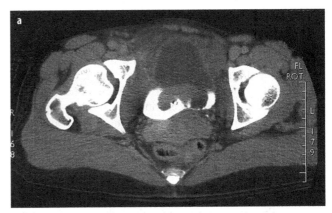

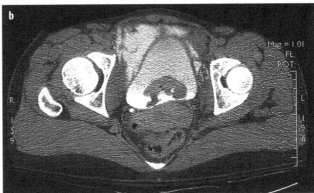

Fig. 6. Gross hematuria following motor vehicle collision resulting in extensive pelvic fractures. **a** Standard CT shows pelvic fluid but no extravasation. **b** CT cystogram documents extraperitoneal bladder rupture (note clot in bladder)

may be due to splenic or other injuries, or pelvic fracture. Extravasation low in the pelvis, not outlining bowel loops (and which may extend up the retroperitoneum) indicates extraperitoneal rupture that most often can be managed conservatively. Extravasation high near the dome outlining bowel loops or extending to the gutters or higher indicates intraperitoneal rupture, and is more often managed surgically [15].

Bowel and Mesenteric Injury

Bowel and mesenteric injury are found in about 5% of patients having surgery for trauma, seen in 0.7% of traumatized patients [1, 16]. Mechanism of injury is direct compressive force, including from seatbelts, although deceleration may play a role. Morbidity and mortality can occur if peritonitis and resulting abscess are missed. Clinical signs and symptoms are non-specific. Although positive diagnostic peritoneal lavage (DPL) or free fluid on sonography may be due to bowel or mesenteric injury, these findings are non-specific [2].

Although some have commented on the difficulty of correct diagnosis by CT, CT is the most accurate diagnostic modality, with a reported sensitivity of 88-96% and a specificity of 80-99% [16-20]. Use of oral contrast,

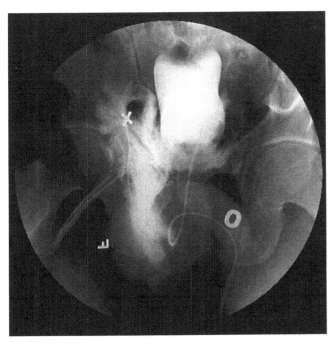

Fig. 5. Gross hematuria after gunshot wound to pelvis. Standard cystogram shows extraperitoneal rupture (*X*, entry site; *O*, exit)

and early scanning after rapid injection of high volume intravenous contrast allows detection of extravasation [21]. Active bleeding is seen as a focal collection with attentuation similar to the aorta at the same level and different from the adjacent organ. Contrast extravasation, whether intravenous contrast from a mesenteric vessel or oral contrast from the bowel lumen, is the most specific sign of mesenteric or bowel injury, but is not common – it was seen in only seven of 26 patients with bowel injury [17]. Free air is thought to be a good sign of perforated bowel, but in fact it has limited value; it is infrequently seen in those patients with bowel injury, and may in fact represent air tracking into the peritoneum from thoracic injuries. Free air was seen in only 28% of true positive CT scans, but in 2% of false positive scans [16]. The commonest finding was unexplained free fluid, even though 70% of those with only unexplained free fluid had no bowel injury. Other findings, such as focal bowel wall thickening, interloop fluid, mesenteric stranding or frank hematoma are often seen (Fig. 7). If a single finding is seen, likelihood of injury is low; a combination of findings, particularly free fluid without an obvious source in combination with focal bowel wall thickening and/or mesenteric stranding is very suggestive of bowel injury and such patients should be further explored or followed very carefully.

Oral contrast presents a risk, although low, of adverse events, including aspiration pneumonia. Given this and the low rate of visible bowel contrast leak, some have questioned the use of oral contrast to detect bowel injury. One study of 1,000 patients [22] and another of 500 [23] showed similar accuracy to previous reports with oral contrast – with a sensitivity of 82-95%, and a specificity of 99%. At our institution, the use of oral contrast has been discontinued in trauma patients with no recognized ill effect.

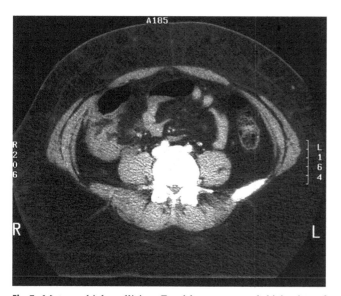

Fig. 7. Motor vehicle collision. Focal hematoma and thickening of cecum; cecal laceration was found at surgery

Splenic Injuries

The spleen is the most frequently injured abdominal organ in blunt trauma. There may be signs of blood loss, or left upper quadrant pain, but the diagnosis largely rests on imaging or surgical exploration. A trend towards non-operative management is supported by evidence that long-term health is better in those who have had splenic function preserved. This necessitates accurate non-invasive diagnosis, and is aided by signs predictive of success or failure of conservative management.

Splenic injuries can cause free fluid, perisplenically or elsewhere, which can readily be detected by sonography. Splenic injury may alter echo texture: lacerations may be anechoic if there is rapid bleeding, but are more commonly more echogenic than normal spleen [2]. With such findings on sonography, the decision whether to further evaluate with CT or to proceed to surgery can be made on clinical grounds (Fig. 1). Splenic injuries may be missed by sonography, particularly if not associated with free fluid. In one large study, there were 43 false negative sonograms, including six splenic ruptures that required surgery [3].

CT is quite sensitive for the detection of splenic injuries [24]. Subcapsular hematoma is seen as a crescentic low attenuation peripheral rim, and intraparenchymal hematoma is seen as a rounded area within the spleen with low attenuation and no enhancement. Lacerations are common, seen as linear or branching low attenuation lesions which often extend to the surface, often associated with perisplenic or free fluid (Fig. 1, 2). Hemoperitoneum tends to be higher attenuation close to the source of the bleeding; thus when the spleen is the source, the collection adjacent to the spleen may be higher in attenuation than elsewhere (Fig. 1), the sentinel clot sign. Lacerations may involve the vasculature. There can be devascularization of the spleen by hilar injury. There may be active extravasation into the peritoneal cavity or a confined area of extravasation – a pseudoaneurysm (Fig. 2). Both types of extravasation indicate that non-operative management may not succeed, although angiographic embolization may control the bleeding and allow splenic salvage [25].

A number of schemes have been devised to grade splenic injury on CT in an attempt to predict outcome, with variable correlation with need for surgery [1]. One of the commonest is the AAST scoring system. In a large study, failure of non-operative management correlated with splenic injury grade: less than 10% failed with grades 1 or 2, while one-third of grade 4 and three-quarters of grade 5 injuries required surgery [26]. Nevertheless, for the individual patient, occasional cases of low-grade injury suffer delayed rupture, and some high-grade injuries are successfully conservatively managed. The additional finding of traumatic pseudoaneurysm or active extravasation (which does not confer to a specific stage in the AAST scoring system) increased the likelihood of failure of non-operative management, whatever the grade [27]. No CT findings are accurate predictors of the need for intervention. Angiographic embolization has similar outcomes and less morbidity compared with surgery [28].

Hepatic Injuries

The liver is the second most frequently injured abdominal organ, accounting for about 20% of abdominal injuries [1, 24]. The right lobe is more often affected than the left, with the posterior right lobe being the most frequently injured segment. Hepatic injuries may be associated with intraperitoneal hemorrhage, but injury may be confined to the liver, or hemorrhage limited by an intact capsule. Laceration of the bare area is associated with extraperitoneal fluid [1]. US may show liver lacerations, which appear similar to splenic injuries, but US has a limited sensitivity of 67%, compared to 93% for CT [29]. This is in part because of the large size of the liver, and the difficulty in clearly imaging all portions by US.

Injuries to the liver include contusion, seen on CT as an ill-defined area of low attenuation; subcapsular hematoma, a crescentic collection limited by the capsule; and intraparenchymal hematoma, a collection of blood within a liver laceration. Laceration is the most common, with linear or branching low attenuation regions, sometimes with jagged margins, that can extend to surface or to vessels. Periportal low attenuation is usually due to edema, but it may represent blood tracking along portal veins. Rarely, this is the only sign of liver injury [1, 24]. The most severe, and rare, injury is avulsion of the hepatic pedicle [30].

Liver injuries may require surgery, but 50-90% can be managed non-operatively. The liver, with a dual blood supply, is relatively resistant to infarction, and has considerable functional reserve. No CT signs or grading schemes have been shown to be reliable predictors of which patients will require intervention. However, active extravasation may predict a need for surgery or angioembolization. The presence of hepatic arterial extravasation or extension of injury into hepatic veins correlates with the need for surgery [31]. Subclassification of extravasation can be useful: extravasation into the peritoneal cavity is highly correlated with the need for surgery, intraparenchymal extravasation with significant hemoperitoneum may require surgery, while extravasation limited within a hepatic hematoma without hemoperitoneum can usually be managed conservatively [21].

References

1. Novelline RA, Rhea JT, Bell T (1999) Helical CT of abdominal trauma. RCNA 37:591-612
2. McKenney KL (1999) Ultrasound of blunt abdominal trauma. RCNA 37:879-893
3. Dolich MO, McKenney MG, Varela JE et al (2001) 2576 Ultrasounds for blunt abdominal trauma. J Trauma 50:108-112
4. Shapiro MJ, Krausz C, Durham RM et al (1999) Overuse of splenic scoring and computed tomographic scans. J Trauma 47:651-658
5. Ochsner MG, Knudson MM, Pachter HL et al (2000) Significance of minimal or no intraperitoneal fluid visible on CT associated with blunt liver and splenic injuries: a multi-center analysis. J Trauma 49:505-510
6. Stassen NA, Lukan JK, Carillo EH et al (2002) Abdominal seat belt marks in the era of focused abdominal sonography for trauma. Arch Surg 137:718-722
7. Goodwin H, Holmes JF, Wisner DH (2001) Abdominal ultrasound examination in pregnant blunt trauma patients. J Trauma 50:689-693
8. Lowdermilk C, Gavant ML, Qaisi W et al (1999) Screening helical CT for evaluation of blunt traumatic injury in the pregnant patient. Radiographics 19:S243-S255
9. McGahan JP, Richards JR, Jones CD et al (1999) Use of ultrasonography in the patient with acute renal trauma. JUM 18:207-213
10. McGahan PJ, Richards JR, Bair AE et al (2005) Ultrasound detection of blunt urological trauma: a 6 year study. Injury 36:762-770
11. Kawashima A, Sandler CM, Corl FM et al (2001) Imaging of renal trauma: a comprehensive review. Radiographics 221:557-574
12. Santucci RA, McAninch JW, Safir M et al (2001) Validation of the American Association for the Surgery of Trauma organ injury severity scale for the kidney. J Trauma 50:195-200
13. Goldman SM, Sandler CM, Corriere JN et al (1997) Blunt urethral trauma: a unified anatomical mechanical classification. J Urol 157:85-89
14. Ali M, Safriel Y, Sclafani SJA et al (2003) CT signs of urethral injury. Radiographics 23:951-963
15. Morgan DM, Nallamalla LK, Kenney PJ et al (2000) CT cystography: radiographic and clinical predictors of bladder rupture. AJR Am J Roentgenol 174:89-95
16. Malhotra AK, Fabian TC, Katsis SB et al (2000) Blunt bowel and mesenteric injuries: the role of screening CT. J Trauma 48:991-998
17. Dowe MF, Shanmuganathan K, Mirvis SE et al (1997) CT findings of mesenteric injury after blunt trauma. AJR Am J Roentgenol 168:425-428
18. Butela ST, Federle MP, Chang PJ et al (2001) Performance of CT in detection of bowel injury. AJR Am J Roentgenol 176:129-135
19. Sharma OP, Oswanski MF, Singer D et al (2004) The role of computed tomography in diagnosis of blunt intestinal and mesenteric trauma. J Emergency Med 27:55-67
20. Elton C, Riaz AA, Young N et al (2005) Accuracy of computed tomography in the detection of blunt bowel and mesenteric injuries. Br J Surgery 92:1024-1028
21. Fang J-F, Chen R-J, Wong Y-C et al (2000) Classification and treatment of pooling of contrast material on CT scan of blunt hepatic trauma. J Trauma 49:1083-1088
22. Stuhlfaut JW, Soto JA, Lucey BC et al (2004) Blunt abdominal trauma: performance of CT without oral contrast material. Radiology 233:689-694
23. Allen TL, Mueller MT, Bonk T et al (2004) Computed tomographic scanning without oral contrast for blunt bowel and mesenteric injuries in abdominal trauma. J Trauma 56:314-322
24. West OC (2000) Intraperitoneal abdominal injuries. In: West OC, Novelline RA, Wilson AJ (eds) Emergency and Trauma Radiology Categorical Course Syllabus, pp 87-98
25. Davis KA, Fabian TC, Croce MA et al (1998) Improved success in nonoperative management of blunt splenic injuries: embolisation of splenic artery pseudoaneurysms. J Trauma 44:1008-1013
26. Peitzman AB, Heil B, Rivera L et al (2000) Blunt splenic injury in adults: multi-institutional study of the Eastern Association for the Surgery of Trauma. J Trauma 49:177-187

27. Gavant ML, Schurr M, Flick PA et al (1997) Predicting clinical outcome of nonsurgical management of blunt splenic injury: using CT to reveal abnormalities of splenic vasculature. AJR Am J Roentgenol 168:207-212

28. Wahl WL, Ahrns KS, Chen S et al (2004) Blunt splenic injury: operation versus angiographic embolization. Surgery 136:891-899

29. Richards JR, McGahan JP, Pali MJ et al (1999) Sonographic detection of blunt hepatic trauma. J Trauma 47:1092-1097

30. Romano L, Giovine S, Guidi Guido et al (2004) Hepatic trauma: CT findings. Eur J Radiol 50:59-66

31. Poletti PA, Mirvis SE, Shanmuganathan K et al (2000) CT criteria for management of blunt liver trauma. Radiology 216:418-427

Trauma of the Abdomen and Pelvis II

S. Ledbetter

Division of Emergency Radiology, Brigham and Women's Hospital, Boston, MA, USA

Introduction

Computed tomography (CT) is the established method for the imaging evaluation of traumatic injury to the abdomen and pelvis. This role has been galvanized in the era of multidetector CT (MDCT) because of the greater speed and flexibility afforded by this modality. MDCT can now image the head, entire spine and torso, often in less time than would be typical for obtaining a standard three-view radiographic trauma series (portable chest, lateral C-spine and AP pelvis). When coupled with its accuracy for detecting multisystem injuries, CT has become the indispensable means by which prompt diagnosis and triage is undertaken for the stable trauma patient. Additionally, the high quality image data sets now obtained from MDCT permit the routine use of post processing techniques such as multiplanar reformation (MPR), maximum intensity projection (MIP) and three-dimensional (3D) image display for improving evaluation and communication of diagnostic results.

MDCT Imaging Techniques

Since most traumatic injury is not isolated to a single anatomic region, abdominal and pelvic imaging is usually undertaken in the context of a complete system evaluation of the multitrauma patient that often includes imaging of the head, entire spine and torso. As previously published by several authors, following a head CT without intravenous contrast material (IVCM), scanning is performed from the circle of Willis, or alternatively, from the thoracic inlet to the symphysis pubis following the intravenous administration of nonionic IVCM (100-150 ml of 300 mg iodine/mL, Ultravist 300) using an injection rate of at least 3 cc/s. Imaging through the abdomen should be timed so that it commences during the portal venous phase of homogeneous parenchymal enhancement. Early or delayed scanning may falsely simulate injury or decrease conspicuity of true injury. At our institution, the emergency radiologist immediately reviews a trauma patient's scans while the patient is on the CT table. When injury is present, delayed imaging is generally performed approximately 3 minutes after the initial IVCM injection, or during the pyelographic phase. Delayed imaging is not performed if no significant injury is detected, thereby reducing radiation exposure for these patients. If immediate review of the initial scan is not an option based on radiologist's availability, or if the incidence of injury is high among a given institution's trauma population, routine acquisition of a delayed scan in every patient may prove a more efficient means of operating procedure. An unenhanced CT is performed in patients with known renal insufficiency or severe contrast allergy, though sensitivity for detecting injury is reduced.

Oral contrast material (OCM) is not routinely used at our trauma center at the time of the initial CT evaluation. Though the use of OCM has been shown to be safe, the perception of providers at our institution is that it delays transit to CT, results in the otherwise unnecessary placement of a nasogastric tube in many patients, and owing to the speed of MDCT, is increasingly of little benefit having rarely progressed beyond the stomach to typical areas of injury by the time CT is performed in most patients. Instead, once immediate life-threatening injuries have been excluded by an initial CT scan, patients with suspected bowel injury based on clinical grounds or results of the initial scan are reimaged after administration of water soluble OCM and a relatively short time for bowel transit, usually about 1 hour.

Rectal contrast material should be administered in all patients with penetrating injuries to the abdomen or flank. Approximately 50 cc of Ultravist 300 (or any IVCM of similar iodine concentration) is injected into a liter of warm saline for use as contrast material. Adequate colonic distention generally involves administration of approximately 500 cc rectal contrast material with the patient in a left lateral decubitus position for suspected left colonic injury, or up to a liter of contrast material with the patient in a right lateral decubitus position for suspected right colonic injury. Use of intravenous, oral and rectal contrast material (i.e., triple contrast CT) has been shown to be a highly accurate means of excluding peritoneal violation in the setting of penetrating trauma to the flank. Additionally, among those patients with peritoneal violation, CT has been reported to accurately predict the need for laparotomy with 100% sensitivity, 96% specificity, 100% negative predictive value, and 97% accuracy.

When bladder injury is suspected, CT cystography is performed. Antegrade filling of the bladder from renal excretion of IVCM is insufficient for excluding bladder injury. Bladder contrast is easily obtained by mixing 50 cc Ultravist 300 in a liter of warm saline. Following the initial scan of the abdomen and pelvis with IVCM, the Foley catheter is unclamped, permitting complete drainage of excreted contrast material. A closed system is used to connect the liter of saline to the indwelling Foley catheter and contrast is instilled in a retrograde fashion with the saline bag approximately 40 cm above the height of the patient's bladder (i.e., the height of the CT table). Bladder contrast is instilled until one of the following: 1) contrast flow stops, 2) 350 to 400 cc of contrast have been instilled, or 3) the patient no longer tolerates contrast instillation. Adequate retrograde distention of the bladder is critical for its proper evaluation. Furthermore, CT cystography should not be performed until after the initial CT scan through the abdomen and pelvis with IVCM. This allows easy discrimination between arterial extravasation and bladder contrast extravasation, both of which are encountered in the setting of pelvic fractures.

Splenic Injury

The spleen is the most commonly injured solid organ in the setting of blunt abdominal trauma, representing approximately 25% of all blunt injuries to the abdominal viscera. The spleen is a highly vascular organ that weighs approximately 75-100 grams in the average adult, contains approximately one unit of blood at any given time and circulates approximately 350 liters of blood per day. With greater recognition of its important immunologic roll, there has been a progressive trend toward the conservative, nonoperative management of splenic injury among hemodynamically stable patients. Today, more than half of all patients with splenic injury are managed nonoperatively.

Splenic injury may be manifest on CT as parenchymal contusion, intraparenchymal or subcapsular hematomas, intrasplenic lacerations, vascular injuries including pseudoaneurysms and arteriovenous fistulas, and active arterial hemorrhage. Parenchymal contusions are seen as poorly defined areas of decreased parenchymal enhancement. Subcapsular hematomas are generally seen as well defined elliptical or crescentic collections of blood that reside immediately below the splenic capsule, may compress the subjacent splenic parenchyma and are of lower attenuation than the enhancing splenic parenchyma. Presence of parenchymal compression helps differentiate subcapsular hematoma from perisplenic hematoma. Intrasplenic lacerations are seen as linear or complex and branching areas of low attenuation coursing through the normally enhancing splenic parenchyma, whereas intra-parenchymal hematomas are seen as intrasplenic low attenuation collections. Active hemorrhage, pseudoaneurysms and arteriovenous fistulas appear as areas of increased density relative to the normally enhancing splenic parenchyma and are of similar attenuation value to an adjacent major artery, generally within 10 Hounsfield units (HU) (i.e., contrast blush [CB]). Traumatic injury may also result in segmental or complete splenic devascularization.

Relying on CT appearance alone to accurately predict those patients requiring splenectomy versus those who can be managed nonoperatively would be highly advantageous. Unfortunately, despite a number of CT grading systems, none has proven reliable in predicting outcome for nonoperative management. Using logistic regression, Schurr et al. showed that CT splenic injury grade had no predictive value for nonoperatively-managed patients. Other studies have shown that CT often underestimates the severity of splenic injury. There is also significant interobserver variability among radiologists in their grading of splenic injury. Despite these limitations, CT has nonetheless greatly facilitated the trend toward nonoperative management, if for no other reason than its contribution toward excluding other injuries that would require surgical exploratory laparotomy.

More recent radiology literature suggests that some CT findings may have strong predictive values for failed nonoperative management. These include: 1) active hemorrhage, 2) post-traumatic pseudoaneurysm, and 3) arteriovenous fistula. All three of these lesions may be seen as a 'contrast blush' on the initial phase of CT scanning. The latter two splenic vascular injuries cannot be further differentiated on contrast-enhanced CT. However, the latter two can be differentiated from active hemorrhage on delayed scanning, at which time the arterial attenuation 'blush' typically decreases to become isodense or minimally hyperdense compared to the normally enhancing splenic parenchyma. Conversely, the arterial 'blush' persists during delayed scanning with active hemorrhage since the contrast material has extravasated from vascular structures and therefore does not 'wash-out'. Furthermore, whereas the splenic vascular injuries of post-traumatic pseudoaneurysm and arteriovenous fistula are always intrasplenic, active hemorrhage may be intrasplenic, subcapsular or freely intraperitoneal (Fig. 1) (Tab. 1).

Among those managed nonoperatively, the majority of failures will occur within 24 hours of admission. Gavant and colleagues reported an 82% failure rate among patients with contrast extravasation or intrasplenic vascular injury (pseudoaneurysm or arteriovenous fistula) who were managed nonoperatively. Other investigators have shown that patients with a CB by CT are 9.2 times more likely to require surgical laparotomy or angiographic embolization. In effect, a CB at CT has a high correlation with failure of nonoperative management. However, to date this finding has not been included in any of the widely used splenic injury grading criteria.

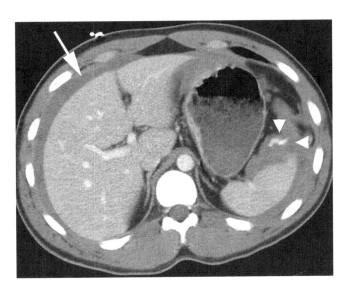

hematomas, intrahepatic lacerations, vascular injuries including pseudoaneurysms and arteriovenous fistulas, and active arterial hemorrhage. Parenchymal contusions are seen as poorly defined areas of decreased parenchymal enhancement. Subcapsular hematomas are generally seen as well defined elliptical or crescentic collections of blood that reside immediately below the hepatic capsule, often compress the subjacent hepatic parenchyma and are of lower attenuation than the enhancing hepatic parenchyma. Presence of parenchymal compression helps differentiate subcapsular hematoma from perihepatic hematoma. Intrahepatic lacerations are seen as linear or complex and branching areas of low attenuation coursing through the normally enhancing hepatic parenchyma, whereas intraparenchymal hematomas are seen as intrahepatic low attenuation collections (Fig. 2).

Fig. 1. Splenic laceration associated with intraperitoneal active arterial extravasation. Axial MDCT images obtained during portal venous phase of scanning show a curvilinear contrast blush adjacent the anterior pole of the spleen (*arrowheads*). Moderate hemoperitoneum (*large arrow*) is present around the liver and spleen. Note that hemoperitoneum adjacent the spleen is of higher attenuation than that adjacent the liver ('sentinel clot')

Table 1. CT splenic injury grading scale

CT Grade I	Laceration(s) < 1 cm deep Subcapsular hematoma < 1 cm diameter
CT Grade II	Laceration(s) 1-3 cm deep Subcapsular or central hematoma 1-3 cm diameter
CT Grade III	Laceration(s) 3-10 cm deep Subcapsular or central hematoma 3-10 cm diameter
CT Grade IV	Laceration(s) > 10 cm deep Subcapsular or central hematoma > 10 cm diameter
CT Grade V	Splenic tissue maceration or devascularization

Modified from Mirvis et al. (1989)

Hepatic Injury

Hepatic injury represents approximately 15-20% of all blunt injuries to the abdominal viscera, placing it as the second most commonly injured solid organ in the setting of blunt abdominal trauma. However, hepatic injury is the most common cause of death following abdominal injury. Historically, most liver injuries were treated surgically despite the fact that as many as 70% had stopped bleeding by that time. Further, a comparison has shown that operative management requires more blood transfusions and results in more complications than does nonoperative management. For these reasons, and given the greater ability to diagnose and monitor hepatic injuries by CT, there has been a progressive trend toward the conservative, nonoperative management of these injuries among hemodynamically stable patients. Today, approximately 80% of all patients with hepatic injury are managed nonoperatively.

Hepatic injury may be manifest on CT as parenchymal contusion, intraparenchymal or subcapsular

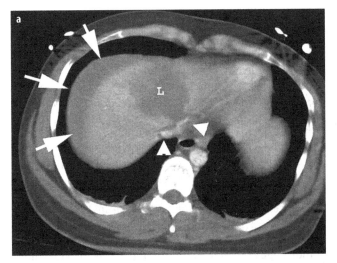

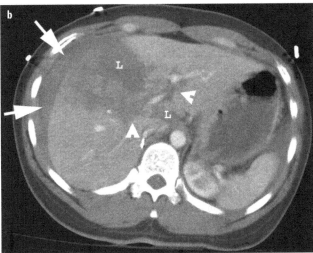

Fig. 2. Complex interlobar hepatic transection (**a, b**) Axial MDCT images obtained during portal venous phase of scanning show a complex laceration (*L*) extending between the right and left hepatic lobes. Moderate hemoperitoneum (*large arrow*) is present. **a** Laceration extends to involve the retrohepatic inferior vena cava (*arrowheads*). **b** More inferiorly, laceration involves the main portal vein with blood tracking along the right and left portal branches (*arrowheads*)

Active hemorrhage, pseudoaneurysms and arteriovenous fistulas appear as areas of increased density relative to the normally enhancing hepatic parenchyma during the portal venous phase, reaching a similar attenuation value to an adjacent major artery, generally within 10 HU (i.e., CB). Traumatic injury may also result in segmental or complete hepatic devascularization.

Though CT grading of hepatic injury has thus far proven to be unreliable in predicting the need for surgery, CT has to be helpful in guiding management, and to have a positive correlation between grade of injury and the increased likelihood of failed nonoperative management. Vascular injuries, including posttraumatic pseudoaneurysm and arteriovenous fistula as well as active extravasation, are strong predictors of failure of nonoperative management. Injuries extending to the regions of the portal and hepatic veins are more likely to require surgery (Fig. 2). Injuries extending to involve the retrohepatic vena cava are particularly lethal, with a mortality rate of 90-100% due to the difficulty in exposing and controlling hemorrhage in this region. Some of these injuries may be further characterized and managed by angiography. At least one major trauma center in the U.S. performs angiography on any of the following: 1) any grade III to V hepatic injury with extension into the region of a portal or hepatic vein, 2) any patient with active hemorrhage or vascular injury (i.e., a CB on portal venous phase) regardless of grade of injury, or 3) in any patient requiring multiple transfusions because of ongoing hepatic hemorrhage (Tab. 2).

Delayed complications may be seen in 10-25% of patients with hepatic injury. Hemorrhage, hepatic abscess and biloma are the most common complications. Delayed hemorrhage is seen in 1.7-5.9% of patients managed nonoperatively. These patients are usually managed with angiography or surgery. Hepatic abscess is seen in 0.6-4% of patients with hepatic injury, but more commonly in those patients managed nonoperatively. These patients are usually managed with percutaneous abscess drainage. Biloma is seen in less than 1% of patients with hepatic injury. Symptomatic patients are usually managed with percutaneous or endoscopic drainage. Asymptomatic patients are managed expectantly since bilomas usually resolve without intervention over the course of weeks to months.

Renal Injury

The kidneys are the third most commonly injured solid organ in the setting of blunt abdominal trauma, representing approximately 10% of all blunt injuries to the abdominal viscera in adults. However, the kidney is the most commonly injured solid organ in the setting of blunt abdominal trauma in children. During the 1950s and 60s, surgical exploration of the injured kidney often led to nephrectomy. As with splenic and hepatic injury, the improved ability to diagnose and monitor renal injuries by CT has facilitated the shift toward nonoperative management of these injuries among hemodynamically stable patients. Absence of hematuria can be reliably used to exclude significant renal injury in the setting of blunt abdominal trauma, but this does not hold true for penetrating trauma. Today, approximately 98% of all patients with renal injury are managed nonoperatively.

Renal injury may be manifest on CT as parenchymal contusion, intraparenchymal, subcapsular or perinephric hematomas, intraparenchymal lacerations, vascular injuries including pseudoaneurysms and arteriovenous fistulas, and active arterial hemorrhage. Additionally, injuries may extend to and disrupt the collecting system, resulting in urinary extravasation (Fig. 3).

Renal contusions are seen as ill-defined round or ovoid hypoattenuating regions on the portal venous phase of scanning, or as persistent contrast staining on delayed images obtained in the pyelographic phase. Subcapsular hematomas are generally seen as well defined elliptical or crescentic collections of blood that reside immediately below the renal capsule, often compress the subjacent renal parenchyma and are of lower attenuation than the enhancing renal parenchyma. Perinephric hematomas are often poorly defined blood attenuating fluid collections contained between the kidney and Gerota's fascia that rarely deform the renal parenchyma. Renal lacerations are seen as linear or complex and branching areas of low attenuation coursing through the normally enhancing renal parenchyma, where as intrarenal hematomas are seen as low attenuation collections within the renal parenchyma. Active hemorrhage, pseudoaneurysms and arteriovenous fistulas appear as areas of increased density relative to the normally enhancing renal parenchyma during the portal venous phase of scanning. The attenuation of these injuries is generally within 10 HU of the renal artery. Traumatic renal injury may also result in segmental or complete renal devascularization.

The organ injury scale (OIS) of the American Association for the Surgery of Trauma (ASTT) is used to calculate the injury severity score (ISS) since the ISS correlates with patient outcome and likelihood of death.

Table 2. CT hepatic injury grading scale

CT Grade I	Laceration(s) < 1 cm deep Subcapsular hematoma < 1 cm diameter
CT Grade II	Laceration(s) 1-3 cm deep Subcapsular or central hematoma 1-3 cm diameter
CT Grade III	Laceration(s) 3-10 cm deep Subcapsular or central hematoma 3-10 cm diameter
CT Grade IV	Laceration(s) > 10 cm deep Subcapsular or central hematoma > 10 cm diameter Lobar maceration or devascularization
CT Grade V	Bilobar tissue maceration or devascularization

Modified from Mirvis et al. (1989)

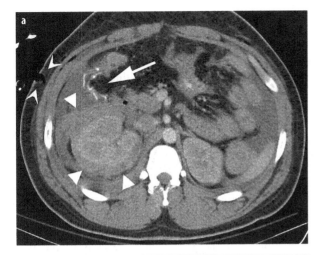

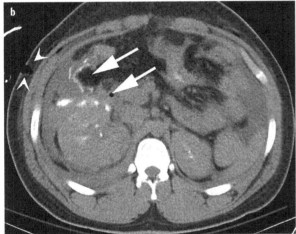

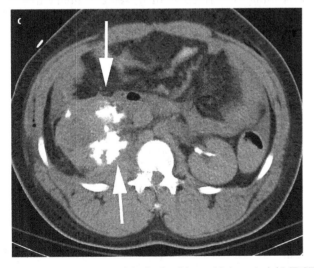

Fig. 3. Gunshot wound to right flank with renal injury. Axial MDCT images obtained during portal venous phase (**a**) and delayed scanning performed during the pyelographic phase (**b, c**). **a, b** Gunshot entry wound is readily identified in the right anterior flank (*concave arrowheads*) with intraperitoneal fluid confirming peritoneal violation. **a** Perinephric hematoma (*arrowheads*) appears contained by Gerota's fascia posteriorly but is less well marginated anteriorly. **a, b** Active arterial extravasation is noted anterior to the right kidney (*large arrows*) with increased contrast accumulation on the delayed phase of scanning. **c** More inferiorly, pyelographic extravasation (*large arrows*) confirms injury to the renal collecting system

However, the CT classification of renal trauma includes important injuries that can be identified at imaging, but that are not explicitly specified in the OIS system. These include: 1) subtotal or segmental renal infarction, 2) traumatic thrombosis of the main renal artery, 3) active extravasation of vascular contrast material, and 4) ureteropelvic junction (UPJ) avulsion.

The majority of renal injuries, approximately 85%, are comprised of grade I and II injuries that are considered relatively minor and do not typically require any intervention. Conversely, grade IV and V renal injuries always require treatment to repair the renal collecting system, arrest hemorrhage, and/or restore renal perfusion. Grade III injuries may or may not require intervention, depending on the presence of CT findings of active bleeding or clinical signs and symptoms suggesting continued bleeding.

Pancreatic Injury

Pancreatic injury is rare. One retrospective review that included 16,188 Level I trauma center admissions over a ten year study period found an incidence of pancreatic injury of 0.4%. In this same study, approximately two thirds (63%) occurred as a result of penetrating trauma, whereas only one third of cases (37%) were due to blunt abdominal trauma. Therefore, the relative incidence of pancreatic injury in penetrating trauma was found to be 1.1% as compared to an incidence of only 0.2% among blunt abdominal trauma patients.

Though CT has been widely used as the primary means of evaluation for blunt abdominal trauma in hemodynamically stable patients, only recently has it begun to gain wider acceptance for evaluation of patients with penetrating mechanisms. Given the low overall incidence of pancreatic injury, coupled with the historically less frequent evaluation of patients with penetrating trauma and the recent advances in MDCT, it remains unclear what role CT may have in excluding or accurately grading pancreatic injury.

Pancreatic injury may be manifest on CT as parenchymal contusion, intraparenchymal or peripancreatic hematomas, intraparenchymal laceration or pancreatic transection (Fig. 4), vascular injuries including post-traumatic pseudoaneurysm, and active arterial hemorrhage. CT has an established role for the evaluation of abdominal trauma, therefore it is most important that the radiologist remain alert to the possibility of pancreatic injury, particularly among those patients with penetrating injuries. Further, among those patients suffering blunt trauma, the relatively protected central position of the pancreas means that pancreatic injury is rarely isolated. Injury to the midline pancreatic body is commonly associated with left hepatic lobe and duodenal injury. Injury to the pancreatic tail is commonly associated with splenic injury. Injury to the pancreatic head is commonly associated with major hepatic, vascular (retrohepatic inferior vena cava, aorta, portal vein and superior mesenteric vessels), and/or duodenal injury. Greater scrutiny of the pancreas when

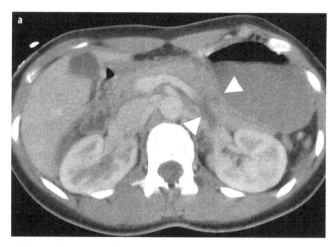

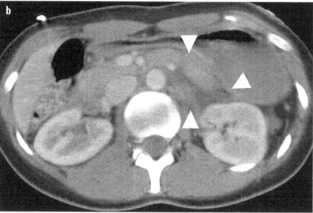

Fig. 4. Pancreatic laceration after motor vehicle collision. **a, b** Axial MDCT images obtained during portal venous phase show a pancreatic laceration near the junction of the pancreatic body and tail (*arrowheads*). Fat stranding is present posterior to the pancreas. A small amount of fluid is present in Morrison's pouch

Unequivocal findings of full thickness bowel injury on MDCT include direct visualization of bowel wall discontinuity with or without extravasation of bowel contents, including oral contrast material. Pneumoperitoneum, though strongly suggestive of full thickness bowel injury in the appropriate clinical setting, is a well-known cause of false positive CT interpretation. Air may be introduced into the peritoneal cavity by alternate means, including diagnostic peritoneal lavage, Foley catheter placement in the setting of intraperitoneal bladder rupture, and translocation of air from the thoracic cavity in the presence of thoracic injury (e.g., pneumothorax or pneumomediastinum). Nonetheless, pneumoperitoneum without an identified source should be considered indicative of full thickness bowel injury until proven otherwise. Focal bowel wall thickening (Fig. 5) usually reflects partial thickness injury (i.e., bowel wall contusion or hematoma) that is most often self-limited in the absence of less equivocal clinical findings (e.g., adjacent pneumoperitoneum or bowel content extravasation). In the absence of solid organ injury, the presence of isolated nonphysiologic quantities of free fluid is associated with an 84.2% incidence of small bowel injury. When coupled with pneumoperitoneum, sensitivity for detecting small bowel perforation increases to 97%. When confronted with nonspecific findings such as focal bowel wall thickening or unexplained free fluid in the setting of blunt abdominal trauma, a thorough CT evaluation of the bowel using water-soluble oral contrast material should be strongly considered among patients for whom surgical exploration is deferred.

Mesenteric injury may or may not be associated with bowel injury. CT findings of mesenteric injury may include ill-defined focal areas of fat stranding that reflect mesenteric contusion, focal collections of blood attenuat-

these associated injuries are present may improve detection of pancreatic injuries. Post-traumatic complications of pancreatic injury may include pancreatitis, pancreatic fistula, pseudocyst or intra-abdominal abscess formation.

Bowel and Mesentery Injury

Bowel and mesenteric injury are relatively rare among patients with blunt abdominal trauma. According to the largest retrospective study to date, the incidence of small bowel injury is 1.1%, and the incidence of colonic injury is 0.3% among these patients. Most frequently injured are the jejunum and ileum at the ligament of Treitz and the ileocecal valve, respectively, as these are sites of transition between fixed and mobile bowel segments, making them prone to the forces of deceleration injury. The next most commonly injured areas are the colon and rectum, followed by the duodenum and stomach. Surgical exploration remains the primary means by which any bowel perforation is treated.

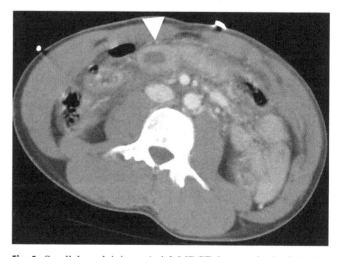

Fig. 5. Small bowel injury. Axial MDCT image obtained during portal venous phase shows circumferential thickening of a small bowel loop in the mid abdomen (*arrowhead*). Interloop fluid is present. Patient went to laparotomy for other intra-abdominal injuries (obviating need for repeat scan with oral contrast material), at which time the small bowel injury was found to be nontransmural

ing mesenteric hematoma or active mesenteric arterial extravasation. Isolated mesenteric contusion is usually managed nonoperatively. Active mesenteric arterial extravasation usually undergoes emergent laparotomy. Mesenteric hematoma management may vary based on its size and association with other injuries. Mesenteric injury can also result in devascularized segments of bowel. As with nonspecific findings of bowel injury, CT evaluation using water-soluble oral contrast material should be strongly considered among patients with mesenteric injury for whom surgical exploration is deferred.

Bladder Injury

Bladder injury is relatively uncommon, with a reported incidence of 1.6% among blunt abdominal trauma patients. Approximately 90% of bladder injuries are the result of motor vehicle collisions or pedestrians struck by car. The remaining 10% are related to falls, pelvic crush injuries (often occupational and/or industrial), and severe blows to the lower abdomen. The likelihood of bladder injury is almost certainly related to its degree of distention at the time of trauma. Hematuria is present in es-

sentially all cases of bladder rupture, and most have gross hematuria.

Bladder rupture can be classified as extraperitoneal (EBR, 57%), intraperitoneal (IBR, 36%), or combined (EBR and IBR, 5-7%). Approximately 7-9% of patients with pelvic fracture will have bladder rupture. Conversely, 83-89% of patients with bladder rupture will have pelvic fracture. Pelvic fracture is almost uniformly present if the bladder rupture is extraperitoneal. Previously, the strong association of EBR with pelvic fracture was mechanistically explained as resulting from direct bladder perforation by bony spicules resulting at the fracture site (Fig. 6a, b). However, at least one study has shown that the site of bladder injury was opposite the fracture site in 65% of cases. More recently, some authors have suggested that shearing forces related to pelvic ring disruption may tear the bladder at its fascial attachments. Whereas EBR more commonly occurs at the low anterior bladder, IBR more commonly occurs at the bladder dome. IBR most commonly results from a direct blow to a distended bladder that increases intravesicular pressure and causes the bladder to burst into the intraperitoneal space. IBR tears are typically much larger (5-10 cm) than those encountered with EBR.

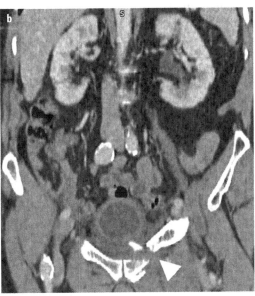

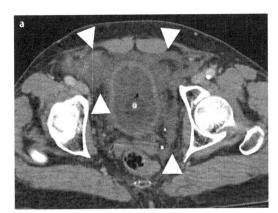

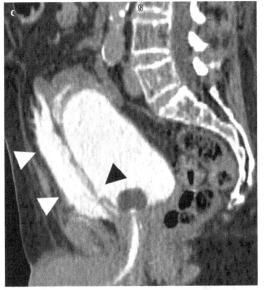

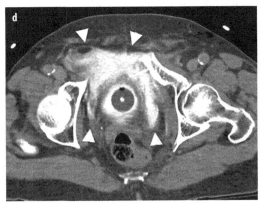

Fig. 6. Extraperitoneal bladder injury. **a** Axial MDCT image obtained during portal venous phase shows low attenuation fluid anterior and lateral to the bladder (*arrowheads*). **b** Coronal reformation shows left superior pubic ramus fracture (*arrowhead*) with a bony spicule directed toward the bladder. Note the absence of free fluid within the peritoneal cavity. **c** Sagittal reformation after retrograde administration of bladder contrast via indwelling Foley catheter shows extraperitoneal extravasation of contrast material into the prevesical space (*white arrowheads*) through a defect (*black arrowhead*) in the low anterior bladder. **d** Axial image obtained at CT cystography shows the 'molar tooth' sign (*arrowheads*) related to extravasation of bladder contrast material anteriorly and laterally. (Images courtesy of Dr. Peter Clarke, Boston)

CT is an excellent means of bladder evaluation when injury is suspected based on mechanism, presence of pelvic fracture and/or hematuria. The standard method for CT cystography, as described earlier, has a reported sensitivity/specificity of 92%/99.6% for IBR, and a sensitivity/specificity of 100%/99.3% for EBR. The most classic finding for EBR is referred to as the 'molar tooth sign' (Fig. 6c, d). This is present when extravasated bladder contrast tracks anteriorly and laterally around the distended bladder, creating the profile of a molar tooth. Extraperitoneal contrast can also track into the anterior abdominal wall, flank, scrotum and thighs. IBR is first suspected by the presence of low attenuation urine ascites during the initial portal venous phase of scanning. Following CT cystography, extravasated bladder contrast resides within the peritoneal cavity and confirms intraperitoneal rupture (Fig. 7).

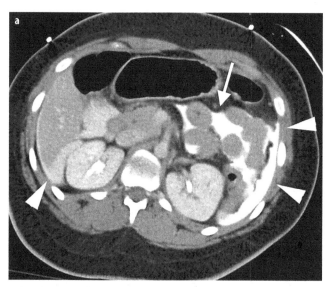

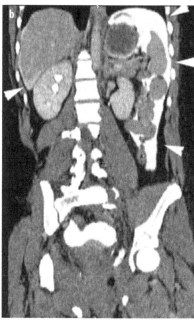

Fig. 7. Intraperitoneal bladder injury in a repeat study performed on a transfer trauma patient whose outside imaging did not accompany them. Axial MD-CT image obtained during portal venous phase (**a**) and coronal MPR (**b**) show a large volume of high-density contrast material pooling in the paracolic gutters (*arrowheads*) and between bowel loops (*large arrow*), confirming intraperitoneal bladder rupture. No solid visceral injury was present. Note absence of oral contrast material within the stomach. (Images courtesy of Dr. Peter Clarke, Boston)

False negatives are known to occur when bladder distention is inadequate for whatever reason (technique, patient tolerance, bladder compression by pelvic hematoma). If CT cystography is not timed correctly in the patient's evaluation, extravasated oral or intravenous contrast material may be mistaken for bladder injury leading to false positive diagnoses.

Intraperitoneal bladder rupture is universally treated by surgical repair. Otherwise, these typically large bladder lacerations continue to decompress and spill urine into the peritoneal cavity where it is resorbed by peritoneal surfaces and leads to uremia. Extraperitoneal bladder rupture is typically managed by catheter drainage. Surgical repair remains an option if adequate drainage cannot be accomplished, injury is in close proximity to the bladder neck, there are associated rectal or vaginal injuries, or the patient undergoes open reduction internal fixation of an anterior pelvic fracture. Approximately 85% of EBR heal by the tenth day, and almost all heal within 3 weeks of injury.

Diaphragmatic Injury

Diaphragmatic injury is present in 1-6% of patients sustaining blunt abdominal trauma. The force required for diaphragmatic injury accounts for the frequent coexistence of other abdominal injuries in 75-100% cases. Diaphragmatic injury is twice as common with penetrating trauma as compared to blunt abdominal trauma. Left diaphragmatic injury is more common than right whether due to blunt (approximately 75%) or penetrating (approximately 56%) mechanisms. Left predominance may be slightly overestimated, since right diaphragmatic injury is more likely to go undiagnosed among nonsurgical cases. Bilateral diaphragmatic injuries occur in 1-5% of patients. The posterolateral aspect of the diaphragm is the most frequent site of injury given the congenital weakness in this region. Diaphragmatic injury is frequently missed in the acute setting.

Diaphragmatic injury may be suspected or diagnosed on the portable chest radiograph obtained as part of a routine trauma series. If gas-containing viscera are identified within the thorax, and particularly if said viscera are constricted at the site of diaphragmatic tear (the 'collar sign'), then diaphragmatic injury can be reasonably assumed. Passage of a nasogastric tube into the stomach can help to confirm its abnormal position in the chest cavity and further establish the diagnosis of diaphragmatic injury.

CT signs that are specific for the diagnosis of diaphragmatic injury include: 1) herniation of abdominal viscera into the thorax (Fig. 8), and 2) focal constriction of the diaphragm around abdominal viscera, the so-called 'CT collar' sign. Nonspecific CT signs of diaphragmatic injury include: 1) discontinuity of the diaphragmatic crus, 2) thickening of the diaphragm, and 3) the 'dependent viscera' sign. Routine use of sagittal and coronal re-

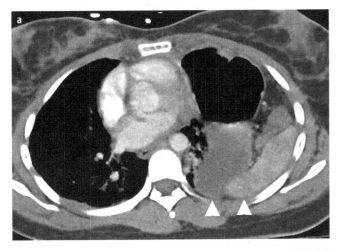

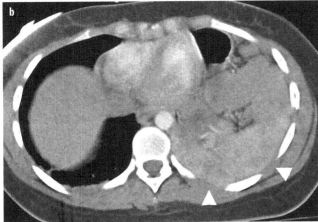

Fig. 8. Left diaphragmatic rupture. **a, b** Axial MDCT images show the stomach within the left hemithorax, and both the stomach and spleen lying dependently on the posterior thoracic wall (*arrowheads*) consistent with the 'dependent viscera' sign. **b** Note the normal suspension on the hepatic dome away from the right posterior thoracic wall owing to the intact right hemidiaphragm

formations in the evaluation of patients sustaining abdominal trauma may improve detection of diaphragmatic injury. Whenever CT is equivocal, MRI may prove helpful in further evaluation.

Suggested Reading

Akhass R, Yaffe MB, Brandt CP et al (1997) Pancreatic trauma: a ten-year old multi-institutional experience. Am Surg 63:598-604

Brody JM, Leighton DB, Murphy BL et al (2000) CT of blunt trauma bowel and mesenteric injury: typical findings and pitfalls in diagnosis. Radiographics 20:1525-1536; discussion 1536-1537

Federle MP, Yagan N, Peitzman AB, Krugh J (1197) Abdominal trauma: use of oral contrast material for CT is safe. Radiology 205(1):91-93

Gavant ML, Schurr M, Flick et al (1997) Predicting clinical outcome of nonsurgical management of blunt splenic injury: using CT to reveal abnormalities in the splenic vasculature. AJR Am J Roentgenol 168:207-212

Killeen KL, Mirvis SE, Shanmuganathan K (1999) Helical CT of diaphragmatic rupture caused by blunt trauma. AJR 173(6):1611-1616

McKenney KL (1999) Ultrasound of blunt abdominal trauma. The Radiology Clinics of North America 37:879-894

Miller LA, Shanmuganathan K (2005) Multidetector CT evaluation of abdominal trauma. Radiol Clin N Am 43:1079-1095

Mirvis SE, Shanmuganathan K (eds) (2003) Imaging in trauma and critical care. WB Saunders, Philadelphia

Mirvis SE, Whitley NO, Vainwright JR, Gens DR (1989) Blunt hepatic trauma in adults: CT-based classification and correlation with prognosis and treatment. Radiology 171:27-32

Morgan AS, Flancbaum K, Esposito D, Cox EF (1986) Blunt injury to the diaphragm: an analysis of 44 patients. J Trauma 26:565-568

Novelline RA, Rhea JT, Bell T (1999) Helical CT of abdominal trauma. The Radiology Clinics of North America 37:591-612

Peitzman AB, Heil B, Rivera L et al (1996) Blunt splenic injury in adults: multi-institutional study of the eastern association for the surgery of trauma. J Trauma 49:177

Poletti PA, Mirvis SE, Shanamuganathan K et al (2000) CT criteria for management of blunt liver trauma: correlation with angiographic and surgical findings. Radiology 216:418-427

Rizzo MJ, Federle MP, Griffiths BG (1989) Bowel and mesenteric injury following blunt abdominal trauma: evaluation with CT. Radiology 173:143-148

Sandler CM, Hall JT, Rodriguez MB, Corriere JN Jr (1986) Bladder injury in blunt pelvic trauma. Radiology 158:633-638

Schurr MJ, Fabian TC, Gavant M et al (1995) Management of blunt splenic trauma: computed tomographic contrast blush predicts failure of nonoperative management. J Trauma 39:507-513

Shanmuganathan K, Killeen K, Mirvis SE, White CS (2000) Imaging of diaphragmatic injuries. J Thorac Imaging 15:104-111

Shanmuganathan K, Mirvis SE, Chiu WC et al (2001) Triple-contrast helical CT in penetrating torso trauma: a prospective study to determine peritoneal violation and the need for laparotomy. AJR Am J Roentgenol 177:1247-1256

Simpson J, Lobo DN, Shah AB, Rowlands BJ (2000) Traumatic diaphragmatic rupture: associated injuries and outcome. J Trauma 82:97-100

Smith JS, Cooney RN, Mucha P (1996) Nonoperative management of the ruptured spleen: a revalidation of criteria. Surgery 120:745-751

Stern EJ (1997) Trauma radiology companion. Lippincott-Raven, Philadelphia

Sutyak JP, Chiu WC, D'Amelio LF et al (1995) Computed tomography is inaccurate in estimating the severity of adult splenic injury. J Trauma 39:514-518

West OC, Jarolimek AM (2000) Abdomen: traumatic emergencies. In: The radiology of ermergency medicine, 4th edn. Lippincott Williams & Wilkins, Philadelphia, pp 689-724

West OC, Novelline RA, Wilson AJ (2000) Categorical course syllabus on emergency and trauma radiology. American Roentgen Ray Society

Variants and Pitfalls in Body Imaging. Abdomen and Pelvis

A. Shirkhoda[1], K. Mortele[2]

[1] Division of Diagnostic Imaging, William Beaumont Hospital, Royal Oak, MI, USA
[2] Department of Radiology, Brigham and Women's Hospital, Boston, MA, USA

Introduction

Computed tomography (CT) and magnetic resonance (MR) imaging are often the primary examinations considered when evaluating patients with a variety of abdominal and pelvic conditions. When these exams are carried out, the radiologist needs to consider the possibility of incidental irrelevant findings or normal anatomic variants, which can mimic pathology. In addition, proper interpretation depends on the quality of the imaging studies, which is dependent on a number of factors. Therefore, optimal protocol and the familiarity of the radiologist with normal variants and pseudo-tumors is essential to correctly interpret such studies. In addition, lack of clinical information such as prior abdominal surgery can contribute to misdiagnoses, leading to erroneous management. For CT, these subjects are discussed in the following three categories.

Procedural Factors

To optimize routine CT examinations of the abdomen, several general principles need to be followed. These include optimization of the technical parameters of the CT scanner for a particular clinical indication, achieving optimal contrast enhancement of the targeted solid organs and surrounding structures and adequate distention of the hollow viscera.

The current technology of spiral (helical) and multidetector CT (MDCT), allow us to scan the entire abdomen and pelvis in one or two breath-holds, often without motion artifact. Thin collimation and a reconstruction interval every 5 mm generally allow adequate CT evaluation. If only axial incremental CT scanning is available, the examination is often optimized by the liberal use of thinner collimation over the area of interest. In MDCT, coronal and sagittal reconstructions will often provide additional diagnostic information and reduce errors and pitfalls.

Administration of oral contrast medium is essential for CT assessment of the abdomen and pelvis. The amount of contrast medium, its density, timely administration and the proper timing of the CT study in relation to the start time of administration are essential elements for the optimal opacification of the gastrointestinal (GI) tract and a reduction in erroneous readings [1]. For evaluation of the pancreas or stomach, water or gas-producing granules prior to CT scanning are often helpful. Inadequate distention or opacification of the hollow viscera can obscure a neoplasm or mimic conditions such as an abscess (Fig. 1, 2).

Intravenous contrast is recommended for CT evaluation of the gastrointestinal tract and it is a requirement for

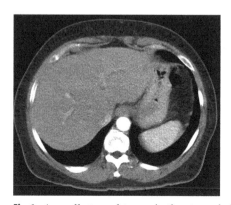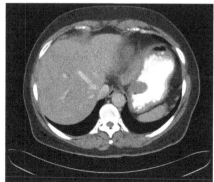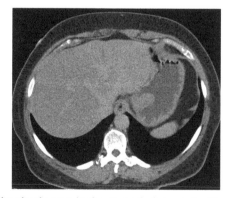

Fig. 1. A small stromal tumor in the stomach (GIST) was missed on the initial study. It can be clearly seen in the stomach distended with dilute barium or water

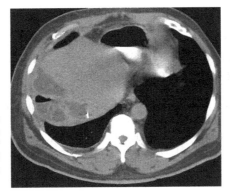
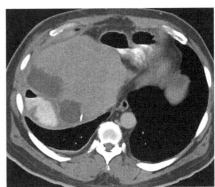

Fig. 2. This febrile patient with recent right hepatic lobectomy was thought to have a multiloculated abscess with probable liver involvement. A repeat CT with oral contrast revealed unopacified bowel loops, which mimicked abscess and intrahepatic bilomas

proper assessment of solid abdominal viscera [3-5]. The wall of the hollow viscera, if well-distended, is easily evaluated by performing contrast CT during the late arterial or early portal-venous phase. For spiral CT, typically 100-120 cc of contrast is injected at a rate of 3-5 cc per second and the data is obtained during both arterial and portal-venous phases. The arterial phase is generally done at a scan delay of 25-30 seconds and reflects enhancement of the solid viscera by their respected arteries. In liver, this will result in little enhancement, as the hepatic artery supplies only 25% of the liver blood. Therefore, there will be minimal enhancement of the hepatic parenchyma, and the portal and particularly hepatic veins often remain unopacified, which can be a source of diagnostic error. Conversely, hypervascular lesions, which are only seen on arterial phase, may not be appreciated if only the venous phase is obtained. Hyper-enhanced areas are occasionally encountered in arterial phase of the liver, referred to as transient hepatic attenuation difference (THAD). This pattern has been described in many conditions that have altered the balance of hepatic arterial and portal-venous blood-flow to a portion of the liver. These include arterial portal shunts, hypervascular tumors, gallbladder inflammation, hepatic congestion, systemic portal shunts, portal vein thrombosis and superior vena cava

obstruction [1]. These intrahepatic areas of attenuation difference may be anatomic and follow a lobar, segmental or subsegmental distribution, or alternatively, in cases such as hepatic congestion, the difference may not follow any obvious anatomic distribution. Such transient patterns can mimic a hypervascular tumor in the liver (Fig. 3). Rarely, THAD can persist in the portal phase and its cause may remain unidentified.

The portal-venous phase of hepatic enhancement allows good detection of hypovascular liver tumors, and is usually performed using an 80 second scan delay.

Spleen displays heterogeneous enhancement patterns during the arterial phase of contrast enhanced CT and MRI. This is related to the variable rate of blood flow to the different histologic components of the spleen. As the terminal arteries transport contrast enhanced blood into the splenic parenchyma, it is first carried into the white pulp before being discharged into the relatively larger volume of red pulp, which is comprised of splenic sinuses and cords. The patterns of heterogeneous enhancement in the spleen have been described as 'serpentine', 'cord-like', 'muddled' or 'striped'. The term 'zebra spleen' has been often applied. By less than two minutes post-injection, the normal spleen should demonstrate a homogeneous enhancing pattern.

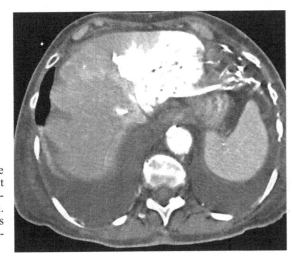
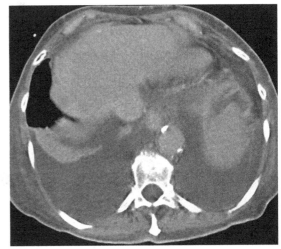

Fig. 3. THAD in the left lobe as a result of patent pericardiophrenic vein. Delayed image does not reveal the enhancing segment

Anatomic Variations

Diaphragm, liver, spleen, pancreas, kidneys, adrenal glands and the GI tract can have numerous anatomic variants. Such findings on sectional imaging occasionally mimic pathologic conditions.

Muscular fibers of the diaphragm, which are primarily in the peripheral region, may invaginate into the adjacent sub-diaphragmatic fat in the upper abdomen and on CT scans or MRI, may be seen as soft tissue nodules (Fig. 4). Deeper diaphragmatic invaginations in the right side can result in accessory liver fissures, which are often seen in the superior aspect of the liver. In the posterior pararenal spaces, the lateral arcuate ligament of diaphragm may be seen as a soft tissue nodule. These diaphragmatic slips are more common in older persons, (nearly 70% frequency in patients older than 70 years, compared with 24% in younger patients) and

are more prominent upon inspiration or in patients with emphysema. The diaphragmatic crura are ligamentous bands that are tendinous at origin. The right crus is longer and larger and often more lobular than the left side. On axial images of CT or MR, thickened areas of the crura can be mistaken for lymphadenopathy or even an adrenal nodule.

The caudate lobe of the liver may be divided in its inferior part into the medial papillary process and the lateral caudate process. If prominent, papillary process may appear similar to an enlarged node at the porta hepatis or simulates a mass in the head of the pancreas [1, 6]. It can extend medially behind the gastric antrum and is separated from the liver on at least one CT scan in about 20% of the patients. With MDCT, reconstruction of images in different planes will solve this issue. Pedunculated accessory hepatic lobe is a rare condition and can mimic an enlarged node or a pancreatic mass (Fig. 5).

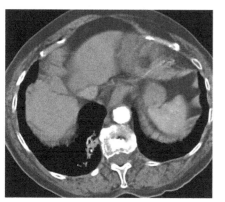 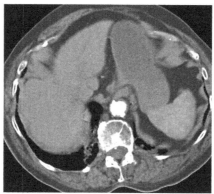 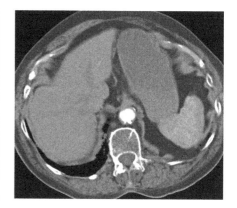

Fig. 4. Prominent invagination of muscular fibers of the diaphragm

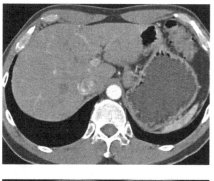 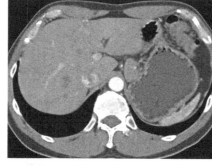 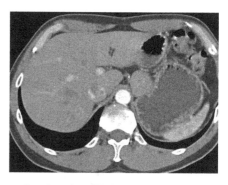

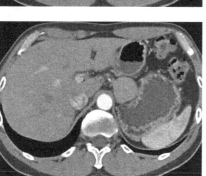 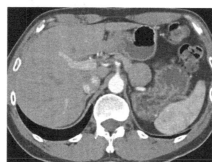 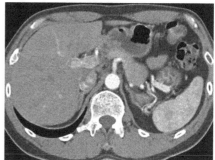

Fig. 5. Pedunculated accessory hepatic lobe. On these six sequential images, one can see the pedicle on the first image. On the subsequent images, while it has the same degree of enhancement as the liver, it mimics a mass in the gastro hepatic ligament or the pancreas

Fatty infiltration of the liver is commonly associated with obesity, diabetes mellitus, Cushing's disease, malnutrition, chronic alcoholic abuse, steroid use or malnutrition related to malignancy or chemotherapy and intravenous hyperalimentation. Differences in perfusion may cause fatty infiltration of the liver to occasionally appear regional or focal and should not be mistaken for mass or infarction. Fatty changes, particularly when patchy, perivascular and multifocal, can be mistaken for liver metastasis on CT scans [7]. However, the presence of an unaltered vascular pattern is a major clue. When focal, in a patient with known malignancy, MRI may occasionally be needed for differentiation from a tumor (Fig. 6). In cases of diffuse fatty infiltration, one or several areas of unaffected liver may remain and represent islands of normal hepatic parenchyma called 'spared areas'.

The spleen has various configurations and positions and its position depends on the length of the splenorenal ligament. Even with normal length, there is some movement to the spleen in supine and prone positions.

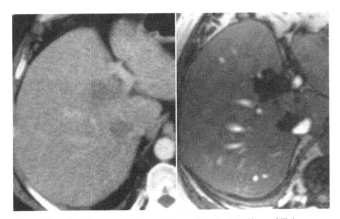

Fig. 6. Two focal areas of low attenuation in the liver CT in a patient with breast carcinoma. Out of phase sequence MR image proves them to represent focal fatty infiltration. Note the normal caliber of a vessel traversing the larger area of low signal

The length of splenorenal ligament can place the spleen in direct contact with, or even dorsal or caudal to the left kidney. Elongated ligament results in *wandering spleen*. In addition, *accessory spleen* and *polysplenia* should not be misdiagnosed as masses. Synchronous and equal enhancement of accessory spleen with the normal spleen is one clue to diagnosis. Patients with history of traumatic splenic rupture who have had a prior splenectomy are prime subjects to develop intra-abdominal splenosis. This condition results in implantation of splenic tissues on the peritoneal surfaces, which grow and mimic small nodules or masses. If the patient develops malignancy at a later age, splenosis should not be mistaken for metastases (Fig. 7).

The pancreas is traditionally divided into five parts, the uncinate process, the head, the neck, the body and the tail. The first four parts are retroperitoneal, while the tail extends into the peritoneum ensheathed in the splenorenal ligament and can have variable configurations. The position of the pancreas is often variable and partly attributes to the increasing laxity in the retroperitoneal connective tissue that accompanies the aging process. The position of the tail also depends on the presence and location of the spleen and the left kidney. Normally, the pancreas has homogeneous density and tapers from the head towards the tail, but there are many variations in contour and density.

Vascular anomalies and normal variants in the retroperitoneum are often related to the inferior vena cava (IVC) and the left renal vein and may be mistaken for a node on unenhanced CT. These include transposition or duplication of the IVC and circumaortic or retroaortic left renal vein.

Fat impingement on IVC can mimic thrombosis. This phenomenon always occurs above the confluence of the hepatic veins and the IVC and relates to the subdiaphragmatic paraesophageal fat extending laterally and superiorly to impinge on the suprahepatic IVC.

Adrenal glands usually have a linear shape, however, on the left side, the adrenal can have a normal triangular

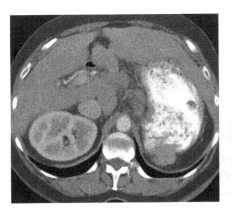
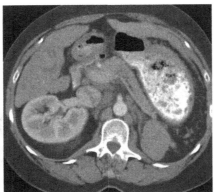
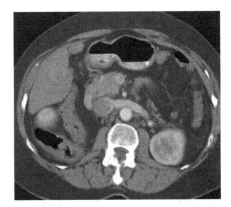

Fig. 7. This 47-year-old woman had a splenectomy after a car accident at the age of 17. A blood transfusion resulted 30 years later in the development of hepatitis C and eventually hepatocellular carcinoma (seen in the middle CT image). Notice the multiple implants that on nuclear study proved to be splenosis

shape (5%) with smooth or concave borders. A gastric diverticulum arising from the gastric cardia, and extending into the left adrenal fossa can mimic an adrenal mass. Oral contrast and scanning in different positions will often clarify the nature of the apparent mass.

Postoperative Pitfalls

Surgery of any type within the abdomen and pelvis may affect the normal orientation of the solid and hollow viscera. This may be due to either organ removal or transplantation, or as a result of an erroneously implanted foreign object, implantation of tissue and prosthesis, or creation of ostomies and pouches.

Pitfalls as the Result of Organ or Tissue Removal

Surgery may be performed in order to remove solid viscera such as a kidney, part of the liver or pelvic organs.

Post-nephrectomy Pitfalls

As the result of nephrectomy, which may be carried out as a treatment for renal cell carcinoma, unopacified bowel loops, pancreas, gallbladder, or spleen may occupy the vacant renal fossa, mimicking tumor recurrence or simulating an abscess, potentially resulting in unnecessary intervention.

Post-hepatic Lobectomy Pitfalls

Regeneration of the remaining liver by hypertrophy, hyperplasia, or both starts to take place immediately after partial hepatectomy. On CT, this is recognized by progressive enlargement and change in contour for six months to one year after resection. As a result, the gallbladder is often displaced to an unusual location, mimicking other pathologic conditions.

Post-cystectomy Pitfalls

Radical cystectomy results in a vacant space, which is usually filled by intestinal loops. Immediate postopera-

tive CT may be carried out in order to rule out an abscess, and follow-up CT is often requested to rule out any recurrent neoplasm. The use of adequate oral contrast agent before CT is important in such patients. Ileostomy, particularly when identified with opacified urine, is recognizable on CT, however a non-opacified continent ileostomy can be mistaken for an abscess or other collections.

Loop electrosurgical excision procedure (LEEP) is a way to test and treat cervical dysplasia. In some cases, it may be used to treat the early stages of cervical cancer. After such a procedure, the CT or ultrasound (US) will show the paucity of cervical tissue as a focal cervical canal dilatation mimicking a cystic lesion (Fig. 8).

Pitfalls as a Result of Abdominoperineal Resection (APR)

After APR for rectal carcinoma, in addition to recurrent tumors, the differential diagnosis of a presacral soft tissue mass should include unopacified bowel loops, relocated pelvic organs such as seminal vesicles or uterus, and postoperative fibrosis [8, 9]. Although the recurrent tumor often needs to be proven by biopsy or follow up, recognition of the other conditions is important to prevent an unnecessary intervention (Fig. 9).

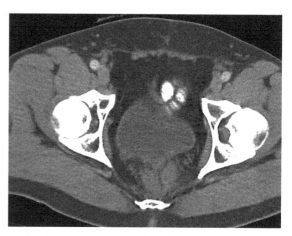

Fig. 9. After APR, the two seminal vesicles are inferiorly displaced

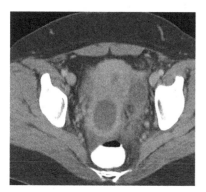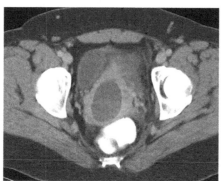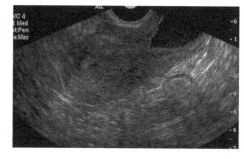

Fig. 8. The cervix after LEEP procedure, mimicking a cystic lesion. Notice the cystic area on the sagittal transvaginal sonogram

Pitfalls as the Result of Implantation of Tissue and Prosthesis

Whenever postoperative radiation therapy is contemplated in the pelvis, one of the limiting factors in its optimization is the low level of radiation tolerance of the small intestine [10]. Omental fat, synthetic absorbable mesh, or occasionally breast implant have been used during surgery to lift the small bowel out of the radiation field in patients treated for gynecologic or colonic cancers. The omental lid is formed into a pedicle flap, based on either the left or the right gastroepiploic artery, and is usually swung down to the left pericolic gutter to cover the denuded pelvic wall. Such a flap serves both as a vascular bed to absorb the serous drainage and as an X-ray barrier for the bowel loops. Without knowledge of such operations, the radiologist may misinterpret the CT images [11].

After localized resection of a renal lesion, such as a cyst, stone-filled caliceal diverticulum, or a small renal cell carcinoma, surgeons have used perinephric fat to tamponade the bleeding cut surface of the kidney before closing the renal capsule over the cortical defect [12]. This may also be done in liver cysts. Such fat can be a source of error in the interpretation of post-operative CT or sonogram. Also when removing large benign liver cyst or hydatid cysts, the surgeon may choose to fill the vacant area with omental fat (Fig. 10).

Pitfalls as the Result of Organ Transplantation

The organs commonly transplanted in the abdomen include the kidney, pancreas, and liver. Ovaries can be reimplanted for the purpose of protecting them from radiation therapy in the pelvis.

Renal Transplantation

In this condition, the transplanted kidney is easily recognizable. Post-operative complications such as infarctions and abscesses, however, may be difficult to diagnose if proper history is not available.

Pancreatic Transplantation

Such surgery is undertaken in selected patients in an attempt to prevent, arrest, or reverse progression of diabetes complications. A whole or segmental graft may have been obtained from a cadaver, and placed in the pelvis, which may appear as a soft tissue mass in pelvic CT.

Oophoropexy

At the time of radical hysterectomy for early-stage cervical carcinoma, the decision to remove or retain grossly normal ovaries in premenopausal patients involves weighing several competing factors. Ovarian conservation and lateral ovarian transplantation may be used when treating such patients [13]. When pelvic irradiation is planned, the ovaries are mobilized at the time of surgery. Then, with their vascular pedicle, they are transplanted near the peritoneum in each pericolic gutter (oophoropexy) and thus are removed from the radiation field. This information is vital to the radiologist so that normal ovaries will not be mistaken for an abnormal mass.

Pitfalls as the Result of Foreign Objects

Topical hemostatic materials are widely used to control bleeding in abdominal surgery. Oxidized regenerated cellulose is often used and is locally absorbed without tissue reaction [14, 15]. However, if left behind, they can mimic an abscess on follow-up CT in a febrile post-operative patient. Erroneously, larger material may be left in the abdomen and can mimic an abscess. Generally, the diagnosis of retained surgical foreign bodies continues to be a problem as long as non-absorbable materials are used (Fig. 11). Cotton sponges are inert, and they do not undergo any specific decomposition or biomedical reaction. Pathologically, however, there may be either an aseptic fibrinous reaction or an exudative response.

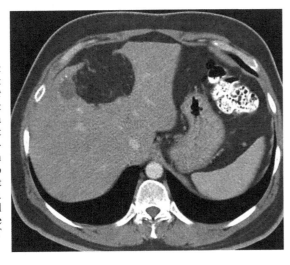 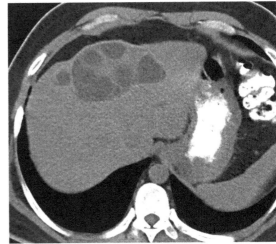

Fig. 10. This patient with hydatid cyst of the liver (*right image*) had a cyst removal about a year previously. At the time of operation, the surgeon used omental fat to fill the vacant space in the liver. Notice a small residual cyst on the post-operative CT scan (*left image*)

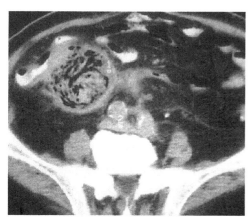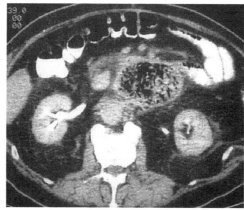

Fig. 11. This patient with history of abdominal aortic aneurysm (AAA) repair was found to have an abnormality extending from left upper quadrant (LUQ) to the right lower quadrant (RLQ). At surgery, a towel was removed

Pitfalls as the Result of Recent Procedures, Pouches, and Ostomies

Changes on CT related to operations such as gastroduodenostomy, gastrojejunostomy, pancreaticojejunostomy, ileocolostomy, and other types of anastomoses in the GI tract or the biliary system, are less likely to be sources of pitfalls. In patients who have had a gastrojejunostomy, however, an unopacified duodenal loop can cause confusion in evaluating the head of the pancreas for mass lesions. Ileostomies and colostomies, particularly when opacified by oral contrast or renal excretion of intravenous contrast, are easily recognizable on CT. A nonopacified continent ileostomy or the reservoir from ileocystostomy, however, can be mistaken for abscesses or other abnormal fluid collections [16].

A Puestow procedure is a surgical procedure performed for patients with chronic pancreatitis [17]. In these patients, the duct within the pancreas becomes dilated and obstructed. During the procedure, the duct is cleared and attached lengthwise to the small intestine. This increases the amount of pancreatic enzymes secreted into the small intestine. A CT scan after such a procedure can reveal an image that may mimic peri-pancreatic cysts.

References

1. Shirkhoda A (1991) Diagnostic pitfalls in abdominal CT. Radiographics 11:969-1002
2. Macari M, Lazarus D, Israel G, Megibow A (2003) Duodenal diverticula mimicking cystic neoplasms of the pancreas: CT and MR imaging findings in seven patients. AJR Am J Roentgenol 180:195-199
3. Marti-Bonmati L, Tabarra E, Manjon JV et al (2003) Comparison of different injection forms in CT examination of the upper abdomen. Abdom Imaging 28:799-804
4. Awai K, Imuta M, Utsunomiya D et al (2004) Contrast enhancement for whole-body screening using multidetector row helical CT: comparison between uniphasic and biphasic injection protocols. Radiat Med 22:303-309
5. Han JK, Kim AY, Lee KY et al (2000) Factors influencing vascular and hepatic enhancement at CT: experimental study on injection protocol using a canine model. J Comput Assist Tomogr 24:400-406
6. Ito K, Honjo K, Fujita T et al (1996) RF Liver neoplasms: diagnostic pitfalls in cross-sectional imaging. Radiographics 16:273-293
7. Hamer OW, Aguirre DA, Casola G et al (2005) Imaging features of perivascular fatty infiltration of the liver: initial observations. Radiology 237:159-169
8. Lee JKT, Stanley RJ, Sagel SS et al (1981) CT appearance of the pelvis after abdominoperineal resection for rectal carcinoma. Radiology 141:737-741
9. Pan G, Shirkhoda A (1987) Pelvic exenteration: role of CT in follow-up. Radiology164:665-670
10. Bakare SC, Shafir M, McElhinney AJ (1987) Exclusion of small bowel from pelvis for postoperative radiotherapy for rectal cancer. J Surg Oncol 35:55-58
11. Shirkhoda A (2000) Abdomen and pelvis; postoperative changes on CT in variants and pitfalls in body imaging. In: Shirkhoda A (ed) Variants and Pitfalls in Body Imaging. Lippincott Williams and Wilkins, Philadelphia, pp 491-503
12. Papanicolaou N, Harbury OL, Pfister RC (1988) Fat-filled postoperative renal cortical defects: sonographic and CT appearance. AJR Am J Roentgenol 151:503-505
13. Parker M, Bosscher J, Barnhill D, Park R (1993) Ovarian management during radical hysterectomy in the premenopausal patient. Obstet Gynecol 82:187-190
14. Kopka L, Fischer U, Gross AJ et al (1996) CT of retained surgical sponges (textilomas): pitfalls in detection and evaluation. J Comput Assist Tomogr 20:919-923
15. Young ST, Paulson EK, McCann RL et al (1993) Appearance of oxidized cellulose (surgical) on post-operative CT scans: similarity to postoperative abscess. Am J Roentgenol AJR 160:275-277
16. Shirkhoda A (1995) Diagnostic pitfalls in abdominal CT relevant to percutaneous interventions. Seminar Intervent Radiol 12:146-162
17. Freed KS, Paulson EK, Frederick MG et al (1997) Abdomen after a Puestow procedure: postoperative CT appearance, complications, and potential pitfalls. Radiology 203:790-794

An Approach to Imaging the Acute Abdomen in Pediatrics

A. Daneman[1], U. Willi[2]

[1] University of Toronto, and Division of General Radiology and Body Imaging, Department of Diagnostic Imaging, The Hospital for Sick Children, Toronto, Ontario, Canada

[2] Department of Radiology, University of Zurich Children's Hospital, Zurich, Switzerland

Introduction

The acute abdomen is a common and often challenging emergency in pediatrics. This chapter will provide an approach to the imaging evaluation of children with acute abdomen, highlighting briefly the more common causes of abdominal pain that may require surgery.

Causes of Acute Abdomen

There is a wide spectrum of pathologies that may give rise to acute abdominal pain. These include congenital and acquired lesions that may present in the immediate neonatal period, or in older infants and children.

The acute abdomen is not uncommon in neonates in Neonatal Intensive Care Units and may be the result of several causes, of which the three most significant are congenital bowel obstruction, complications of mid-gut malrotation and necrotizing enterocolitis (NEC).

In older infants and children the common causes of acute abdominal pain that may require surgery include acute appendicitis, complications of malrotation, intussusception, and Meckel diverticulum. Inflammatory bowel diseases may also present with acute abdominal symptomatology.

Although the above-mentioned causes of acute abdominal pain are due to lesions involving the gastrointestinal (GI) tract, there are many causes of the acute abdomen that are due to abnormalities of other viscera, including gynecological abnormalities such as ovarian torsion; omental lesions such as omental infarcts; obstructions of the biliary and urinary tracts due to stones; and inflammatory processes such as pancreatitis or hepatitis.

It has to be emphasized that abdominal pain may also be due to referred pain from extra-abdominal pathologies such as pneumonia or pleural effusion. Diseases such as sickle cell disease, Henoch-Schonlein purpura and hemolytic uremic syndrome may also cause significant acute abdominal pain. During imaging of the child with acute abdominal pain these other pathologies should also be considered.

Abdominal trauma may also cause acute abdomen. Occasionally, mild abdominal trauma may cause abdominal pain out of proportion to the degree of trauma and imaging in these children may reveal an underlying abnormality such as a neoplasm (Fig. 1) or an anomaly such as uretero-pelvic obstruction. Furthermore, one should

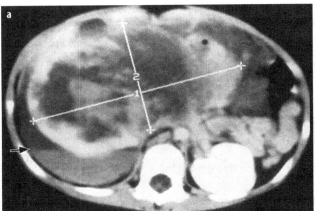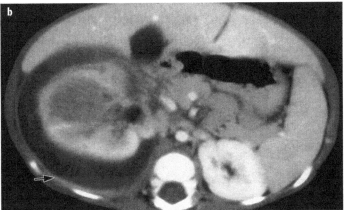

Fig. 1. CT scan after intravenous contrast injection in a 3 year old boy with minor abdominal trauma. **a** Scan shows large solid mass (outlined by electronic cursors). Fluid is noted in the right flank with a fluid fluid level (*arrow*). **b** The right kidney is displaced forward by a large perinephric fluid collection with a fluid fluid level (*arrow*). The mass is noted to arise in the kidney. This is an example of a marked amount of hemorrhage occurring following minor trauma to the abdomen in a patient with an underlying Wilms' tumour

consider non-accidental injury or abuse when certain traumatic lesions, such as hematomas of the left lobe of the liver and duodenum or pancreatitis are found, especially if these are present in combination.

Modalities

(i) Sonography Ultrasound (US) has come to play an increasingly important role in the management of children with acute abdominal pain, and has replaced the plain abdominal radiograph as the initial modality of choice in many clinical situations. The major advantages of US are that it does not utilize ionizing radiation, it is relatively inexpensive and the abdominal viscera including the bowel can be well-delineated. This allows the confirmation or exclusion of many pathological entities.

(ii) The plain abdominal radiograph (AXR) remains a standard method for the evaluation of the acute abdomen in some clinical situations. It is essential when peritonitis is present and perforation is suspected.

All neonates with an acute abdomen are evaluated with AXR. This modality is essential for the evaluation of conditions such as NEC and congenital bowel obstruction. In the former the AXR may be diagnostic and in the latter the findings guide the choice of subsequent contrast examinations of the gastrointestinal tract. Views with a horizontal beam are essential to exclude the presence of free air due to bowel perforation and can be performed with the neonate in the dorsal or lateral decubitus positions.

In older children the diagnosis of intestinal obstruction can often be made on the supine film alone. A search for air fluid levels on the upright view does not always add extra information and a search for free air in the abdomen is often more easily achieved using a lower radiation dose with a single upright view of the chest, which also serves to exclude lung pathology.

However, AXR findings are often non-specific in both the neonate and older child, limiting its utility.

(iii) Contrast studies of the GI tract are essential in certain conditions such as suspected mid-gut malrotation and congenital bowel obstruction. In the latter situation the contrast enema is important for diagnosis and therapy in some patients.

(iv) Computed tomography (CT) is reserved for more complicated imaging situations where US may not provide all the information required, e.g. in children with appendicitis when gas obscures the right lower quadrant, in older, obese children, or in children with abscesses. CT without contrast injection is also extremely helpful for the delineation of urinary stones that are not clear on US.

(v) Magnetic resonance (MR) has a very limited role in children with acute abdominal pain. However, it can depict anatomy exceptionally well in certain conditions, where it may be used to complement findings on US. Such conditions include biliary and pancreatic duct anomalies as well as gynecological disorders such as complex anomalies associated with hydrocolpos.

Acute Appendicitis

Acute appendicitis is a common clinical entity in pediatrics. In many patients clinical diagnosis can be easily made and no imaging is required prior to appendicectomy. However, imaging is extremely important in children who present with non-specific features. We use US as the modality of initial choice and try to reserve CT for those patients in whom US examination is inconclusive. We also use CT in patients with abscesses, in order to better define the extent of the abscesses prior to drainage by the interventional radiology team.

The diagnosis of appendicitis is made on US when the diameter of the appendix is greater than 6 mm and the appendix is non-compressible (Fig. 2). However, this should not be considered an absolute measurement and other features should be considered, including edema of the

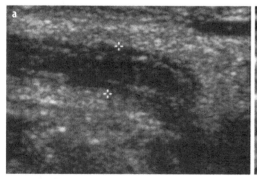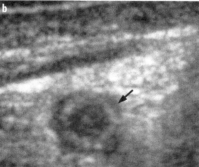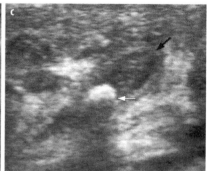

Fig. 2. Sonograms showing examples of acute appendicitis. **a** Longitudinal scan through the appendix shows distention of the appendix (distance between cursors measured 0.8 cm). The appendix was non-compressible and there is echogenic tissue surrounding the appendix due to edema of the surrounding mesentery. **b** Transverse scan through the appendix (*arrow*) shows a distended non-compressible appendix with surrounding edema of the soft tissues. **c** Example of appendicitis involving only the tip of the appendix. The tip of the appendix is distended to well above 0.6 cm (*black arrow*). The white arrow indicates the presence of an echogenic appendicolith with posterior shadowing. This example illustrates the importance of searching for the tip of the appendix

mesentery, hyperemia of the wall of the appendix on color or power Doppler examination, the presence of an appendicolith and local fluid collections or abscess formation. There are other conditions that may cause the appendix to become thick-walled and dilatated, including cystic fibrosis, Henoch-Schonlein purpura and inflammatory bowel diseases.

Malrotation

The radiologist plays an exceptionally important role in the diagnosis of this condition, which can potentially lead to bowel necrosis requiring extensive bowel resection and may even be fatal.

During development, the midgut undergoes a process of growth and elongation involving:
(i)   *Herniation* of the midgut into the umbilical cord along the axis of the superior mesenteric artery (SMA)
(ii) *Rotation* of 270 degrees in an anticlockwise direction
(iii) *Reduction* of the midgut into the abdomen by 12 weeks gestation and
(iv) *Fixation* of parts of the midgut by peritoneum.

The normal process of rotation and fixation is essential for the midgut to assume its normal mature position in the abdomen. However, abnormalities due to the arrest of rotation and/or fixation may occur at any phase of the above process and may involve only part or all of the midgut. This may, therefore, lead to a number of variations of malrotation and/or malfixation. The vast majority of these variations are associated with clinical symptoms that usually present within the first few months of life and may be life-threatening. Others may be associated with few or no symptoms and are incidentally found.

Malrotation usually leads to obstruction of the duodenum by (i) peritoneal (Ladd) bands that anchor the cecum to the retroperitoneum across the duodenum in the right upper quadrant, (ii) midgut volvulus due to the narrowed base of the mesentery or more rarely, (iii) internal hernia.

The clinical picture and imaging appearances depend on the nature and degree of obstruction as well as the presence or absence of vascular compromise.

Variety of Imaging Appearances of Malrotation

(i) Plain abdominal radiograph: In typical cases there is gaseous distension of the duodenum (Fig. 3), but the appearance may often be non-specific or even normal. In some patients the duodenum may be filled with fluid and not visible and only the stomach is distended with air. In children with severe vascular compromise due to volvulus, the entire small bowel is dilated (with air fluid levels), and resembles a low bowel obstruction or ileus (Fig. 4). One should therefore never rely on plain film findings to rule out malrotation. In any child where there is a suspicion of malrotation, particularly those with bilious vomiting, contrast studies of the GI tract or sonography should be carried out.

(ii) Contrast studies of the GI tract: In the past there was much debate about whether the upper GI series or contrast enema is the most effective way to diagnose malrotation. Today most institutions rely more on the upper GI series but if in doubt – do both! On the upper GI series the duodenojejunal flexure is absent and the proximal small bowel typically lies in the midline (Fig. 5). Rarely an internal hernia may be delineated. On the contrast enema the cecum is usually in the right upper quadrant and the ascending colon and hepatic flexure are not correctly positioned. One pitfall in diagnosis is the variation in position that the above structures may assume normally or with malrotation. Meticulous technique is critical to either type of study in order to delineate these structures accurately. The use of too much or too little contrast material may render the study undiagnostic.

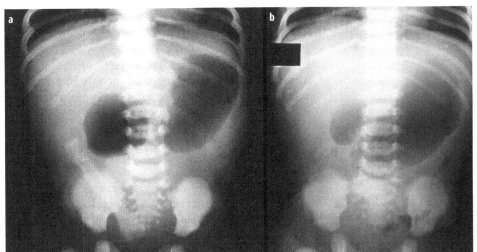

Fig. 3. Examples of high gastrointestinal obstruction in newborns. **a** A double bubble appearance is present due to distention of the stomach and duodenum by gas. There is no gas distally. The findings are typical of a duodenal atresia. **b** A double bubble is again noted due to gaseous distention of the stomach and duodenum. However, small amounts of gas are noted distally. Although this suggests the presence of a duodenal stenosis, this appearance is more likely due to a malrotation with obstruction of the duodenum usually due to Ladd's bands. Rarely, this appearance may be seen with a duodenal atresia when air passes around the atresia through distended ducts in the pancreas

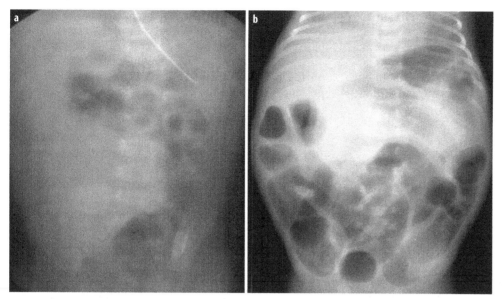

Fig. 4. Abdominal radiographs in two newborns with malrotation and volvulus. **a** Bowel gas is slightly distended and there is a soft tissue mass in the right hemi-abdomen due to fluid filled loops involved in the volvulus. At surgery the loops were viable. **b** Marked bowel gas distention throughout the abdomen. This is a non-specific appearance that may resemble a low congenital bowel obstruction or an ileus. There are some fluid-filled loops in the upper abdomen causing a small mass effect. At surgery there was malrotation with a volvulus and extensive necrotic bowel

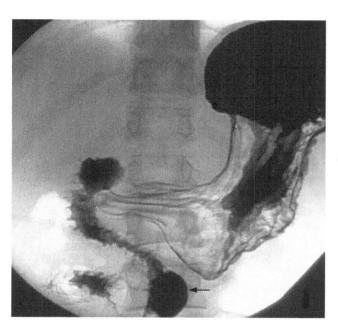

Fig. 5. Upper GI series in a 14-year-old boy presenting with vomiting and abdominal pain. The stomach is normal. The third part of the duodenum passes only to the midline and then inferiorly (*arrow*) and then to the right. This is a typical appearance of midgut malrotation. The duodenojejunal junction is absent from its normal position in the left upper quadrant

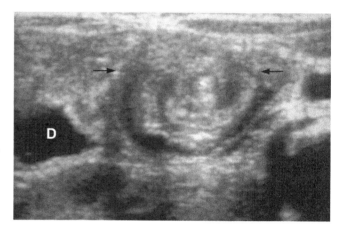

Fig. 6. A transverse sonogram of the upper abdomen in a neonate with bilious vomiting and abdominal tenderness. The duodenum (*D*) is distended with fluid and has a beak shape. In the mid abdomen there is a mass noted with concentric circles (*arrows*). This is typical of the whirlpool sign seen in midgut malrotation and volvulus

(iii) Sonography: Sonographic signs have been recently described in malrotation, but a normal sonogram does not exclude malrotation. Abnormalities that have been described include: (a) fluid distention of the duodenum, (b) inversion of the superior mesenteric artery and vein relationship – unfortunately this can be seen in a small proportion of asymptomatic, normal individuals, and (c) the whirlpool sign seen with midgut volvulus (Fig. 6). Rarely, ascites may be present in neonates.

Necrotizing Enterocolitis

NEC usually presents in infants in the Neonatal Intensive Care Unit – and is found more commonly in premature neonates. The classic presentation includes abdominal distention and blood in the stool. The radiologist plays an important role at the time of diagnosis of this condition, during follow-up and in the detection of later complications such as strictures.

(i) AXR: At the time of diagnosis there are three abnormalities that may be present on AXR, including bowel dilatation, intramural gas and portal venous gas.

Bowel dilatation is present in almost 100% of the patients with NEC and the degree of distention of the bowel usually correlates well with the clinical severity. Follow-up AXR may show asymmetric dilatation and fixed loops in those infants whose status deteriorates.

Intramural gas is not present in 100% of patients and the amount of intramural gas does not always correlate well with the degree of clinical severity (Fig. 7). *Portal venous gas* is usually present in patients with severe NEC. Disappearance of intramural gas and portal venous gas does not always correlate with clinical improvement, as the gas eventually disappears even in those children who deteriorate clinically.

(ii) US is an extremely useful modality for investigating patients with NEC, as it can provide information regarding the presence of intraperitoneal fluid, bowel wall thickness and bowel perfusion (using color or power Doppler sonography) (Fig. 8).

US is more accurate than AXR for documenting the presence of free and focal intra-peritoneal fluid and can also define the character of this fluid. It is well known that not all patients with NEC will show free air on AXR following perforation, and may present only with the presence of free fluid.

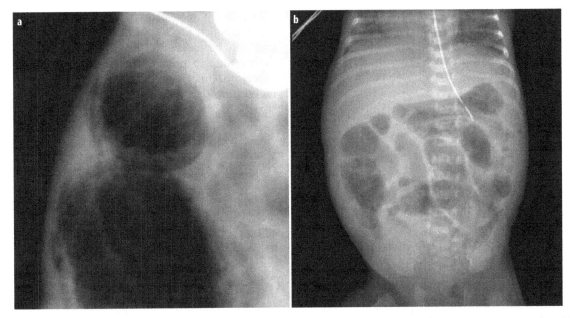

Fig. 7. Necrotizing enterocolitis in two newborns. **a** Bowel in the right flank shows marked distention with gas and evidence of intramural gas. Intramural gas is most commonly seen in newborns with necrotizing enterocolitis. **b** In another neonate there is moderate bowel gas distention. A bubbly appearance in the flanks suggests the presence of intramural air

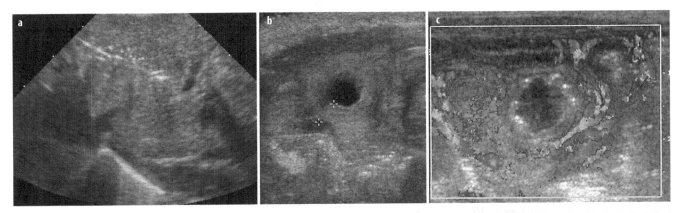

Fig. 8. Sonograms of the abdomen in three neonates with necrotizing enterocolitis. **a** Scan through the liver shows hyperechoic foci that have a linear or punctate configuration within the liver due to the presence of portal venous gas. Sonography is more sensitive for depicting the presence of portal venous gas than abdominal radiographs. **b** Loop of bowel showing marked thickening of the wall (between electronic cursors). Although this is seen commonly in necrotizing enterocolitis, thickening of the bowel wall is non-specific and can be seen in any cause of bowel edema. There is no intramural gas in the wall of this loop. **c** Color Doppler sonogram of the bowel shows two loops of bowel that are hyperemic, indicating that they are viable. The loops are found one on each side of another loop of bowel, which is distended with fluid and has hyperechoic foci in the bowel wall. The hyperechoic foci represent areas of intramural gas. There is no blood flow noted in this loop, suggesting that it is necrotic. Necrosis in this loop was confirmed at surgery

We have shown in the early phases of NEC that the bowel wall is quite thickened, while in more severely affected patients the mucosa and submucosa of the bowel sloughs into the lumen of the bowel, leaving a markedly thinned bowel wall, more prone to perforation. Thinning of the bowel wall can be documented with sonography. We have shown that in NEC the bowel (particularly thickened bowel) becomes markedly hyperemic and this indicates the presence of viable bowel. However, absence of bowel perfusion in single or multiple loops of bowel (particularly when the bowel wall is thinned) indicates the presence of necrosis and may warrant surgical intervention even if there is no free air present on the plain radiograph.

Sonography comes to play a more important role in the follow-up of patients that do not respond to medical management and those who deteriorate clinically. In these patients US may provide information that is not depicted with AXR.

Meckel Diverticulum

Meckel diverticulum most commonly presents as painless rectal bleeding due to ulceration caused by the presence of ectopic gastric mucosa. These patients are usually adequately diagnosed and managed following a radionuclide scan.

In under 50% of the children presenting with Meckel diverticulum clinical findings are more complex, with a combination of abdominal pain, vomiting and occasionally, rectal bleeding. In children with acute pain the diagnosis is often difficult and non-specific. US can be used successfully to document the presence of an inflamed or hemorrhagic Meckel diverticulum. In this situation the Meckel diverticulum has a variable appearance and may simulate the presence of an inflamed duplication cyst, appendicitis and sometimes a small intussusception. When this somewhat atypical appearance is present on US one should consider the diagnosis of a complicated Meckel diverticulum rather than the other pathologies it simulates.

Intussusception

See the chapter, 'Intussusception: An Approach to Management' for a review of this important cause of acute abdomen in Pediatrics.

Congenital Bowel Obstruction in the Neonate

Obstruction due to congenital lesions may occur at all levels of the GI tract and are, from a practical point of view, divided into 'high' or 'low' lesions. The high obstructions denote lesions of the esophagus, stomach, duodenum and upper small bowel. The low obstructions include lesions of the lower small bowel and large bowel, and anorectal malformations.

The distribution of dilated bowel loops on plain radiographs usually enables relatively easy differentiation of high from low obstruction, by evaluating the number of visible gas-filled loops. Fluid-filled loops may be difficult to visualize on plain radiographs and may masquerade as free fluid or masses; thus, they occasionally complicate the picture. It should be emphasized that the differentiation of dilated gas-filled small from large bowel loops may be impossible in neonates. Free air is not usually evident in these patients unless the diagnosis is delayed. Intramural air (and even portal venous gas) may be seen proximal to high grade obstruction, but it is much more commonly seen in NEC. Calcification may be present in the peritoneum (meconium peritonitis) due to prenatal perforation, in the wall of the bowel proximal due to an atresia, or in the bowel content within the lumen occasionally proximal to low obstruction.

Most complete high obstructions are easily diagnosed on plain radiographs. If the diagnosis is in doubt, air can be injected slowly via a feeding tube into the lumen of the GI tract to confirm or exclude an obstruction. In incomplete obstructions (e.g. malrotation and stenoses), positive water-soluble contrast agents are required to confirm the level and nature of obstruction.

Low obstructions include ileal and colonic atresias, meconium ileus, functional immaturity of the large bowel, Hirschsprung's disease and anorectal malformations. Although there are some features on plain radiographs that might suggest any of the above conditions, radiographic findings are often non-specific. Differentiation of these conditions, therefore, will depend on other factors such as clinical history and physical examination. Invariably, these conditions require the use of a water-soluble contrast enema to define the distal colon and ileum for a more confident diagnosis. The contrast enema may also prove therapeutic in patients with meconium ileus or meconium plugging in the colon.

Suggested Reading

Ang A, Chong NK, Daneman A (2001) Pediatric appendicitis in 'real-time': the value of sonography in diagnosis and treatment. Pediatr Emerg Care 17:334-340

Ashley LM, Allen S, Teele RL (2001) A normal sonogram does not exclude malrotation. Pediatr Radiol 31:354-356

Baldisserotto M, Marchiori E (2000) Accuracy of noncompressive sonography of children with appendicitis according to the potential positions of the appendix. AJR Am J Roentgenol 175:1387-1392

Bombelburg T, Von Lengerke HJ (1992) Sonographic findings in infants with suspected necrotizing enterocolitis. European J Radiol 15:149-153

Buonomo C (1999) The radiology of necrotizing enterocolitis. RCNA 37(6):1187-1198

Chao HC, Kong MS, Chen JY et al (2000) Sonographic features related to volvulus in neonatal intestinal malrotation. J Ultrasound Med 19:371-376

Daneman A, Lobo E, Alton DJ, Shuckett B (1998) The value of sonography, CT and air enema for detection of complicated Meckel diverticulum in children with nonspecific clinical presentation. Pediatr Radiol 28:928-932

Daneman A, Myers M, Shuckett B, Alton DJ (1997) Sonographic appearances of inverted Meckel diverticulum with intussusception. Pediatr Radiol 27:295-298

Donnolly LF, Rencken IO, deLorimier AA, Gooding CA (1996) Left paraduodenal hernia leading to ileal obstruction. Pediatr Radiol 26:534-536

Doria AS, Amernic H, Dick P et al (2005) Cost-effectiveness analysis of weekday and weeknight or weekend shifts for assessment of appendicitis. Pediatr Radiol 35:1186-1195

Dufour D, Delaet MH, Dassonville M et al (1992) Midgut malrotation, the reliability of sonographic diagnosis. Pediatr Radiol 22:21-23

Faingold R, Daneman A, Tomlinson G et al (2005) Bowel viability assessment by colour doppler sonography in necrotizing enterocolitis. Radiology 235:587-594

Fotter R, Sorantin E (1994) Diagnostic imaging in necrotizing enterocolitis. Acta Paediatr Supp 396:41-44

Fujii Y, Hata J, Futagami K et al (2000) Ultrasonography improves diagnostic accuracy of acute appendicitis and provides cost savings to hospitals in Japan. J Ultrasound Med 19:409-414

Katz ME, Siegel MJ, Shackelford GD, McAlister WH (1987) The position and mobility of the duodenum in children. AJR Am J Roentgenol 148:947-951

Kim G, Daneman A, Alton DJ et al (1997) The appearance of inverted Meckel diverticulum with intussusception on air enema. Pediatr Radiol 27:647-650

Kosloske AM, Love CL, Rohrer JE et al (2004) The diagnosis of appendicitis in children: outcomes of a strategy based on pediatric surgical evaluation. Pediatrics 113:29-34

Levy AD, Hobbs CM (2004) From the Archives of the AFIP. Meckel diverticulum: radiologic features with pathologic correlation. Radiographics 24:565-587

Long FR, Kramer SS, Markowitz RI et al (1996) Intestinal malrotation in children: tutorial on radiographic diagnosis in difficult cases. Radiology 198:775-780

Long FR, Kramer SS, Markowitz RI, Taylor GE (1996) radiographic patterns of intestinal malrotation in children. Radiographics 16:547-556

Loyer E, Eggli KD (1989) Sonographic evaluation of superior mesenteric vascular relationship in malrotation. Pediatr Radiol 19:173-175

Manji R, Warnock GL (2000) Left paraduodenal hernia: an unusual cause of small-bowel obstruction. Can J Surg 44:455-457

Miller SF, Seibert JJ, Kinder DL, Wilson AR (1993) Use of ultrasound in detection of occult bowel perforation in neonates. JU Med 12:531-535

O'Hara SM (1996) Pediatric gastrointestinal nuclear medicine. Radiol Clin North Am 34:845-862

Pena BMG, Taylor GA, Fishman SJ, Mandl KD (2002) Effect of an imaging protocol on clinical outcomes among pediatric patients with appendicitis. Pediatrics 110:1088-1093

Poortman P, Lohle PNM, Schoemaker CMC et al (2003) Comparison of CT and sonography in the diagnosis of acute appendicitis: a blinded prospective study. AJR Am J Roentgenol 181:1355-1359

Puylaert JB (1986) Acute appendicitis: US evaluation using graded compression. Radiology 158:355-360

Shimanuki Y, Aihara T, Takano H et al (1996) Clockwise whirlpool sign at color Doppler US: an objective and definite sign of midgut volvulus. Radiology 199:261-264

Sivit CJ (2004) Imaging the child with right lower quadrant pain and suspected appendicitis: current concepts. Pediatr Radiol 34:447-453

Taylor GA (2004) Suspected appendicitis in children: in search of the single best diagnostic test. Radiology 231:293-295

Weinberger E, Winters WD, Liddell RM et al (1992) Sonographic diagnosis of intestinal malrotation in infants: importance of the relative positions of the superior mesenteric vein and artery. AJR Am J Roentgenol 159:825-828

Wilson SR (1998) The gastrointestinal tract. In: Rumack CM, Wilson SR, Charboneau JW (eds) Diagnostic ultrasound, 2nd edn. Mosby, St. Louis, pp 279-327

Yoo SJ, Park KW, Cho SY et al (1999) Definitive diagnosis of intestinal volvulus in utero. Ultrasound Obstet Gynecol 13:200-203

Impairments of Swallowing: Diagnosis by Cineradiography

W. Brühlmann

Institut für Röntgendiagnostic, Stadtspital Triemli, Zurich, Switzerland

Topic and Learning Objective

This seminar concentrates on dynamic examination carried out using videofluoroscopy or digital cinematography.

After a short introduction on topographic and functional anatomy, radiographic anatomy, physiology and examination technique, cineradiographic sequences of normal deglutition, dysfunction of the pharyngoesophageal sphincter and typical examples of neuromuscular diseases affecting deglutition will be analyzed in detail.

After this seminar, participants should be able to correctly analyze impairments of swallowing and, with the help of a decision tree (Fig. 1) and a differential diagnostic table (Table 1), be able to allocate an individual case to the correct group of differential diagnoses.

Examination Technique

Liquid barium sulfate suspension is utilized for routine examinations. Semi-solid or solid (tablets) preparations may also be used in specific instances. Water-soluble contrast media are used where perforation is suspected. When used in patients with suspected aspiration, the preparations must be non-ionic and of low osmolarity, as aspiration of ionic contrast agent can lead to severe lung edema.

The ideal imaging modality available is digital cineradiography, but videofluorography represents a feasible alternative. It is less expensive and exposes the patient to less radiation; however, its use results in compromises in resolution and handling, especially for frame-by-frame analyses. The oral and pharyngeal phases are recorded with at least 30 frames per second, starting in the upright position. Oral cavity, pharynx and pharyngo-esophageal segments should be in the field of vision; the image intensifier should be kept stationary. At least one swallow is filmed in the antero-posterior (a.-p.) and in the lateral position. In the a.-p. position, head and body should be perfectly aligned; any relative rotation will cause unilateral passage of the bolus through the hypopharynx and may thus simulate palsy or a tumor. One swallow should be examined in the lateral decubitus position, eliminating the effect of gravity and making weakness of propulsion more evident. Finally, one swallow is followed from the mouth to the stomach in the left posterior oblique (LPO) prone position. Here, digital recording of fluoroscopy

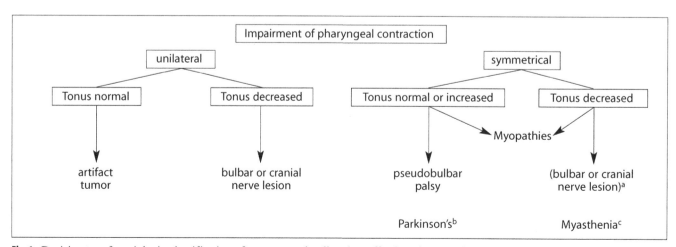

Fig. 1. Decision tree for etiologic classification of neuromuscular disorders affecting pharyngeal motility
[a] Rigor, mainly of the tongue, resulting in 'piecemeal deglutition'; [b] bilateral lesions lead to complete aphagia, making radiologic examination impossible; [c] 'fatigue' phenomenon: progressive impairment with repeated swallows

Table 1. Systematic classification of neuromuscular lesions and their effects on deglutition

Site of lesion	Typical representative	Phase affected	Asymmetry	Tonus	Aspiration primary	Aspiration secondary	Frequent or specific symptoms
Psychogenic	anxious depression	1	–	normal	–	–	apraxia
Cortical (tumor, cortical infarct)		1	–	normal	–	apraxia	
Corticobulbar tracts (brain stem)	pseudobulbar palsy	1 + 2	–	normal or +	–	+	PES[a]
Extrapyramidal system	Parkinson's disease	1 (+ 2)	–	normal	–	–	rigor, piecemeal deglutition
Cerebellum	tumor, metastasis	1	+	normal	–	–	
	cerebellar atrophy	1	–	normal	–	–	
Nuclei, cranial nerves	tumor or surgery post. fossa/skull base	1, 2, 1 + 2 (depending on nerves affected)	+	–	+	+	
End plates	myasthenia	1 + 2	–	(–)[b]	–	+	fatigue phenomenon nasal regurgitation
Striated muscle[c]	polymyositis	1 + 2	–	normal or –	–	+	
Smooth muscle[c]	systemic sclerosis	3	–	–	–	+	reflux (LES incompetence)

[a] Incomplete relaxation of pharyngoesophageal sphincter
[b] May be normal at beginning of examination
[c] Often combined (overlap syndromes)

with a pulse rate of 12 to 15 pps can be used, which exposes the patient to less radiation. During the entire bolus passage through the esophagus, the patient should not swallow, as this would immediately interrupt peristalsis.

Anatomy and Physiology

Topography and radiographic anatomy will not be dealt with in this abstract. Functional muscular anatomy divides the pharyngeal musculature into three groups: the *elevators*, the *constrictors* and the *pharyngoesophageal sphincter*. The *elevators* insert at the base of the skull, the jaw, the hyoid bone and the thyroid cartilage. These muscles move the laryngopharynx upward and forwards at the beginning of the pharyngeal phase. The *constrictors*, consisting of the ceratopharyngeus, the thyreopharyngeus and the oblique part of the cricopharyngeus muscle, propel the bolus through the pharyngeal cavity by their peristaltic activity in conjunction with the tongue rolling backward and downwards over the hyoid bone. The *pharyngoesophageal sphincter*, consisting of the transverse portion of the cricopharyngeus muscle and adjacent transverse fibers of the esophageal musculature, maintains a tonic contraction between swallows. As soon as peristaltic contraction of the constrictors begins, the sphincter relaxes completely

and will not contract again until complete passage of the ingested bolus into the esophagus.

Deglutition can be divided into an oral, a pharyngeal and an esophageal phase.

The *oral phase (phase 1)* is under full voluntary control. First, the taste, texture and temperature of the bolus are analyzed. The voluntary act of swallowing is prepared by premotor activity of cortical areas in the cingulate gyrus, the insula and the inferior frontal gyrus.

When a bolus has been recognized as edible and palatable, the motor activities in the oral phase are controlled by the precentral gyrus. After mastication, the bolus is loaded onto the back of the tongue. It is held there in the form of a spoon, between the back of the tongue and the soft palate and pharyngopalatine arch.

The *pharyngeal phase (phase 2)*, starts with a voluntary upward movement of the soft palate, allowing the bolus to flow into the mesopharynx, where it comes into contact with tactile receptors of the mucosa. This triggers the *swallowing reflex* via afferent fibres mainly from the cranial nerves IX and X, which run within the solitary tract. From here on, swallowing cannot be influenced by voluntary control. It is 'organized' and controlled by the *medullary swallowing center*, which consists of the nucleus tractus solitarii, the nucleus ambiguus and surrounding parts of the formatio reticularis. Efferent pathways run within the cranial nerves V and VI, and, mainly, through the cranial nerves X and XII and their nuclei. Nerves X and XII anastomose to form the plexus pharyngeus. During passage of the bolus through the hypopharynx, the airways have to be sealed to avoid aspiration. The entrance of the larynx is closed by axial compression of its vestibule during elevation of the larynx against the base of the tongue, while the glottis itself is closed by the action of the external and internal laryngeal musculature innervated by cranial nerve X.

The *esophageal phase (phase 3)* is also initiated by the medullary swallowing center. Peristaltic contraction of the striated musculature within the first centimeters of the esophagus is innervated by 'early motoneurons' within the nucleus ambiguus, while the activity of the more distal smooth musculature is influenced by 'late motoneurons' within the nucleus of the vagus nerve. Here, peristaltic activity can also be induced by local distension, independent of the medullary center.

Cineradiography: Normal Appearance

During phase 1, the tongue collects a liquid bolus from the floor of the mouth with a symmetrical movement. The bolus is then contained within the oral cavity by the closed portal formed by the soft palate and the pharyngopalatine arch. Phase 2 is immediately initiated after opening of the portal. The soft palate is pulled up and backwards, until it comes into contact with the posterior pharyngeal wall and completely seals the passage between epipharynx and mesopharynx. The tongue rolls back and downwards over the elevated hyoid bone, initiating propulsion of the bolus, which is assisted and completed by peristaltic contraction of the pharyngeal constrictor. This is best seen in the lateral projection as a 'stripping wave', which moves downwards along the posterior pharyngeal wall. During passage of the entire bolus, the posterior aspect of the pharyngoesophageal junction is smooth. However, a slight bulge of the posterior wall amounting to less than one third of the sagittal diameter of the lumen, caused by some residual contraction of the pharyngoesophageal sphincter, is, especially in older patients, still considered as normal. At the beginning of phase 2, the larynx is elevated and compressed under the base of the tongue. The laryngeal vestibule, seen as an air-filled cavity before the beginning of phase 2, collapses completely. The epiglottis is tilted backwards and downwards over the aditus laryngis. A small amount of contrast agent may initially penetrate under the epiglottis into the laryngeal vestibule. It will, however, be completely ejected during further passage of the bolus. The glottis is closed during phase 2.

In the resting state after a barium swallow, the pharynx shows only a thin contrast coating of its walls. No resid-

ual material should be pooled in the valleculae or the pyriform recesses. The aspect of the barium-coated pharynx should be symmetrical in the a.-p. projection; both pyriform recesses are at the same height and have a pointed lower aspect with an acute angle between the lateral hypopharyngeal wall and the 'floor' of the hypopharynx.

Pathologic Phenomena

Apraxia is characterized by difficulty or inability to initialize the pharyngeal phase of swallowing. A bolus that has been loaded on the back of the tongue is held there, then released to the floor of the mouth, then gathered and loaded again by the tongue etc., until the patient finally 'decides' to swallow. Phase 2 and 3 are usually normal. Apraxia occurs with cortical (mainly precentral) lesions, with psychogenic disorders (namely, anxious depression) or after long-time gastric tube or parenteral feeding.

Impairments of phase 1 are usually due to impaired motility of the tongue. Lesions of the cranial nerve XII or its nucleus will lead to lax paralysis of the tongue, while lesions of the corticobulbar tracts lead to symmetric, spastic paralysis. Both types of lesions make gathering and loading of the bolus onto the back of the tongue difficult or impossible. Often, the bolus will have to be passively 'decanted' into the pharynx by tilting the head backwards. Parkinson's disease causes rigor or 'stiffness' of the tongue. The bolus is gathered from the floor of the mouth and swallowed in very small fractions ('piecemeal deglutition'). In patients with myasthenia gravis, tongue motility decreases with repeated swallows. Due to reduced tonus of the muscles inserting into the hyoid bone, the tongue sinks down into the floor of the mouth. *Impairment of pharyngeal motility* can be unilateral or symmetric, lax or spastic.

Unilateral impairment is usually due to bulbar or cranial nerve lesions (X and XII), leading to lax paralysis. The bolus will pass mainly through the intact side of the pharynx, while the affected side passively bulges out. In the resting state after a swallow, the pyriform recess of the affected side contains a pool of residual material. Its floor is at a lower level than its counterpart and forms a more obtuse angle with the lateral pharyngeal wall. *Bilateral, symmetric impairment* can be caused by pseudobulbar palsy, by fibrous encasement ('frozen neck' after radiotherapy) or by myopathies. The muscle tone in the resting state is normal or increased. *Bilateral laxity*, with sagging and residual contrast pooling of both pyriform recesses develops after repeated swallows in patients with myasthenia gravis ('fatigue phenomenon'). *Nasal regurgitation* occurs mainly with myasthenia gravis. It is usually possible to compensate for unilateral palsy of the velum palatinum after lesions of cranial nerve XII. *Aspiration* can occur in two forms, which are entirely different with respect to their mechanism and their severity. *Primary as-*

piration is due to a defective closure of the larynx during swallowing. The first protective mechanism is closure of the aditus laryngis by axial compression of the vestibulum under the base of the tongue. This mechanism can be impaired by palsy of the elevator muscles inserted into the hyoid bone (nerves VII und IX), of the tongue itself (nerve X), and by postoperative defects at the base of the tongue and the supraglottic part of the larynx. If glottic closure is still intact, only a small part of the bolus penetrates into the laryngeal vestibule during deglutition and is held there until reopening of the glottis after deglutition, when it is aspirated into the trachea. The second and last barrier against aspiration is closure of the glottis by apposition of the true and false cords of the two sides. If this mechanism fails, too, a part of the ingested bolus is aspirated directly into the airways. This very serious and life-threatening event can be produced by lesions of cranial nerve X at or above the ganglion nodosum (above the origin of the superior laryngeal nerve), by defects at the glottis itself, or by severe sensory impairment preventing the initiation of the swallowing reflex after penetration of the bolus from the oral cavity into the pharynx.

In *secondary aspiration*, the laryngeal closure mechanisms are intact. Aspiration occurs because of a spillover of material retained in the pyriform recesses. The material penetrates into the larynx, which reopens after the pharyngeal phase of swallowing. This form of aspiration can occur with any disease that causes severe impairment in pharyngeal motility. The amount of aspirated material is limited to the amount of material retained in the pharynx. The risk of aspiration can be reduced by repeatedly swallowing after ingestion of a bolus.

A systematic overview of the neuromuscular disorders that may cause impairment in swallowing is given in Table 1 and Fig. 1. Frequently, a specific diagnosis has already been established before the patient is referred for cineradiographic examination of swallowing difficulties. However, dysphagia or aspiration may be the first or most prominent symptom of a neurologic or muscular disorder. Here, the radiologist should not only describe the pathologic phenomena he has observed, but also give a differential diagnosis of the diseases that could be responsible.

Dysfunctions of the pharyngoesophageal sphincter can be classified into alterations of its resting tonus and impairments of relaxation. *Spasm* (increased resting tonus) can only be diagnosed by manometry, and not by radiologic methods, but only by. *Chalasia* (decreased or absent resting tonus) is a phenomenon that has only been observed in myotonic dystrophy or after myotomy of the sphincter. In conjunction with esophageal motility disorders, it can lead to reflux of esophageal and gastric contents into the pharynx and cause secondary aspiration. *Incomplete relaxation (Achalasia), delayed opening and premature closure* of the sphincter can occur without an evident underlying disease (idiopathic form) or sec-

ondary to a variety of diseases. An overview of the incidence and etiology of sphincter dysfunctions is given in Tables 2 and 3.

The only effective therapy for sphincter dysfunctions, except those secondary to a curable underlying disease, is myotomy of the sphincter. Here, cineradiographic examination serves not only to diagnose the dysfunction, but also to establish indications for and contraindications against myotomy. A good result after surgery can only be expected if pharyngeal propulsion of the bolus is not severly impaired. In severe gastroesophageal reflux, myotomy is contraindicated as the pharyngoesophageal sphincter is the last barrier against reflux into the pharynx and aspiration of gastric contents. *Zenker's diverticula* invariably have their origin within Killian's triangle, between the pharyngoesophageal sphincter and the pharyngeal constrictor muscles. They are very frequently associated with dysfunctions of the sphincter, mostly with premature closure. Although the transition from a mere dysfunction of the sphincter into the formation of a diverticulum has not yet been demonstrated in a patient, a causative role of impaired sphincter relaxation is very probable. *Lateral diverticula* of the pharynx are very rare. Acquired diverticula can have their origin in a weak point of the thyreohyoid membrane or at the lateral wall of the pharyngoesophageal segment, between the cricopharyngeal muscle and the circular muscle fibers of the esophagus. Congenital diverticula are communicating branchiogenic cysts. Their pharyngeal orifice is situated at the tonsillar fossa or the vallecula (2nd branchial cleft remnants) or at the lateral wall of the pyriform recessus (3rd and 4th branchial cleft remnants).

Table 2. Incidence of impaired pharyngoesophageal sphincter relaxation in 600 patients with dysphagia

Total	110	(18%)
incomplete relaxation		40%
dyscoordination	delayed relaxation	10%
	premature contraction	30%
combined dysfunctions		20%

Table 3. Etiology of pharyngoesophageal sphincter dysfunction in 100 patients

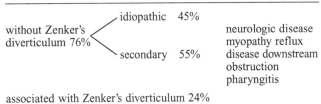

without Zenker's diverticulum 76%	idiopathic 45%	neurologic disease myopathy reflux disease downstream obstruction pharyngitis
	secondary 55%	

associated with Zenker's diverticulum 24%

Suggested Reading

Brühlmann W (1990) Röntgendiagnostik des pharyngo-oe- sophagealen Ueberganges. Archives of Oto-Rhino-Larnyg- ology (Suppl I):87-106

Brühlmann W (1991) Die ätiologische Differenzierung von neuro- muskulär bedingten Schluckstörungen mittels Röntgenkine- matographie Fortschr. Röntgenstr 155:556-561

Daniel St, Brailey K, Foundas A (1999) Lingual discoordination and dysphagia following acute stroke: analyses of lesion loca- tion. Dysphagia 14:85-92

Dodds W, Stewart E, Logemann J (1990) Physiology and radiolo- gy of the normal and pharyngeal phases of swallowing. AJR Am J Roentgenol 154:953-963

Ekberg O, Feinberg M (1991) Altered swallowing function in el- derly patients without dysphagia: radiologic findings in 56 cases. AJR Am J Roentgenol 156:1181-1184

Jones B (2003) Normal and abnormal swallowing imaging in diagno- sis and therapy, 2nd ed. Springer, Berlin, Heidelberg, New York

Watanabe Y, Abe S, Ishikawa T et al (2004) Cortical regulation dur- ing the early stage of initiation of voluntary swallows in Humans. Dysphagia 19:100-108

Diseases of the Esophagus

M.S. Levine

Gastrointestinal Radiology, Department of Radiology, University of Pennsylvania Medical Center, Philadelphia, PA, USA

Introduction

This syllabus reviews the findings on esophagography for a variety of esophageal diseases, including reflux esophagitis, Barrett's esophagus, other types of esophagitis, benign and malignant esophageal tumors, varices, lower esophageal rings, esophageal intramural pseudodiverticulosis, and esophageal motility disorders.

Reflux Esophagitis

Reflux esophagitis is by far the most common inflammatory disease involving the esophagus. The single most common sign of reflux esophagitis on double-contrast esophagrams is a finely nodular or granular appearance in the distal third of the esophagus, with poorly defined radiolucencies that fade peripherally due to edema and inflammation of the mucosa [1]. In other patients, barium studies may reveal shallow ulcers and erosions in the distal esophagus contiguous with the gastroesophageal junction [2]. Reflux esophagitis may also be manifested by thickened longitudinal folds due to edema and inflammation that extend into the submucosa. However, thickened folds should be recognized as a nonspecific finding of esophagitis. Other patients with reflux esophagitis may have a single enlarged, chronically inflamed fold that arises at the gastric cardia and extends into the distal esophagus as a smooth protuberance, also known as an inflammatory esophagogastric polyp [3]. These lesions have no malignant potential, so endoscopy is not warranted when barium studies reveal typical findings of an inflammatory polyp in the distal esophagus.

Scarring from reflux esophagitis can lead to the development of a reflux-induced stricture (i.e., 'peptic' stricture) in the distal esophagus, almost always above a hiatal hernia. Such strictures typically appear as smooth, tapered segments of concentric narrowing, but asymmetric scarring can lead to asymmetric narrowing with focal sacculation or ballooning of the esophageal wall between areas of fibrosis. Other peptic strictures may be manifested by short, ring-like areas of narrowing that could be mistaken for Schatzki rings in patients with dysphagia [4]. Scarring from reflux esophagitis can also lead to longitudinal shortening of the esophagus and the development of fixed transverse folds, producing a 'stepladder' appearance due to pooling of barium between the folds [5]. These folds should be differentiated from the thin transverse striations (i.e., 'feline' esophagus) often seen as a transient finding at fluoroscopy due to contraction of the longitudinally oriented muscularis mucosae [6].

Barrett's Esophagus

Barrett's esophagus is a premalignant condition in which there is progressive columnar metaplasia of the distal esophagus due to chronic reflux and reflux esophagitis. Barrett's esophagus is thought to develop in about 10% of all patients with reflux esophagitis. Double-contrast esophagrams can be used to classify patients with reflux symptoms at high, moderate, or low risk for Barrett's esophagus, based on specific radiologic criteria [7]. Patients are classified at high risk when double-contrast esophagrams reveal a mid-esophageal stricture or ulcer, or a reticular mucosal pattern (usually associated with a hiatal hernia and/or gastroesophageal reflux) [7]. In such cases, endoscopy and biopsy should be performed for a definitive diagnosis. Patients are classified at moderate risk for Barrett's esophagus when double-contrast studies reveal reflux esophagitis or peptic strictures in the distal esophagus [7]. The decision for endoscopy in this group should be based on the severity of symptoms, age, and overall health of the patients. Finally, patients are classified at low risk for Barrett's esophagus when double-contrast studies reveal no structural abnormalities. The majority of patients are found to be in this category, and the prevalence of Barrett's esophagus is so low that they can be treated empirically for their reflux symptoms, without need for endoscopy [7].

Infectious Esophagitis

Candida Esophagitis

Candida albicans is the most common cause of infectious esophagitis. It usually occurs as an opportunistic infection in immunocompromised patients, particularly AIDS patients. Only about 50% of patients with *Candida* esophagitis are found to have thrush, so the absence of oropharyngeal disease in no way excludes this diagnosis.

Candida esophagitis is usually manifested on double-contrast studies by multiple discrete plaque-like lesions that tend to be oriented longitudinally and are separated by normal mucosa [8]. Double-contrast esophagrams have a sensitivity of 90% in detecting *Candida* esophagitis [8], primarily because of their ability to demonstrate these mucosal plaques. During the past two decades, a much more fulminant form of candidiasis has been encountered in patients with AIDS, who may present with a grossly irregular or 'shaggy' esophagus caused by innumerable coalescent pseudomembranes and plaques with trapping of barium between these lesions (Fig. 1) [9]. Other patients with achalasia or scleroderma may develop a 'foamy' esophagus with innumerable tiny bubbles layering out in the barium column; this phenomenon presumably results from the yeast form of fungal infection [10]. When typical findings of *Candida* esophagitis are encountered on double-contrast esophagrams, these patients can be treated with antifungal agents without the need for endoscopy.

Herpes Esophagitis

The herpes simplex virus type 1 is another common cause of infectious esophagitis. Most affected patients are immunocompromised, but herpes esophagitis may occasionally develop as an acute, self-limited disease in otherwise healthy individuals [11]. Viral infection initially leads to the development of small vesicles that rupture to form discrete, punched-out ulcers on the mucosa. As a result, herpes esophagitis may be manifested on double-contrast studies by multiple superficial ulcers on a normal background mucosa (Fig. 2) [12]. In the appropriate

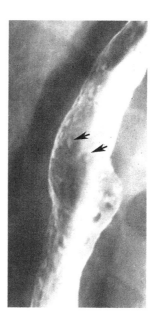

Fig. 2. Herpes esophagitis. Double-contrast esophagram shows multiple small, discrete ulcers with surrounding mounds of edema (*arrows*) in mid-esophagus

clinical setting, small, discrete ulcers without plaques should be highly suggestive of herpes esophagitis, as ulceration in candidiasis almost always occurs on a background of diffuse plaque formation. As the disease progresses, however, herpes esophagitis may be manifested by a combination of ulcers and plaques, mimicking *Candida* esophagitis [12].

Cytomegalovirus Esophagitis

Cytomegalovirus (CMV) is another cause of infectious esophagitis that occurs in patients with AIDS. CMV esophagitis may be manifested on double-contrast studies by multiple small ulcers or, even more commonly, by one or more giant, flat ulcers that are several centimeters or more in length [13]. Herpetic ulcers rarely become this large, so the presence of one or more giant ulcers should suggest CMV esophagitis in patients with AIDS. However, the differential diagnosis also includes giant human immunodeficiency virus (HIV) ulcers in the esophagus (see next section). Because CMV is treated with toxic antiviral agents such as ganciclovir, endoscopy is required to confirm the presence of CMV before treating these patients.

Human Immunodeficiency Virus Esophagitis

HIV infection can lead to the development of giant esophageal ulcers indistinguishable from those caused by CMV. Double-contrast esophagrams typically reveal one or more giant ulcers surrounded by a radiolucent rim of edema, sometimes associated with a cluster of small satellite ulcers (Fig. 3) [14]. Occasionally, these individuals may have associated palatal ulcers or a characteristic rash on the upper body. The diagnosis is established by obtaining endoscopic biopsy specimens, brushings, or cultures to rule out CMV esophagitis as the cause of the ulcers. Unlike CMV ulcers, HIV-related esophageal ul-

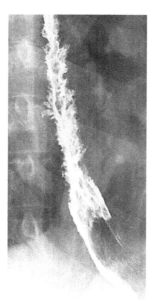

Fig. 1. Advanced *Candida* esophagitis in a patient with AIDS. Double-contrast esophagram shows 'shaggy' esophagus of fulminant esophageal candidiasis due to innumerable plaques and pseudomembranes with trapping of barium between lesions

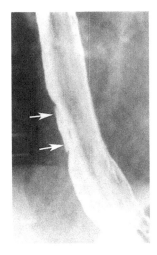

Fig. 3. HIV ulcer in a patient with AIDS. Double-contrast esophagram shows large, flat ulcer in profile (*arrows*) in distal esophagus. Although CMV esophagitis could produce identical findings, endoscopic brushings and biopsies revealed no evidence of CMV

cers usually heal dramatically on treatment with oral steroids [14]. Thus, endoscopy is required in HIV-positive patients with giant esophageal ulcers to differentiate esophagitis caused by HIV and CMV, so appropriate therapy can be instituted in these patients.

Drug-induced Esophagitis

Tetracycline and doxycycline are the two most common causes of drug-induced esophagitis in the United States, but other offending agents include potassium chloride, quinidine, aspirin or other nonsteroidal antiinflammatory drugs (NSAIDs), and alendronate sodium [15]. Affected individuals typically ingest the medication with little or no water immediately before going to bed. The capsules or pills usually become lodged in the mid-esophagus where it is compressed by the adjacent aortic arch or left main bronchus. Prolonged contact of the esophageal mucosa with these medications presumably causes an irritant contact esophagitis. Affected individuals may present with severe odynophagia, but marked clinical improvement usually occurs after withdrawal of the offending agent.

The radiographic findings depend on the offending medication. Tetracycline and doxycycline are associated with the development of small, shallow ulcers in the upper or mid-esophagus indistinguishable from those in herpes esophagitis [15]. These ulcers almost always heal without scarring because of their superficial nature. In contrast, potassium chloride, quinidine, NSAIDs, and alendronate sodium may cause more severe esophageal injury, sometimes leading to the development of larger ulcers and strictures [15].

Idiopathic Eosinophilic Esophagitis

Idiopathic eosinophilic esophagitis (IEE) is a chronic form of esophagitis characterized by an increased number of intraepithelial eosinophils (more than 20 per high power field) on endoscopic biopsy specimens [16]. The etiol-

ogy is uncertain, but this condition most likely develops as a result of an inflammatory response to ingested food allergens. Most adults with IEE are young men with longstanding dysphagia and recurrent food impactions [16]. They classically have an atopic history (e.g., asthma, allergic rhinitis) and peripheral eosinophilia, but IEE frequently occurs as an isolated condition [16]. Affected individuals are treated with topical steroids (swallowing metered doses of aerosolized steroid preparations) and protein-free diets with varying degrees of success.

IEE may be manifested on esophagography by segmental strictures in the esophagus. The strictures often contain distinctive ring-like indentations, resulting in a so-called 'ringed' esophagus [16]. Other patients with IEE may have diffuse esophageal narrowing, resulting in a 'small-caliber' esophagus [16]. A ringed esophagus has also been described in congenital esophageal stenosis. Affected individuals may develop strictures with multiple concentric rings indistinguishable from those in IEE (Fig. 4) [17]. Although congenital esophageal stenosis is usually not associated with an allergic history or peripheral eosinophilia, this condition also occurs in young men with longstanding dysphagia, and biopsies from the esophagus may also reveal increased numbers of intra-epithelial eosinophils [17]. Due to the similarities in the clinical, radiographic, and pathologic findings of these conditions, the symptoms of some of the patients with reported congenital esophageal stenosis may have been due to IEE.

Benign Tumors

Squamous papillomas are the most common benign mucosal tumors in the esophagus, usually appearing on

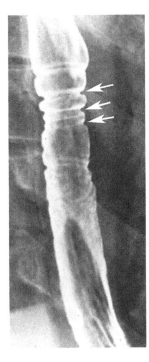

Fig. 4. Congenital esophageal stenosis. Double-contrast esophagram shows mild narrowing of midesophagus with distinctive ring-like constrictions (*arrows*), most likely due to cartilaginous rings in wall of esophagus

double-contrast esophagrams as small, sessile polyps with a smooth or slightly lobulated contour. In contrast, leiomyomas are the most common benign submucosal tumors in the esophagus, appearing on esophagography as intramural masses with the typical features of the submucosal lesions found elsewhere in the gastrointestinal tract.

Fibrovascular polyps are rare, benign tumors consisting of fibrovascular and adipose tissue covered by squamous epithelium [18]. Fibrovascular polyps usually arise near the cricopharyngeus, gradually elongating over a period of years as they are dragged inferiorly by esophageal peristalsis. Rarely, these patients may have a spectacular clinical presentation with regurgitation of a fleshy mass into the mouth or even asphyxia and sudden death if the regurgitated polyp occludes the larynx [18]. Fibrovascular polyps typically appear on barium studies as smooth, expansile, sausage-shaped masses in the esophagus (Fig. 5) [18]. Polyps composed predominantly of adipose tissue may appear as fat-density lesions on CT (Fig. 6a), whereas polyps containing adipose and fibrovascular tissue may have a more heterogeneous appearance with areas of fat juxtaposed with areas of soft-tissue density (Fig. 6b) [18].

Esophageal Carcinoma

Double-contrast esophagography has a sensitivity of greater than 95% for the detection of esophageal cancer [19]. Early esophageal cancers are usually small, protruded lesions less than 3.5 cm in size. These tumors may be manifested on double-contrast studies by plaque-like lesions, by sessile polyps with a smooth or slightly lobulated contour, or by focal irregularity of the esophageal wall [20]. Early adenocarcinomas may also be manifested by a localized area of wall flattening or irregularity

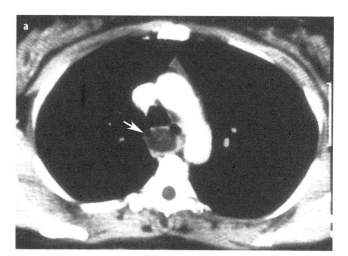

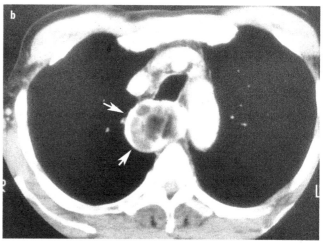

Fig. 6. a Giant fibrovascular polyps on CT scan shows expansile mass (*arrow*) of fat density in mid-esophagus. This finding is seen when a polyp is composed predominantly of adipose tissue. **b** CT scan in another patient shows expansile, heterogeneous mass (*arrows*) in esophagus. This finding is seen when lesion contains adipose and fibrovascular tissue

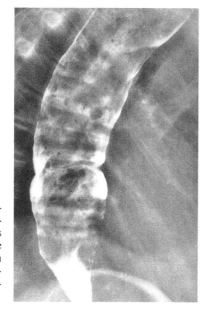

Fig. 5. Giant fibrovascular polyp. Double-contrast esophagram shows long, smooth, expansile mass extending from proximal esophagus distally to near gastroesophageal junction

within a pre-existing peptic stricture [20]. Superficial spreading carcinoma is another form of early esophageal cancer characterized by poorly defined nodules or plaques that merge with one another, producing a confluent area of disease [20].

Advanced esophageal carcinomas usually appear on barium studies as infiltrating (Fig. 7), polypoid, ulcerative (Fig. 8), or varicoid lesions that mimic the appearance of varices due to submucosal spread of tumor [20]. Squamous cell carcinomas and adenocarcinomas of the esophagus cannot be reliably differentiated on barium studies. Nevertheless, squamous cell carcinomas tend to involve the upper or mid-esophagus, whereas adenocarcinomas are located predominantly in the distal esophagus. Unlike squamous carcinomas, adenocarcinomas also have a marked tendency to invade the gastric cardia or fundus, comprising as many as 50% of all malignant tumors involving the gastroesophageal junction [20].

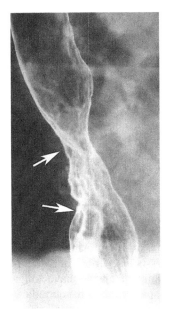

Fig. 7. Adenocarcinoma arising in Barrett's esophagus. Double-contrast esophagram shows advanced infiltrating carcinoma (*arrows*) as an irregular area of luminal narrowing with mucosal nodularity and ulceration in distal esophagus above hiatal hernia

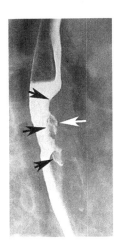

Fig. 8. Squamous cell carcinoma of esophagus. Double-contrast esophagram shows polypoid mass (*black arrows*) with central area of ulceration (*white arrow*) in mid-esophagus

Other Malignant Tumors

Esophageal lymphoma may be manifested on barium studies by submucosal masses, polypoid lesions, enlarged folds, or strictures. Spindle cell carcinoma (formerly known as carcinosarcoma) is another rare malignant tumor characterized by bulky, polypoid intraluminal masses that expand the lumen of the esophagus without causing obstruction. Other rare malignant tumors involving the esophagus include leiomyosarcoma and malignant melanoma.

Varices

Uphill varices are usually caused by portal hypertension with hepatofugal flow through dilated esophageal collaterals to the superior vena cava. Uphill varices appear on barium studies as serpentine longitudinal filling de-

fects in the distal thoracic esophagus. They are best seen on mucosal relief views of the collapsed esophagus using a barium paste or high-density barium suspension. In contrast, downhill varices are caused by superior vena cava obstruction with downward flow via dilated esophageal collaterals to the portal venous system. Most patients with downhill varices present clinically with the superior vena cava syndrome. Downhill varices also appear as serpentine longitudinal filling defects, but these varices are almost always confined to the upper or mid-esophagus.

Lower Esophageal Rings

The term Schatzki ring is reserved for symptomatic patients with lower esophageal rings who present with intermittent dysphagia for solids, especially meat. The rings appear on barium studies as smooth, symmetric ring-like constrictions at the gastroesophageal junction, almost always located above a hiatal hernia (Fig. 9a) [21]. The rings can be missed if the distal esophagus is not adequately distended at fluoroscopy (Fig. 9b), so it is important to obtain prone views of the esophagus during continuous drinking of a low-density barium suspension [21]. Conversely, rings can also be missed if the hiatal hernia is over-distended, resulting in overlap of the distal esophagus and hernia that obscures the ring [22]. Rings with a maximal luminal diameter of more than 20 mm rarely cause dysphagia, whereas rings with a maximal diameter of less than 13 mm almost always cause dysphagia [23].

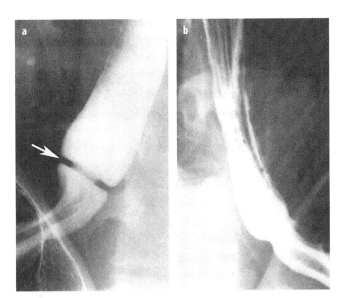

Fig. 9. Schatzki ring. **a** Prone, single-contrast esophagram shows smooth, symmetric, ring-like constriction (*white arrow*) in distal esophagus directly above hiatal hernia. **b** Ring is not seen on upright, double-contrast esophagram from same examination because of inadequate distention of this region

Esophageal Intramural Pseudodiverticulosis

Esophageal intramural pseudodiverticula consist of dilated excretory ducts of deep mucous glands in the esophagus. The pseudodiverticula typically appear on esophagography as flask-shaped outpouchings in rows parallel to the long axis of the esophagus (Fig. 10) [24]. When viewed *en face* on double-contrast esophagrams, the pseudodiverticula can be mistaken for tiny ulcers. When viewed in profile, however, they often appear to be 'floating' outside the wall of the esophagus without apparent communication with the lumen [24]. Barium studies often reveal an isolated cluster of pseudodiverticula in the distal esophagus in the region of a peptic stricture, so they presumably occur as a sequela of scarring from reflux esophagitis [24]. Less frequently, the pseudodiverticula have a diffuse distribution and are associated with high strictures, or they occur as an isolated finding [24]. When strictures are present, these patients may present with dysphagia, but the pseudodiverticula themselves rarely cause symptoms.

Esophageal Motility Disorders

Achalasia

Primary achalasia is an idiopathic condition, whereas secondary achalasia is caused by other underlying conditions, most commonly malignant tumors involving the gastroesophageal junction (especially carcinoma of the gastric cardia). Primary achalasia is characterized by absent primary peristalsis in the esophagus and incomplete relaxation of the lower esophageal sphincter, manifested

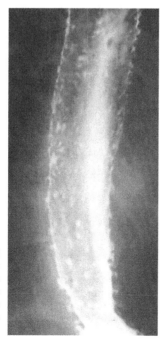

Fig. 10. Esophageal intramural pseudodiverticulosis. Double-contrast esophagram shows multiple outpouchings in longitudinal rows parallel to the long axis of esophagus, which was otherwise normal

on barium studies by tapered, beak-like narrowing of the distal esophagus adjacent to the gastroesophageal junction. In advanced disease, the esophagus can become massively dilated and tortuous distally (i.e., a 'sigmoid' esophagus).

Secondary achalasia is also characterized by absent peristalsis in the esophagus and beak-like narrowing near the gastroesophageal junction. In secondary achalasia caused by a tumor at the gastroesophageal junction, however, the length of the narrowed segment is often greater than that in primary achalasia because of spread of tumor into the distal esophagus [25]. The narrowed segment may also be asymmetric, nodular, or ulcerated because of tumor infiltrating this region. In some cases, barium studies may reveal other signs of malignancy at the cardia with distortion or obliteration of the normal cardiac rosette [25]. The clinical history is also important, as patients with primary achalasia almost always have longstanding dysphagia, whereas patients with secondary achalasia are usually older individuals (over the age of 60) with recent onset of dysphagia (less than six months) and weight loss [25].

Diffuse Esophageal Spasm

Symptomatic diffuse esophageal spasm (DES) may be manifested on barium studies by intermittently weakened or absent primary peristalsis with repetitive, lumen-obliterating nonperistaltic contractions, producing a classic 'cork-screw' esophagus [26]. More commonly, however, these patients have multiple nonperistaltic contractions of mild to moderate severity without a corkscrew appearance [26]. The majority of patients with DES have also been found to have impaired opening of the lower esophageal sphincter on barium studies, with beak-like narrowing of the distal esophagus similar to that seen in achalasia [26]. It should therefore be recognized that DES is characterized radiographically by frequent LES dysfunction with nonperistaltic contractions of varying severity, rather than a classic corkscrew appearance.

References

1. Dibble C, Levine MS, Rubesin SE et al (2004) Detection of reflux esophagitis on double-contrast esophagrams and endoscopy using the histologic findings as the gold standard. Abdom Imaging 29:421-425
2. Levine MS (2000) Gastroesophageal reflux disease. In: Gore RM, Levine MS (eds) Textbook of Gastrointestinal Radiology, 2nd edn. WB Saunders, Philadelphia, pp 329-349
3. Styles RA, Gibb SP, Tarshis A et al (1985) Esophagogastric polyps: radiographic and endoscopic findings. Radiology 154:307-311
4. Gupta S, Levine MS, Rubesin SE et al (2003) Usefulness of barium studies for differentiating benign and malignant strictures of the esophagus. AJR Am J Roentgenol 180:737-744
5. Levine MS, Goldstein HM (1984) Fixed transverse folds in the esophagus: a sign of reflux esophagitis. AJR Am J Roentgenol 143:275-278

6. Furth EE, Rubesin SE, Rose D (1995) Feline esophagus. AJR Am J Roentgenol 164:900
7. Gilchrist AM, Levine MS, Carr RF et al (1988) Barrett's esophagus: diagnosis by double-contrast esophagography. AJR Am J Roentgenol 150:97-102
8. Levine MS, Macones AJ, Laufer I (1985) Candida esophagitis: accuracy of radiographic diagnosis. Radiology 154:581-587
9. Levine MS, Woldenberg R, Herlinger H, Laufer I (1987) Opportunistic esophagitis in AIDS: radiographic diagnosis. Radiology 165:815-820
10. Sam JW, Levine MS, Rubesin SE, Laufer I (2000) The 'foamy' esophagus: a radiographic sign of Candida esophagitis. AJR Am J Roentgenol 174:999-1002
11. Shortsleeve MJ, Levine MS (1992) Herpes esophagitis in otherwise healthy patients: clinical and radiographic findings. Radiology 182:859-861
12. Levine MS, Loevner LA, Saul SH et al (1988) Herpes esophagitis: sensitivity of double-contrast esophagography. AJR Am J Roentgenol 151:57-62
13. Balthazar EM, Megibow AJ, Hulnick D et al (1987) Cytomegalovirus esophagitis in AIDS: radiographic features in 16 patients. AJR Am J Roentgenol 149:919-923
14. Sor S, Levine MS, Kowalski TE et al (1995) Giant ulcers of the esophagus in patients with human immunodeficiency virus: clinical, radiographic, and pathologic findings. Radiology 194:447-451
15. Levine MS (2000) Other esophagitides. In: Gore RM, Levine MS (eds) Textbook of Gastrointestinal Radiology, 2nd edn. WB Saunders, Philadelphia, pp 364-386
16. Zimmerman SL, Levine MS, Rubesin SE et al (2005) Idiopathic eosinophilic esophagitis in adults: the ringed esophagus. Radiology 236:159-165
17. Oh CH, Levine MS, Katzka DA et al (2001) Congenital esophageal stenosis in adults: clinical and radiographic findings in seven patients. AJR Am J Roentgenol 176:1179-1182
18. Levine MS, Buck JL, Pantongrag-Brown L et al (1996) Fibrovascular polyps of the esophagus: clinical, radiographic, and pathologic findings in 16 patients. AJR Am J Roentgenol 166:781-787
19. Levine MS, Chu P, Furth EE et al (1997) Carcinoma of the esophagus and esophagogastric junction: sensitivity of radiographic diagnosis. AJR Am J Roentgenol 168:1423-1426
20. Levine MS (2000) Carcinoma of the esophagus. In: Gore RM, Levine MS (eds) Textbook of Gastrointestinal Radiology, 2nd edn. WB Saunders, Philadelphia, pp 403-433
21. Ott DJ, Chen YM, Wu WC et al (1986) Radiographic and endoscopic sensitivity in detecting lower esophageal mucosal ring. AJR Am J Roentgenol 147:261-265
22. Hsu WC, Levine MS, Rubesin SE (2003) Overlap phenomenon: a potential pitfall in the radiographic detection of lower esophageal rings. AJR Am J Roentgenol 180:745-747
23. Schatzki RE (1963) The lower esophageal ring: long term follow-up of symptomatic and asymptomatic rings. AJR Am J Roentgenol 90:805-810
24. Levine MS, Moolten DN, Herlinger H, Laufer I (1986) Esophageal intramural pseudodiverticulosis: a reevaluation. AJR Am J Roentgenol 147:1165-1170
25. Woodfield CA, Levine MS, Rubesin SE et al (2000) Diagnosis of primary versus secondary achalasia: reassessment of clinical and radiographic criteria. AJR Am J Roentgenol 175:727-731
26. Prabhakar AM, Levine MS, Rubesin SE et al (2004) Relationship between diffuse esophageal spasm and lower esophageal sphincter dysfunction on barium studies and manometry in 14 patients. AJR Am J Roentgenol 183:409-413

Diseases of the Stomach and Duodenum: Basics of Radiologic-Pathologic Correlation

J.E. Lichtenstein[1], F.J. Scholz[2]

[1] Department of Radiology, University of Washington Medical Center, Seattle, WA, USA
[2] Department of Radiology, Lahey Clinic Medical Center, Burlington, MA, USA

Introduction

The purpose of this workshop is to apply basic principles of radiologic-pathologic correlation to the differential diagnosis of diseases of the stomach and duodenum. Tumors and inflammatory or reactive processes will be emphasized and used as illustrative examples in the syllabus.

The stomach and duodenum are violent places, with hostile pH levels and endocrine and exocrine glands with feedback loops that are in constant battle. The end result is that both are prone to diseases of excess acid or alkali, or diseases of diminished resistance to these caustics. In addition, hormonal influences affect the structure and function of stomach and duodenum; gastrin is the most famous hormone associated with the stomach. In addition to stimulating gastric parietal cell acid production, gastrin also stimulates all neuroendocrine glands of the alimentary tract to some degree. Carcinoid glandular hyperplasia of the stomach occurs with high persistent gastrin levels, as seen in Zollinger Ellison Syndrome, atrophic gastritis, and with acid suppression medications. Recent controversy has arisen about the possible relationship of acid suppression therapy with hyperplastic gastric polyps and atrophic gastritis.

'Radiologic-pathologic correlation' employs knowledge of pathological processes (along with physiology and anatomy) for the analysis of radiologic abnormalities to enhance differential diagnosis [1, 2]. The dictionary defines pathology as: 'The study of the essential nature of diseases and, especially, the structural and functional changes produced by them.' In this sense, the radiologist is truly a pathologist who sees the changes in vivo, when there is still an opportunity to intervene.

It is common teaching practice to classify disease by pathologic diagnoses. In practice, the patient seldom presents with a known diagnosis, but with non-specific complaints. Diagnosis is suggested by analyzing morphologic changes seen radiologically. Incorporating knowledge of pathology with clinical information should aid in the formation of a rational differential diagnosis, while avoiding rote memorization of exhaustive lists and 'gamuts'. Pathologic correlation is especially useful in the gastrointestinal (GI) tract where diagnosis depends heavily on determining the layer of the bowel wall involved, and on patterns of filling defects, strictures, fold abnormalities and ulcers.

Normal Structure

A brief review of normal bowel structure may aid in the appreciation of pathologic alterations. The bowel varies in structure and function from region to region, but many anatomic features are common throughout. The gut is a stratified tube that is organized into four main layers: mucosa, submucosa, muscularis and an outer adventitial covering (Fig. 1, 2).

The mucosa, in turn, has three layers. The luminal lining of squamous or columnar epithelial cells provides a protective surface involved in absorption and mucus production. The lamina propria is a supportive layer of mesenchyme containing capillaries and nerves. A thin layer of smooth muscle, the muscularis mucosae, separates the mucosa from the submucosa. Lymphoid follicles tend to lie near, or bridge across, the muscularis mucosae.

The submucosa is a layer of soft fibroconnective tissue containing the main blood vessels, lymphatics and nerves that supply the mucosa. The main muscular wall, the mus-

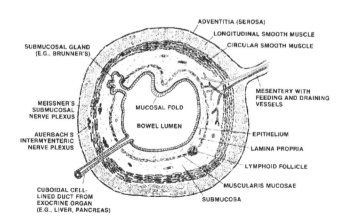

Fig. 1. Diagram of an idealized cross-section of normal bowel showing the major components found in the upper GI tract

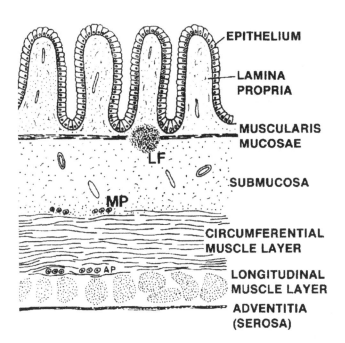

Fig. 2. Diagram showing representative features seen in photomicrographs of normal bowel. Relative proportions and details of epithelium vary with organ and location. (*LF*, lymphoid follicle; *AP*, Auerbach's autonomic myenteric nerve plexus; *MP*, Meissner's submucosal nerve plexus)

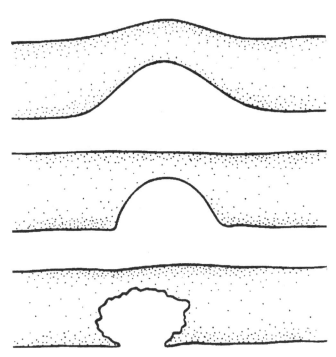

Fig. 3. Drawings of classic effects of masses on bowel which are determined by location of lesion: extrinsic (*top*), submucosal (*middle*), and mucosal (*bottom*)

cularis propria, generally has an inner circular and outer longitudinal layer. Auerbach's autonomic nerve plexus, which controls peristalsis, is located between the two layers. 'Adventia' is a general term for whatever surrounds the gut. Much of the GI tract is surrounded by delicate fibrofatty mesenchyme supporting a continuous thin fibrous layer, the serosa. The esophagus and retroperitoneal portions of the duodenum and colon lack a defined serosa. The continuity of the adventia with surrounding tissue can facilitate spread of inflammatory and neoplastic disease.

Morphology of Lesions

The radiographic morphology of lesions almost always gives important clues about the pathologic diagnosis (Fig. 3, 4). Overgrowths of the luminal surface epithelium can cause hyperplasias, adenomas, or carcinomas, depending on the degree of histologic atypia. Epithelial polyps and tumors tend to protrude into the lumen, have irregular surface texture, form acute angles with the surrounding surface, and usually do not displace the centerline of the gut unless they become quite large. Benign lesions tend to grow slowly, are often small, rounded and, if growing into the lumen, have time to be drawn out onto stalks by peristaltic action. Aggressive lesions spread out and involve adjacent structures. They are likely to be broad-based and tethered to deeper mural structures. They become large more rapidly and are more likely to outgrow their blood supply and become necrotic. Non-uniform, multi-centric growth tends to cause irregular contours and lobulation.

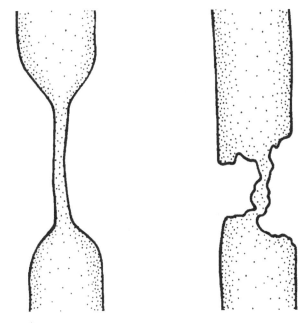

Fig. 4. Drawings of strictures illustrating classic distinction between smoothly tapered benign process on left and abrupt-edged, irregular-surfaced, malignant lesion on right

Any of the subepithelial mesenchymal tissues may lead to benign or malignant overgrowths, the malignant forms being termed sarcomas. Submucosal lesions also tend to grow toward the lumen, being restrained by the firm, rubbery muscularis propria. The displaced mucosal surface tends to be smooth with obtuse angles at the edges. Masses arising in the muscle wall (e.g., gastrointestinal stromal tumors (GISTs), leiomyomas and leiomyosarcomas) may grow either towards the lumen (endoenteric) or away from it (exoenteric), or in a combination of patterns. Extrinsic masses sometimes bulge into the lumen, but they typically have very obtuse angles at the margins and tend to displace the lumen centerline earlier than intrinsic lesions.

Hamartomas are mixed arrangements of otherwise normal tissues. They are generally benign and usually contain both epithelial and mesenchymal elements.

Most *strictures* result from scarring or from cellular infiltration. With scarring, the narrowing has smooth margins, whereas with infiltration, the contour depends on the nature of the process and its location within the wall. Healing of many types of injury results in scarring and stricture formation. Strictures from widespread inflammation, as in caustic ingestion or radiation, are likely to be elongated. When the injury is old and the epithelium has healed, the luminal surface will be smooth with tapering edges (Fig. 4).

Irregularity of the luminal surface of a stricture indicates involvement of the epithelium. It may be caused either by ulceration or a primary epithelial process such as carcinoma, the infiltration of which produces the stricture. Frequently the stricture is caused more by fibrous reaction to the tumor cells than by the mass of neoplastic cells *per se*. Mucin-producing adenocarcinoma is especially likely to exhibit this tendency. Benign strictures are often long and smoothly tapered, whereas malignant strictures tend to produce focal, relatively short, irregular strictures with abrupt edges.

Strictures may be due to compression by extrinsic encircling masses. While uncommon in the stomach, annular pancreas provides a classic example in the duodenum (Fig. 5) [3]. The mucosa and submucosa are unaffected except for being smoothly stretched over the lesion, providing a smooth contour.

Dilatation in hollow peristaltic organs occurs either because of distal obstruction or because of intrinsic neural, or muscular, abnormality. Excluding a mechanical obstruction, the most common cause of dilatation is adynamic ileus. The precise mechanism is often unclear. It can result from local irritation, apparently involving the autonomic nerve plexi in the bowel wall. Dilatation caused by intrinsic structural changes in the bowel is relatively uncommon. Achalasia is a classic prototype in which deficiency of ganglion cells in Auerbach's plexus of the esophagus results in hypotonia and progressive dilatation. Gastroparesis from diabetic neuropathy and smooth muscle atony and atrophy in scleroderma (progressive systemic sclerosis) due to collagen vascular disease are other examples.

Thickening of the mucosal folds lining the gut is a common pattern, especially in the stomach and duodenum. Inflammation is very common but the radiographic findings, such as spasm and irritability, and fold irregularity and

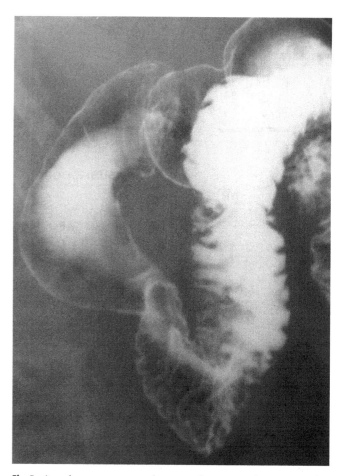

Fig. 5. Annular pancreas causing smooth, concentric, compressive narrowing of descending duodenum

thickening are often non-specific and difficult to distinguish from normal variation when relatively mild. Erosions through the epithelium that do not breach the muscularis mucosae, separating the mucosa from the submucosa, may be detected with double contrast barium technique (Fig. 6). Aphthous lesions suggest granulomatous disease, especially Crohn's disease, but are not specific.

Hyperplasia of normal structures, or infiltration or deposition of cells or foreign material may cause thickening. Examples of diffuse epithelial overgrowth include Menetrier disease in which gastric fundal folds are markedly thickened by proliferation of the superficial mucus-producing cells (Fig. 7). Zollinger-Ellison Syndrome is another classic example in which an ectopic gastrin source stimulates gastric acid production and marked hyperplasia of parietal cells in the deep mucosal glands of the gastric fundus. Excess fluid is found with both entities, but inflammation and ulcers due to excess acid are found only in Zollinger-Ellison Syndrome. Both of these conditions are classically distinguished from other inflammatory disease in which fold thickening is usually more distal.

Ulcers are holes in the normal protective epithelial barrier lining the gut. They result in protrusions of contrast be-

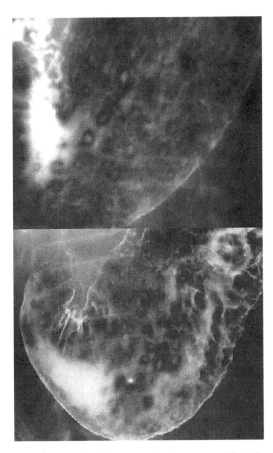

Fig. 6. Erosive gastritis. Air contrast barium upper GI study showing contrast pooling in multiple shallow gastric erosions surrounded by lucent edema

yond the expected margin of the lumen of the organ. They may be caused by noxious agents in the bowel lumen or by insults such as mucosal ischemia or inflammation in the mucosa itself. Infection with *Helicobacter pylori* is now recognized as the etiology for most upper GI tract ulceration. Once the surface is breached, the erosion can extend more deeply. In a benign ulcer, the surrounding epithelium remains relatively resistant and intact, although inflamed. Destruction of the less resistant submucosa undermines mucosa, which tends to overhang the crater edge. The firm, rubbery muscularis mucosae is relatively resistant and forms a temporary barrier. The resulting flat-bottomed defect has narrow communication with the lumen and a characteristic 'collar button' shape. Surrounding mucosal folds extend all the way in to the edge of the ulcer.

In contrast, adenocarcinoma typically produces a nodular, irregular epithelium. An ulcer in this surface has irregular edges that tend to be eroded along with underlying tissue without undermining. Erosion into an extensive tumor mass produces an irregular, saucer-shaped hole rather than a flat bottom. Ulceration into a submucosal tumor such as a GIST or lymphoma nodule produces a variably shaped crater, but because the epithelium is not primarily involved, its edge is often sharply defined.

Tumors are usually seen as combinations of filling defects and strictures. Carcinoma is, by definition, an epithelial lesion. Its mucosal origin is generally reflected by the presence of ulcers and luminal nodules. Its poor prognosis can be explained, in part, by a propensity for sub-

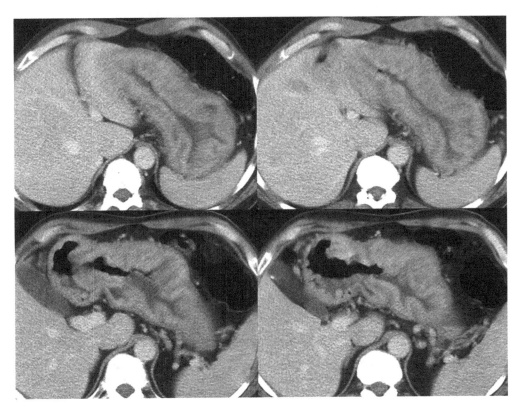

Fig. 7. Menetrier disease. CT showing grossly enlarged gastric folds in the fundus due to hyperplasia of secretory cells in the superficial layers of the mucosa

mucosal extension and for spread through the wall. Benign hyperplastic and adenomatous tumors also arise in the epithelium and this is reflected in their roentgen appearance, often allowing their differentiation. Other tumors arise in the submucosal mesenchyme. Many of these are slow growing and benign. They present radiographically as rounded intramural lesions with smooth overlying mucosa. As such lesions become large, however, the epithelium may ulcerate.

The normal histologic components vary with the region of the gut and so do their tendencies for pathologic growth. One must know the local 'track record' for successful prediction. For example, the stratified squamous esophageal epithelium commonly transforms to squamous cell carcinoma after long exposure to smoke and alcohol. Flat, glandular, columnar epithelium frequently becomes metaplastic, leading to adenocarcinoma at the esophagogastric junction, but only rarely does so in the small bowel. Solid mural tumors of the esophagus are likely to be benign spindle-cell, stromal tumors, regardless of their size. Similar lesions in the stomach are likely to be malignant, especially if larger than a few centimeters. Polyps in the duodenum are likely to be hyperplasias of Brunner's glands or hamartomas including pancreatic tissue. Those entities would be rare elsewhere and similar gross morphology would prompt different considerations.

Malignant Gastric and Duodenal Tumors

Adenocarcinoma

Gastric carcinoma is decreasing in frequency in Western counties and duodenal carcinoma is rare. By the time they become markedly symptomatic, the tumors are often advanced and beyond cure. The role of the radiologist at that point is to locate and stage the tumor. However, radiographic studies performed for other reasons provide the potential for detection of asymptomatic early gastric carcinoma.

Sometimes epithelial malignancies grow into the lumen as a mainly cellular mass of tissue with little fibrosis. Such a lesion is more often well-differentiated. Typically, the surface is lobulated or ulcerated, as opposed to the usually smooth surface of benign lesions (Fig. 8).

Mucin-producing tumors have a tendency to infiltrate widely and incite a great deal fibrotic reaction. Fold thickening may result, and often the wall is thickened and appears stiff and constricted, producing the classic 'leather bottle' appearance. The lesion may extend around the lumen in an annular manner (Fig. 9) [4, 5].

Other Malignancies

Lymphoma is a mesenchymal process, but has many possible appearances. Typically lesions are lobulated. The mucosa may be intact until late, but ulceration into the soft, cellular tumors is often extensive.

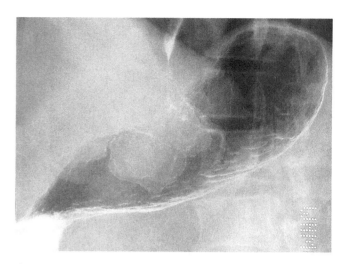

Fig. 8. Multilobulated polypoid gastric adenocarcinoma growing into the lumen

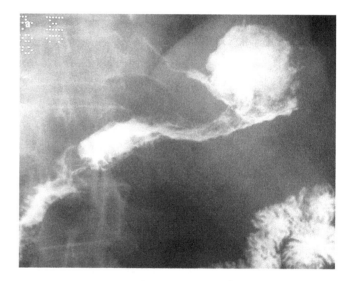

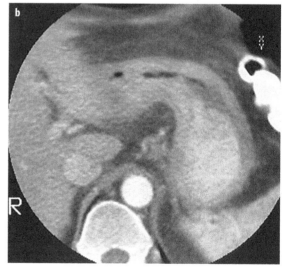

Fig. 9. Infiltrating schirrous gastric carcinoma causing marked thickening and stiffening of the stomach and constricting the lumen. **a** Single contrast barium upper GI. **b** CT of same case

Metastases are frequently multiple but can have many appearances, depending upon the primary tumor and whether the lesions are submucosal or serosal. Metastasized breast cancer, in particular, has a tendency to resemble sclerosing mucin-producing adenocarcinoma. Kaposi sarcoma, a soft biphasic mixture of vascular and stromal tissue, tends to form rounded subepithelial nodules in the stomach of HIV positive patients.

Benign Tumors

The incidence of benign tumors is difficult to define since, if they are small or produce little effect on the lumen, they are often asymptomatic and escape attention. They are relatively common among clinically evident tumors, but the absolute incidence is probably much higher and probably exceeds that of malignancy [6].

Epithelial hyperplasias and adenomas may form sessile or pedunculated nodules. Adenomas are neoplastic, usually polypoid, excrescences due to proliferation of dysplastic epithelial cells. Excluding polyposis syndromes, they are usually solitary and are uncommon in the duodenum.

Villous tumors imply more severe dysplasia, with more aggressive growth. The lesions tend to be more sessile, larger, and have more irregular surface texture.

Barium trapped in the interstices of the villous surface gives a striated, reticulated, or 'soap bubbly' appearance (Fig. 10). In the duodenum they are usually found near the papilla and frequently harbor foci of carcinoma, especially if large [7, 8]. It is tempting to speculate that the dysplasia results from the irritating effect of bile or pancreatic secretions.

Mesenchymal tumors arise in the deeper layers. Thus, initially, their overlying epithelial layer of the mucosa is intact. The smooth luminal surface provides a convenient means of predicting the nature of such tumors (Fig. 11). Other aspects of appearance depend upon the consistency of the tumor tissue and its site of origin within the wall. Virtually any type of mesenchymal cell in the bowel wall may occasionally give rise to neoplastic or hamartomatous tumors, but only a very few occur frequently enough to warrant serious consideration.

Spindle Cell/Stromal Tumors

Gastrointestinal stromal tumors (GISTs) and leiomyomas are by far the most common benign mesenchymal tumors of the GI tract [9]. Leiomyomas are thought to usually arise from the smooth muscle of the wall. GISTs are now considered to arise from the interstitial cells of

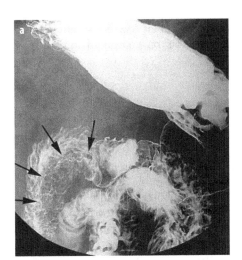

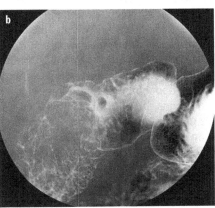

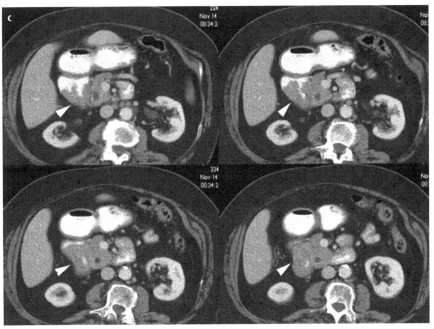

Fig. 10. Villous adenoma in proximal duodenum containing foci of adenocarcinoma. **a, b** Barium upper GI showing filling defect in lumen (*arrows*, **a**; *arrowheads* indicate tumor in duodenum). Irregular texture correlates with fronds of dysplastic surface epithelium. **c** CT of same case

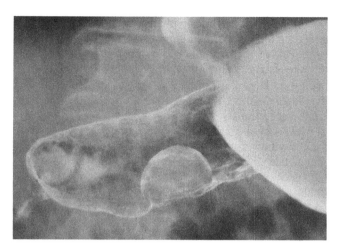

Fig. 11. Submucosal, benign, spindle cell tumor of the gastric antrum protruding into the lumen with a very smooth covering surface of stretched, but otherwise intact, surface epithelium

Cajal, which are stem cells similar to the pacemaker cells of the bowel wall. They are characterized by expression of a tyrosine kinase growth factor receptor, KIT (CD117). The pathologic criteria for malignancy in both smooth muscle cell tumors and GISTs are somewhat arbitrary. They depend upon averaging the number of mitotic figures in multiple high power microscopic fields and assessing cellularity and pleomorphism [10, 11]. The tumors tend to grow slowly. Although often small and difficult to detect, occasionally such tumors may become huge.

Malignancy in stromal tumors correlates well with size, except in the esophagus where the vast majority are benign, even when very large. Stromal tumors tend to grow as firm, rubbery, rounded masses of compact intertwined bundles of spindle cells. The tumors have no true capsules but are usually easily shelled out from surrounding compressed tissue. Their roentgen appearance depends upon their site of origin, size and direction of growth.

Tumors arising in the outer layers of the wall tend to grow outward into the surrounding tissue. If small, they cause no symptoms and the majority are probably never detected. When larger, they may appear as extrinsic masses. Lesions arising on the inner aspect of the muscle wall or muscularis mucosae more easily displace the pliable submucosa and mucosa than the firmer muscle wall. Thus they grow toward the lumen and tend to cause symptoms relatively early. Ordinarily the epithelium is stretched smoothly over such submucosal masses, often with obtuse angles at the periphery. If such lesions become large enough, however, they may protrude into the lumen and develop short pedicles. In that case the mucosa will be tucked around the lesion with acute angles at the borders, a limitation of the so-called 'sulcus sign' sometimes used to distinguish mucosal from submucosal or extrinsic lesions. While the covering mucosa is initially intact, the protruding submucosal mass exposes it to trauma from luminal contents and may compromise its

blood supply. Superficial ulceration, thus, is an expected complication of any such lesion and may be its mode of presentation. Vascularity within GISTs and smooth muscle lesions is variable, often being rather sparse. Frequently, however, there are prominent arteries in the superficial layers of such tumors and these can be the source of sudden, dramatic hemorrhage when eroded by ulcers. Such behavior is well known with gastric GISTs where the luminal acid is ulcerogenic and where the lesions can become larger without luminal compromise.

GISTs are usually solitary, but may also be multiple in a small number of cases. Calcification is rare in GI tract leiomyomas, as opposed to the situation in the uterus. When it occasionally occurs, it can be a useful radiographic clue to the diagnosis.

Lipoma

Lipomas are rare, uniformly benign, localized proliferations of submucosal fat. Like leiomyomas, they grow by slow compression of surrounding tissue and usually no true capsule can be defined. Their soft texture and submucosal origin dictate that the tumors grow almost entirely into the lumen with relatively little effect on the muscle wall. As they become large they may form pedunculated, intraluminal, polypoid masses and may cause intussusception. The overlying mucosa is initially intact but may eventually breakdown and ulceration is one means of presentation. Their low X-ray attenuation allows a confident diagnosis on computed tomography (CT) (Fig. 12).

The Duodenum

The duodenum, although subject to the above generalities, is one of the most unique and dynamic parts of the body [12-16]. It has both intra- and retro-peritoneal portions. Being centrally located in the abdomen, it is often affected by diseases in neighboring organs. It is a battleground of acids and alkalis relating to drainage from three of the body's major sources of digestive chemicals: the liver via the biliary tree; the pancreas, draining alkaline secretions and powerful enzymes through the major and minor papillae; and the stomach, producing caustic acids. It has a complex embryology involving development of adjacent organs and numerous anomalies. As a consequence of location, embryology, histology, surrounding structures and the adjacent organs draining into it, the pathology of the duodenum differs from that of other alimentary tract organs. Inch for inch and ounce for ounce, more distinct pathologies occur here than in any other abdominal organ.

Developmental phenomena give rise to annular pancreas, webs and choledochoceles, and account for ectopias. Anatomy dictates patterns of obstruction and spread of disease from adjacent organs, as well as patterns of rupture

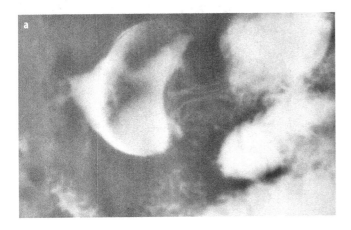

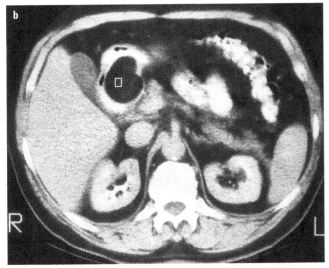

Fig. 12. Lipoma in the duodenal bulb. **a** Smooth filling defect displacing contrast in bulb on barium upper GI study. **b** CT in same case showing smooth, intraluminal mass in duodenal bulb with very low attenuation measured in the rectangular area of interest

and hematoma formation in blunt trauma. Exposure to gastric acid leads to ulcers and hyperplasias. Influx of bile and pancreatic juice is thought to determine some types and sites of mucosal neoplasia. The examples presented here will stress radiologic-pathologic correlation.

References

1. Theros E (1969) The value of radiologic-pathologic correlation in the education of the radiologist. AJR Am J Roentgenol 107:235-257
2. Lichtenstein JE (1986) (Revised 1991 and again revised by Gore R 1994) Basics of radiologic pathologic correlation in the GI tract. In: Tavaras JM, Ferrucci JT Jr (eds) Radiology: diagnosis/imaging/intervention. Vol 4, Chp 4, Lippincott, Philadelphia, pp 1-19
3. Ladd AP, Madura JA (2001) Congenital duodenal anomalies in the adult. Arch Surg 136:576-584
4. Gore RM, Levine MS, Ghahremani GG, Miller FH (1970) Gastric cancer. Radiologic diagnosis. Radiol Clin North Am 35:311-329
5. Levine MS, Megibow AJ, Kochman ML (2000) Carcinoma of the stomach and duodenum. In: Gore RM, Levine MS (eds) Textbook of gastrointestinal radiology, 2nd ed. Saunders, Philadelphia, pp 601-626
6. Perez A, Saltzman JR, Carr-Locke DL et al (2003) Benign non-ampullary duodenal neoplasms. J Gastrointest Surg 7:536-541
7. Buck JL, Elsayed AM (1993) Ampullary tumors: radiologic-pathologic correlation. Radiographics 13:193-212
8. Jean M, Dua K (2003) Tumors of the ampulla of Vater. Curr Gastroenterol Rep 5:171-175
9. Levy AD, Remotti HE, Thompson WM et al (2003) Gastrointestinal stromal tumors: radiologic features with pathologic correlation. Radiographics 23:283-304
10. Fletcher CD, Berman JJ, Corless C et al (2002) Diagnosis of gastrointestinal stromal tumors: a consensus approach. Hum Pathol 33:459-465
11. Miettinen M, El-Rafai W, Sobin LH, Lasota J (2002) Evaluation of malignancy and prognosis of gastrointestinal stromal tumors: a review. Hum Pathol 33: 478-483
12. Jayaraman MV, Mayo-Smith WW, Movson JS et al (2001) CT of the duodenum: an overlooked segment gets its due. Radiographics Spec No:S147-S160
13. Lichtenstein JE, Scholz FJ (2005) Duodenum: basics of radiologic-pathologic correlations. In: Ros PR, Gourtsoyiannis NC (eds) Radiologic-pathologic correlation from head to toe. Springer-Verlag, Berlin-Heidelberg, pp 253-272
14. Michelassi F, Erroi F, Dawson PJ et al (1989) Experience with 647 consecutive tumors of the duodenum, ampulla, head of the pancreas, and distal common bile duct. Ann Surg 210:544-554, discussion 554-556
15. Reeders JWAJ, Rosenbusch G (1994) Radiology of benign and malignant diseases of the duodenum. In: Freeny PC, Stevenson GW (eds) Margulis and Burhenne's alimentary tract radiology. Mosby, St. Louis, 467-511
16. Scholz FJ (1981) Duodenum in surgical radiology. In: Teplick JG, Haskin ME (eds) Surgical Radiology: A complement in radiology and imaging to the Sabiston Davis Christopher Textbook of Surgery. Saunders, Philadelphia, pp 502-537

Suggested Reading

Fenoglio-Preiser CM, Lantz PE, Listrom MB et al (1999) Gastrointestinal pathology: an atlas and text, 2nd ed. Lippincott-Raven, Philadelphia

Lichtenstein JE (1993) Inflammatory conditions of the stomach and duodenum. Radiology Clinics of North America 31:1315-1333

Levine MS (1994) Stomach and duodenum. In: Gore RN, Levine MS (eds) Textbook of gastrointestinal radiology, 2nd ed. Saunders, Philadelphia, pp 514-702

Levy A (2005) Neoplastic and non neoplastic diseases of the stomach. In: Ros PR, Gourtsoyiannis NC (eds) Radiologic-pathologic correlation from head to toe. Springer-Verlag, Berlin-Heidelberg, pp 237-251

Lewin KJ, Appleman HD (1996) Tumors of the esophagus and stomach. Third series, fascicle 18. Armed Forces Institute of Pathology, Washington DC

Morson BC, Dawson IMP (1979) Gastrointestinal pathology, 2nd ed. Blackwell Scientific Publications, Oxford, pp 3-63

Nelson SW, Rohrmann CA Jr (1994) Nonneoplastic diseases of the stomach. In: Freeny PC, Stevenson GW (eds) Margulis and Burhenne's alimentary tract radiology. Mosby, St Louis, pp 318-372

Small Bowel Imaging

N. Gourtsoyiannis

Department of Radiology, University of Crete, Heraklion, Greece

Introduction

The mesenteric small intestine is a difficult organ to examine. Long-term experience has shown that there are no shortcuts to achieving a reliable examination, and several parameters need to be respected if a confident diagnosis is to be made. These include: selection of patients, closely supervised studies, background data, image quality, familiarity with imaging findings and utilization of radiologic-pathologic correlations.

Thoughtful *selection of patients* by clinicians is essential to make radiologic examination cost-effective. *Closed supervised studies*, incorporating an adequate index of clinical suspicion, co-operation between a focused radiologist and a keen physician, expertise, and time are important. *Familiarity with imaging findings* and *image quality*, are necessary to guarantee demonstration of fine surface mucosal detail and transitional morphological changes. Applying the principles of *radiologic-pathologic correlation* to the interpretation of radiological findings offers a certain advantage and in association with the *background data* available, including localization and distribution of changes, extent of involvement, the solitary or multiple nature of the lesions present and the clinical history, enable a confident differential diagnosis.

Based on its long-term follow-up results and its high negative predictive value, *enteroclysis* has been shown as a most reliable screening examination for the assessment of possible small bowel disease.

Enteroclysis combined with computed tomography (CT) offers the advantages of both techniques. Distention of small bowel lumen and cross-sectional display are proven imaging qualities gained with CT enteroclysis. Available prospective data suggest that the technique is advisable in patients with obstructive symptoms, in patients with known or suspected malignancy and when assessing complications of small bowel Crohn's disease.

Magnetic resonance enteroclysis (MRE), a combined functional and morphological imaging method, has only recently been performed routinely in clinical practice with adequate image quality and sufficient small bowel distention (Fig. 1). Thus far, results have shown that the

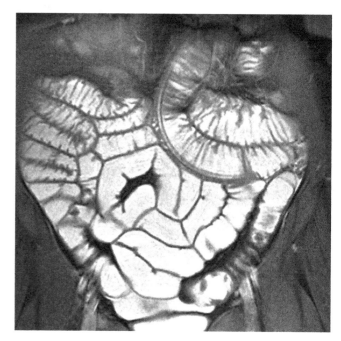

Fig. 1. Coronal true FISP section demonstrating small bowel at its entire length. The use of an iso-osmotic water solution as an intra-luminal contrast agent resulted in homogeneous opacification of the bowel lumen. Note the increased conspicuity of the normal bowel wall due to the high resolution capabilities and total absence of motion

functional information provided by MRE equals that of enteroclysis alone, whereas the inherent advantages of an MR imaging approach over enteroclysis include detection of extra-luminal pathologic conditions, and detailed morphological evaluation of the bowel wall, as well as of the entire abdomen. Moreover, MRE has a distinct advantage over the currently available CT enteroclysis technique, due to its ability to provide real-time functional information.

Clinical entities that may require radiological investigation of the small intestine most frequently include Crohn's disease, small bowel neoplasms and Meckel's diverticulum.

Crohn's Disease

The most characteristic features of Crohn's disease of the small intestine are the variety of its radiological appearances and the multiplicity of radiological features often present in the majority of patients. Categorization of these radiological features has been defined in terms of stenotic and non-stenotic forms, active and chronic, early and late or advanced, or into superficial, transmural and extramural changes.

Most information on the sequence of progression of the pathological lesions in Crohn's disease is derived from radiological descriptions. The early lesions of Crohn's disease are: blunting, flattening, thickening, distortion and straightening of the valvulae conniventes. These changes are followed by discrete ulcers and by longitudinal and transverse ulcers. The stenotic phase eventually develops and the involved segment is transformed into a rigid, cast-like tube; fistulae may be seen at this stage. Deep ulcers precede sinuses and fistulae to other organs.

Discrete ulcers are seen as small collections of barium with surrounding radiolucent margins. Fissure ulcers are seen in profile and may penetrate deep into the thickened intestinal wall; small abscess cavities are occasionally seen at the base of deep fissure ulcers. Longitudinal ulcers running along the mesenteric border of the ileum are a characteristic feature of Crohn's disease, although they are only occasionally present. Cobblestoning is caused mostly by a combination of longitudinal and traverse ulceration. Discontinuous involvement of the intestinal wall shows either as skip lesions or asymmetry. Asymmetrical involvement of the intestinal wall produces the characteristic 'pseudodiverticulae' appearance. The pseudodiverticulae represent small patches of normal intestine in an otherwise severely involved segment. The involved segment contracts and the normal areas become pseudodiverticula. Inflammatory polyps (pseudopolyps) are occasionally seen in Crohn's disease and are seen as small discrete filling defects in a severely involved segment.

Cross-sectional imaging modalities offer an important complementary diagnostic perspective in patients with Crohn's disease, due to their ability to directly image the intestinal wall and surrounding mesentery and therefore to determine the extramucosal extent and spread of the disease process.

CT is being performed with increasing frequency and has been shown to be extremely valuable in documenting mesenteric disease, including fibrofatty proliferation, abscess or phlegmon formation, microadenopathy and in adequately evaluating perirectal and/or perianal extension of Crohn's disease. It has also been suggested that CT is the most sensitive means of demonstrating an enterovesical fistula. In addition, the ability of CT to simultaneously evaluate extraintestinal organs may allow the detection of concurrent hepatobilliary, urinary or musculoskeletal complications, that may well lead to significant changes in the management of the individual patient.

MRE is emerging as a valuable technique for the evaluation of small bowel in patients with Crohn's disease. Administration of 1.5-2 liters of iso-osmotic water solution through a nasojejunal catheter ensures bowel distention and facilitates identification of bowel wall abnormalities. True fast imaging steady-state free precession (FISP), half-acquisition Fourier-transformed single shot turbo spin echo (HASTE) and post-gadolinium T1-weighted 3D FLASH sequences can be employed in a comprehensive and integrated MRE examination protocol. The characteristic transmural lesions of Crohn's disease, such as bowel wall thickening, linear and fissure ulcers, and cobblestoning are accurately depicted by MRE, especially when using true FISP sequence (Fig. 2, 3). MRE is of equal value with conventional enteroclysis in assessing the number and extent of involved small bowel segments and in disclosing lumen narrowing and/or prestenotic dilatation. MRE has a clear advantage over conventional enteroclysis in demonstrating extramural manifestations and/or complications of Crohn's disease, including fibrofatty proliferation, mesenteric lymphadenopathy, sinus tracts and fistulae or abscesses. Disease activity may be accurately appreciated by contrast-enhanced 3D FLASH images, by gadolinium uptake in the wall of the involved seg-

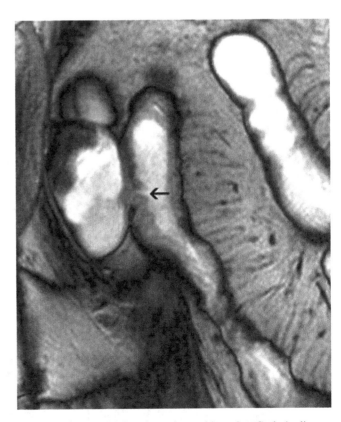

Fig. 2. A 23-year-old female patient with active Crohn's disease (CDAI = 196). Coronal true FISP spot view demonstrates a distal ileum transmural involvement with a fissure ulcer (*arrow*). Increased mesenteric vascularity and fibrofatty proliferation is also noted

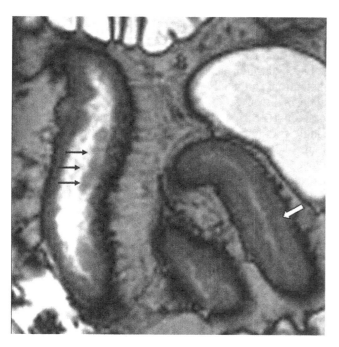

Fig. 3. Coronal true FISP spot view in a patient with Crohn's disease. Extensive wall thickening is demonstrated (*white arrow*) in an ileal loop, while cobblestoning is depicted as patchy areas of high signal intensity, sharply demarcated, along an adjacent affected segment (*arrows*)

ment (Fig. 4), while increased mesenteric vascularity is easily depicted on true FISP and 3D FLASH images. The clinical utility of MRE in Crohn's disease has not been widely established. At present, the method may be

suggested as a complementary diagnostic tool with advancing perspectives.

Neoplasms

Small intestinal neoplasms are surprisingly and universally rare. Documented rarity, further complicated by non-specific clinical presentation and a small index of clinical suspicion make their detection a challenge for both the physician and the radiologist. A mean symptoms-diagnosis interval up to three years for benign tumors and two years for malignant neoplasms has been reported. Inadequate radiologic examination or incorrect interpretation of radiological findings is estimated to account for an average of twelve months delay in diagnosing primary malignancies of the small intestine. Radiological appearances of these neoplasms, however, shown with enteroclysis and CT or MR imaging correlates almost perfectly with the morphological changes recognized in the gross pathology specimens. This ability to accurately image small intestinal neoplasms, independently of their size, anatomic localization and growth tendency, represents a major improvement in their diagnosis and management.

Adenocarcinoma

Adenocarcinoma appears to be the most common malignant neoplasm of the small intestine. It is a solitary lesion mostly located in the proximal small intestine. It is al-

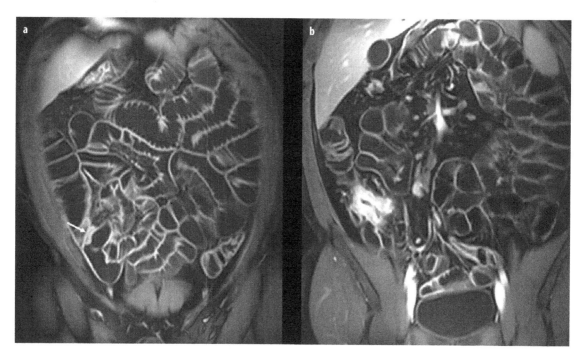

Fig. 4. Coronal FLASH image with fat saturation acquired 75 seconds after intravenous injection of gadolinium. Iso-osmotic water solution renders the lumen with low signal intensity, while normal intestinal wall presents with high signal intensity (*left*). In case of a hyperemic lesion (*right*), local increased gadolinium uptake generates this light bulb appearance

most always symptomatic, with non-specific clinical presentation and a dismal prognosis, mainly due to a late diagnosis. Its appearances on enteroclysis reflect its pattern of growth and include annular constricting lesions, filling defects, polypoid and/or ulcerated masses, or a combination of the above. Infiltrative adenocarcinomas are the most common type. Adenocarcinoma appears on CT as a solitary, focal, sharply outlined mass, causing thickening of the intestinal wall and narrowing of its lumen. The tumor may be homogeneous or heterogeneous when ulcerated and shows moderate contrast enhancement. Infiltration of the mesentery is seen with advanced disease, whereas associated lymphadenopathy is found in almost 50% of patients at presentation. Predominantly ulcerated adenocarcinomas may simulate lymphomas, malignant gastorintestinal stromal tumors (GISTs) or metastatic melanomas, whereas annular-type lesions will need to be differentiated from secondary adenocarcinoma, carcinoid, tuberculosis or Crohn's disease.

Lymphoma

Lymphoma represents 20% of primary small intestinal malignancies. Clinical presentation is variable, depending on whether involvement is primary or secondary, or whether it is preceded by other disorders, such as adult celiac disease, immunoproliferative disease or immunodeficiency syndromes. Radiological appearances mirror the pattern of growth. Enteroclysis can define a wide spectrum of features, including luminal narrowing with mucosal destruction, multiple intra-luminal polypoid filling defects, broad-based ulceration, aneurysmal dilatation, a large excavated mass and fistula formation. Infiltrative lymphomas may cause thickening of the intestinal wall without eliciting a desmoplastic reaction. A combination of different signs is rather frequent and multi-centricity of involvement is seen in almost one fourth of patients. CT appearances of intestinal lymphoma are also variable and may be categorized as aneurysmal, nodular, ulcerative and constrictive, while mesenteric involvement will usually feature as a conglomerate mass of mesenteric/retroperitoneal tissue, or a 'Sandwich-like' complex, due to encasement of vessels from enlarged mesenteric lymph nodes. Radiologic differential diagnosis include adenocarcinoma, Crohn's disease, and, less often, malignant GIST and metastatic melanoma.

Carcinoid

Carcinoid tumor is the most common neoplasm of the small intestine found at autopsy or incidentally during laparotomy. Almost 90% of lesions are located in the distal ileum, they may be multiple in approximately one third of cases, while coexistence with other primary malignancies is estimated to occur in another third of cases. The radio-

logical findings mirror the stage that the pathological process has reached at the time of examination. Primary ileal carcinoids usually feature as solitary, round, sharply-demarcated intramural filling defects. Luminal narrowing, usually asymmetrical, is present less often, whereas intestinal obstruction or intussusception is uncommon. Submucosal extension of the tumor will result in thickening of the valvulae conniventes and intestinal wall thickening. In the presence of extensive mesenteric fibrosis, diffuse luminal narrowing, fixation, angulation or kinking of intestinal loop(s) are also demonstrated. Carcinoid tumors are best recognized on CT on the basis of mesenteric findings. These include a discrete, uniform, soft tissue mass occasionally associated with linear soft tissue strands radiating into the surrounding mesentery in a stellate pattern, while displacing adjacent intestinal loops. Segmental intestinal wall thickening, ascites, hypervascular liver metastases, that are usually hypodense on precontrast scans, and occasionally dystrophic calcification in metastatic nodes or in liver metastases, may be also encountered.

Gastrointestinal Stromal Tumors (GISTs)

Histologically, GISTs are typically spindle cell tumors that have a prominent, nerve sheath tumor-like nuclear palisading pattern. Other GISTs may show prominent perinuclear vacuoles. GISTs may also have an epithelioid appearance, containing cells with round nuclei and abundant cytoplasm. It is now believed that GISTs are derived from the intestinal cells of Cajal. Recent application of immunohistochemical studies has revealed strong and uniform expression of the KIT (CD117, stem cell factor receptor) protein and CD34 in GISTs. This offers the possibility to accurately diagnose these tumors and separate them from other mesenchymal tumors of GI tract.

Benign GIST is the most common symptomatic benign neoplasm. Its type of growth is reflected in its radiological appearances. A broad-based, round or semi-lunar filling defect is usually seen with intraluminal tumors, while a mass effect on neighboring loops is seen with extraluminal benign GISTs. Dumb-bell type tumors combine features of both. Deformity of the intestinal wall, mucosal ulceration and signs of intussusception may also be seen. Despite their distinctive tendency to bleed, ulceration is rather infrequently demonstrated in intestinal benign GISTs, on enteroclysis. When seen, ulcerations are usually single, small, well-defined and round or linear in shape. Intussusception may be an additional feature of a benign GIST, easily depicted by either CT or enteroclysis. Besides enteroclysis, CT may contribute to the preoperative diagnosis of such neoplasms, by detecting unsuspected pathology and localizing it within the small bowel, or additionally characterizing pathology detected on barium studies. On CT, benign GISTs usually present as round, smoothly-outlined, homogeneous soft tissue masses, associated with the intestinal wall, while showing marked contrast enhancement. When large, such lesions may displace or deform adjacent small bowel loops.

Malignant GISTs grow slowly, predominantly extra-luminally and eccentrically, and are prone to develop degenerative changes such as necrosis, hemorrhage, calcification, fistula or secondary infection. Determination of the malignant potential of GISTs is based on factors such as location, tumor size, degree of cellularity and pleomorphism, and presence or absence of necrosis. Small intestinal GISTs sized less than 5 cm are usually benign, regardless of their cellularity. However, GISTs greater than 10 cm in size and/or with mitotic counts greater than 5/50 high power field usually behave in a malignant fashion. Such tumors have a high risk for liver metastases and/or diffuse intra-abdominal spread. Bone and lung metastases are rare.

The radiologic appearances of malignant GISTs are fairly characteristic. On barium studies the main feature is frequently a large, extrinsic, non-obstructing mass displacing or distorting adjacent barium-filled loops of intestine. This may be associated with ulceration, cavitation or fistula formation. Less often, a GIST may appear as a large cavity filled with barium and it may be difficult to identify the connection between the small intestine and the cavity.

A CT scan may add considerably to the pre-operative evaluation of these tumors. CT can accurately demonstrate the size, shape and extent of the lesion, uniformity of densities and enhancing patterns, and it can depict the presence of liver, peritoneal or other metastases. CT is useful in the differentiation from other malignant tumors that often have a predominantly submucosal location and/or appear largely excavated, such as lymphoma or metastatic melanoma. The main differential diagnosis of malignant GISTs, however, includes their benign counterparts, benign smooth muscle or neurogenic tumors. CT criteria favoring malignancy include an irregular, lobulated, large-sized mass, heterogeneous tissue density, central liquefactive necrosis, seen as water density with or without air fluid level, ulceration or fistula formation. Liver metastases from malignant GISTs are large, necrotic or cystic in nature with peripheral or 'rim' enhancement, whereas peritoneal metastases may appear as widely distributed, multiple, round, smoothly-outlined, homogeneous satellite masses.

The signal intensity on MRI suggests that GISTs usually have no fibrotic component, and that the inner portion of these tumors does not usually contain blood products. Their signal intensity on MRI has been reported to be hyperintense compared to fat on T1-weighted image. They also show intense enhancement after gadolinium-chelate injection (Fig. 5).

GISTs are distinctive compared to other malignant small intestinal neoplasms as they have a greater tendency to grow extra-luminally, to develop large ulcers and therefore to bleed, and attain a large size without obstruction. They do not normally metastasize to the regional lymph node and they have a larger survival rate, even despite metastases.

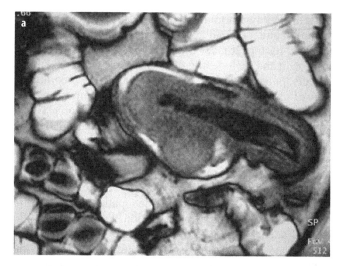

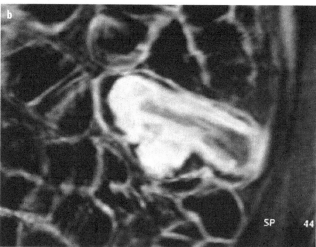

Fig. 5. MR enteroclysis showing jejunal intussusception due to a benign GIST tumor. A round well-circumscribed mass of intermediate signal intensity is shown in a coronal true FISP image (**a**). Post gadolinium coronal 3D FLASH image (**b**) demonstrates marked homogeneous enhancement of both the tumor mass and the viable intestinal wall

Meckel's Diverticulum

Meckel's diverticulum is the most common congenital anomaly of the small intestine, occurring in 1-3% of the population. It is mostly asymptomatic. One of the most common complications is lower gastrointestinal bleeding, which may be acute, life-threatening, chronic or intermittent, and is mostly due to ectopic gastric mucosa and peptic ulceration. Ectopic gastric mucosa is found in 15-20% of cases, in almost 90% of those who present with bleeding of the pediatric age group, but in only 7% of similar cases in adults.

Pre-operative radiological diagnosis of Meckel's diverticulum ranges from difficult to very difficult. Radionuclide imaging, the Meckel's scan, based on the affinity of the isotope technetium-99m pertechnetate for functioning ectopic gastric mucosa, has long been considered a most sensitive study. However, sensitivity varies with technique and age, and it is estimated to be around 60% for adults. False positive results do occur, at a disturbing frequency, in a number of conditions, whereas false negative results usually occur with symptomatic diverticula without ectopic gastric mucosa or acutely hemorrhaging diverticula.

Enteroclysis has been also suggested as a most reliable imaging technique for the pre-operative diagnosis of a Meckel's diverticulum. It usually shows a blindly ending sac of variable size, arising from the antimesenteric border of ileum. Additional characteristic findings include a gastric rugal pattern or a triangular fold pattern, at the base of the diverticulum. Careful fluoroscopy with compression is essential.

However, unsuccessful demonstration of a Meckel's diverticulum on enteroclysis despite a detailed examination is not unusual. The reasons for this include stenosis of the ostium, filling with intestinal contents, rapid emptying, or small size. CT has been reported to be of value in Meckel's diverticulitis and infracted Meckel's diverticulum.

Selective angiography is a well-established method for both non-hemorrhaging-negative scintigraphic, and for massively bleeding, diverticula. Extravasation of contrast into the bowel lumen is an expected angiographic finding in a patient with active bleeding. Very recently the importance of visualization and identification of the vitelline artery for the diagnosis of a Meckel's diverticulum itself, with or without active hemorrhage, has again been stressed.

Characteristic angiographic findings of selective or superselective catheterization will include: a) an abnormal elongated vessel, originating from the ileal artery, without anastomotic branches to the ileal artery branches; and b) a group of dilated tortuous vessels at the distal portion of this artery, without branches.

References

1. Gourtsoyiannis N, Nolan D (1997) Imaging of Small Bowel Neoplasms. Elsevier, Amsterdam
2. Rossi P, Courtsoyiannis N, Bezzi M et al (1996) Meckel's diverticulum: imaging diagnosis. AJR Am J Roentgenol 166:567-573
3. Dixon PM, Roulston ME, Nolan DJ (1993) The small bowel enema: a 10-year review. Clin Radiol 4:46-48
4. Barloon TJ, Lu CC, Honda H et al (1994) Does a normal small bowel enteroclysis exclude small bowel disease? A long term follow-up of consecutive normal studies. Abdom Imaging 19:113-115
5. Bender GN, Maglinte DT, Kloeppel VR et al (1999) CT-Enteroclysis: a superfluous diagnostic procedure or valuable when investigating small bowel disease. AJR Am J Roentgenol 172:373-378
6. Gourtsoyiannis N, Papanikolaou N, Grammatikakis J et al (2000) MR Imaging of the small bowel with a true-FISP sequence after enteroclysis with water solution. Invest Radiol 35:707-711
7. Umschaden HW, Szolar D, Gasser J et al (2000) Small-bowel disease: comparison of MR enteroclysis images with conventional enteroclysis and surgical findings. Radiology 215:717-725
8. Gourtsoyiannis N, Papanikolaou N, Grammatikakis J et al (2001) MR enteroclysis protocol optimization: comparison between 3D FLASH with fat saturation after intravenous gadolinium injection and true FISP sequences. Eur Radiol 11:908-913

Essentials and Clinical Applications of CT Enteroclysis

D.D. Maglinte

Department of Radiology, Indiana University Hospital, Indiana University School of Medicine, Indianapolis, IN, USA

Introduction

Technologic advances have made small bowel imaging a rapidly changing field and a challenge to radiology. Radiological investigations dominated small bowel imaging for all of the last century until the advent of wireless capsule endoscopy (WCE) [1]. Although traditionally the simplicity, availability and low cost of small bowel follow through (SBFT) made it the most commonly performed examination, barium enteroclysis has been shown to have overall higher accuracy and reliability. However, this is at the expense of increased invasiveness and decreased patient tolerance without the use of conscious sedation [2, 3]. The disadvantage of all barium small bowel examinations is their inability to provide any extraluminal information that may have important clinical implications for patients with diseases of the small bowel. Much of the diagnostic information from barium studies was derived from the indirect mucosal and mural changes produced by lesions within or outside the lumen, allowing for substantial intra- and interobserver variation and difficulty in interpreting equivocal or even overt findings. This has become particularly apparent with the increased use of contrast-enhanced computed tomography (CT) studies [4-6]. A comparison of barium enteroclysis and abdominal CT done on the same patients with small bowel Crohn's disease has demonstrated a much higher success of CT in revealing mural and extraluminal manifestations of disease, including abscesses, while enteroclysis was superior for luminal abnormalities, including bowel obstruction (especially low-grade), sinus tracts, fistulae, and ulcerations, mainly as a result of the enteral volume challenge generated by the controlled infusion of the contrast agent [7]. It was only a matter of time until computed tomographic enteroclysis (CTE) was developed to overcome the individual deficiencies of these techniques and to combine the advantages of both examinations into one technique. Initially reported by Kloppel et al. in 1992 [8], CTE was shown to be highly accurate for the depiction of mucosal abnormalities as well as bowel thickening, fistulae, and other extraintestinal complications of Crohn's disease. The first North American report performed studies in patients with suspected small bowel obstruction [9]. Bender et al.

showed that CT enteroclysis was superior to conventional CT for the diagnosis of lower grades of bowel obstruction and was also able to reveal the nature of the obstructive lesion. Notably, in these patients, adhesions were inferred on conventional CT when no mass, inflammatory changes or any other significant pathology were seen at the point of obstruction.

The introduction of multislice CT technology with its ability to scan larger volumes at a faster speed and the use of thinner section collimation allowing acquisition of near isotropic voxels, have made high resolution reformatting in different planes a simple and practical procedure with newer software. This technology has also resulted in improved performance and feasibility of CT enteroclysis, leading to an increased use of this method around the world [10-13]. At the same time, progress in endoscopy has been remarkable. Wireless capsule endoscopy (WCE) and very recently, double-balloon enteroscopy have allowed full exploration of the small bowel, the latter completed with interventional capabilities previously only available through intra-operative enteroscopy [14, 15]. This update examines the various modifications made to CTE that have evolved since its original description more than ten years ago, presents an overview of its clinical applications and analyzes its role in the investigation of small bowel diseases in the era of complementary endoscopy studies.

Technical Modifications

Since the original reports using dilute positive enteral contrast, CT enteroclysis has evolved into two distinct modifications, one using neutral enteral contrast with intravenous (iv) contrast enhancement and the other using positive enteral contrast [16-19]. Each modification has technical differences, and these will be described separately. For both modifications, bowel preparation includes a low residue diet, ample fluids, a laxative on the day prior to the examination, and nothing by mouth on the day of the examination. As with barium enteroclysis, patients using a 13 F enteroclysis catheter (MEC Cook Inc. Bloomington IN) are given the option to have conscious sedation, as has been previously suggested [16].

CTE with Neutral Enteral and iv Contrast

The enteral contrast agents used with CTE are water, 0.5% methyl cellulose and dilute barium (VoLumen®, EZ EM Inc., Westbury, NY). All of these agents have been used successfully by many practitioners. Methyl cellulose was used initially by some radiologists because of its perceived slower absorption compared to water [20]. We also initially used methyl cellulose, but currently prefer water. Water is not absorbed has fast that a collapsed small bowel results, and is eliminated quickly. In a busy tertiary care facility practice, performing an average of four CTE a day, we have not yet had a patient develop complications with the use of water. VoLumen® has a flavoring agent and additives to decrease absorption. Taste is not an issue with enteroclysis. The spread of acquisition with multislice CT technology has caused the development of fast rate of enteral infusion using an hypotonic agent to keep the small intestine distended. The lower attenuation of water compared with methyl cellulose and VoLumen® contrasts well with the mucosal enhancement produced by the iv contrast agent and allows a global look at all abdominal and pelvic organs (Fig. 1). Both methyl cellulose and VoLumen® (which also contains gum and dilute barium) have a slightly higher attenuation than water. All have been used successfully without complications. We prefer

VoLumen® for the oral hyperhydration method (CT enterography – a non-enteral volumed challenged examination). We prefer water for CTE because of its viscosity, which allows us to infuse faster at a slower infusion rate, decreasing the incidence of vomiting. Its lower attenuation and cost are additional factors. The amount and rate of administration of iv contrast depends on the radiologist's individual preference. We prefer CT acquisition during the late arterial/early portal venous phase where maximum intestinal mucosal enhancement occurs [21].

Catheter Tip Position

A small balloon catheter is used for CTE because of the lack of viscosity of water and the low viscosity of the other neutral enteral agents, (9 F MCTE catheter, EZ EM Inc., Westbury NY). This small soft catheter obviates the need for conscious sedation. The balloon and catheter tip are ideally positioned distal to the crossing of the superior mesenteric artery. The balloon is inflated with 30-40 ml of air. A 60 ml syringe of air is injected into the infusion lumen and additional air is injected into the balloon if air refluxes proximally. This also allows us to see if the catheter tip is in a diverticulum. Our technique of performing CTE with neutral enteral and iv contrast is summarized in Table 1.

We observe the position of the balloon and gauge the response of the patient to the rate of initial infusion (100 ml/min). If the balloon is pushed back to the descending segment at this rate, we decrease the infusion rate to 80 ml/min. In some patients, particularly those with irritable bowel syndrome, patients complain of abdominal pain at this rate even if the balloon is not pushed back, in which case we decrease the rate to 60 ml/min. This is also done when patients complain of nausea. We raise the rate by 20 ml from the fluoroscopic rate at the CT table. If the patient evacuates some of the water when no CT unit is immediately available, we infuse 2 l on the CT table before iv contrast is given. In patients with prior surgery that involved the ileocecal valve, we decrease the amount infused at CT to 1 l but increase the infusion rate to 150 ml/min, if possible. The high rate of infusion keep the

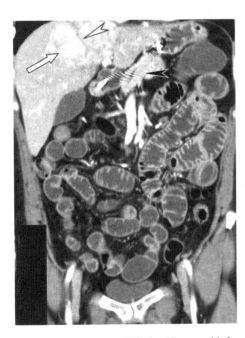

Fig. 1. Neutral enteral contrast CTE in 47-year-old female with Crohn's disease and abdominal pain. Coronal reformatting of isotropic resolution acquisition showed no small bowel abnormality. Incidental hypervascular liver mass (*arrow*) with scar (*white arrowhead*) was demonstrated, later proven to be focal nodular hyperplasia. Note dark and bright stripes (*black arrowhead*) adjacent to the nasoduodenal tube. This (Feldkamp) artifact is due to the off-center modulation of pixel noise in the z position when dealing with a wide cone beam (40-channel CT was used in this study). The artifact is most obvious on coronal or sagittal reformats at sites where X-ray attenuation changes rapidly along the z direction

Table 1. CT enteroclysis with neutral enteral/iv contrast

Fluoroscopic Phase
a. Balloon positioned in distal duodenum to the left of the spine
b. 0.3 mg glucagon iv
c. Infuse 2 l of water at 100 ml/min – adjust as described
   Transfer patient to CT table

CT Phase
d. Give 0.3 mg glucagon iv
e. Infuse 1.5 l of water at 120 ml/min
f. iv contrast: 4 ml/sec, total 150 ml
   CT acquired at 50 sec delay
g. Balloon deflated and catheter retracted to level of black marker, refluxed water in stomach decompressed before catheter withdrawn

small bowel distended for a longer time. The glucagon (or buscopan) keeps the small bowel aperistaltic and allows the patient to hold the large amount of contrast in the small bowel and colon. We give the glucagon in two small doses to diminish the nausea that is common with higher doses and to prolong its effect.

CT Enteroclysis with Positive Enteral Constrast

The enteral contrast chosen has varied from a 4-15% water soluble contrast solution, to dilute 6% barium solution [14]. The concentration used mostly depends on the preference of the radiologist.

Catheter Balloon Tip Position

The balloon and catheter tip can be positioned initially in the descending duodenum because infusion of enteral contrast is done under fluoroscopic control. A 13 Fr diagnostic enteroclysis catheter, or a 13.5 decompression/enteroclysis catheter are used (MEC or MDEC, Cook, Inc., Bloomington, IN) because of the viscosity of the contrast material. After the balloon is inflated with 30-40 ml of air, a syringe of air is injected into the infusion lumen. Air is added to the balloon if backflow occurs. If, at the start of infusion with slower infusion rates, the balloon is pushed back or contrast refluxes proximal to the balloon, the infusion is stopped and the catheter tip is advanced to the distal duodenum or proximal jejunum and the balloon is inflated. In asthenic patients the catheter tip and balloon should be immediately advanced to the distal duodenum or, when using the long decompression/enteroclysis catheter, to the proximal jejunum. Table 2 shows our CTE protocol with positive enteral contrast.

The amount infused at CT should be increased to 1.5 liters before CT acquisition if the patient eliminates contrast while waiting for a CT table. Otherwise, the amount infused at CT will depend on the amount seen at fluoroscopy, in order to reach the pelvic segments of small bowel or when an abnormality (mass or gradient) is seen fluoroscopically. Determination of optimal infu-

sion rates during the fluoroscopic phase is important when using positive enteral contrast, as this is the main factor that keeps the small intestine distended during CT acquisition (Fig. 2). Newer digital fluoroscopic units allow improved post processing of fluoroscopic images obtained during optimum distention and result in diagnostic single-contrast examinations when using a 12% solution of sodium diatrizoate. In some instances, subtle gradients of low-grade partial obstruction may be observed during the fluoroscopic phase and not on the CT images. The etiology of obstruction may not be seen fluoroscopically. When combined with the CT images, fluoroscopic observations recorded on the spot radiographs add confidence to the diagnosis.

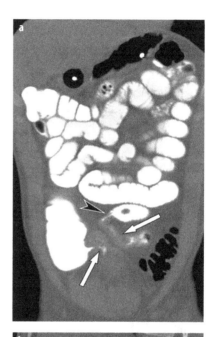

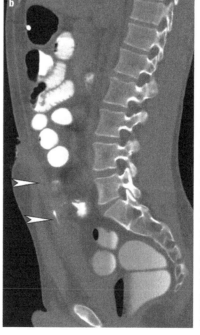

Fig. 2. Positive contrast CTE in 29-year-old male with Crohn's disease with allergy to iv contrast. **a** Coronal reformat showed low-grade small bowel obstruction with sharp transition point (*black arrowhead*). The cause of the obstruction was a long segment of fibrostenosis (*arrows*). **b** Sagittal reformat showed enteric fistula (*white arrowheads*). In view of fibrostenosis, patient was not treated with infliximab (inhibitor of tumor necrosis factor-alpha)

Table 2. CTE with positive enteral contrast

Fluoroscopic phase:
a. Balloon catheter tip in descending or distal duodenum
b. 12% water soluble contrast: 2l plus infusion rate at 55-150 ml/min (adjusted for optimal enteral volume challenge)
c. Limited fluoro and radiography to cecum
   Transfer patient to CT

CT Phase:
d. Infuse 500 ml to 1 l on CT table with infusion continued during scanning. Infusion rate increased by 10 ml/min from fluoroscopically determined infusion rate. Amount determined at fluoroscopy
e. Withdraw enteroclysis catheter to stomach (black marker) - suction refluxed contrast then withdraw catheter

CT Parameters

Table 3 lists our CT parameters using 4, 16, 40, and 64 multi-detector channels.

Routine soft tissue viewing and post processing in CT enteroclysis.

(WW = 360 H WL = 40 H) with neutral enteral and iv contrast. Small bowel windows (WW = 1200 H WL = 200 H) are used for viewing positive enteral contrast CT.

The small bowel window settings used can be adjusted to individual preference (Fig. 2a, b).

The large number of projection data images collected when acquiring near isotropic or isotropic voxels with multislice CT means that practical handling of the source data or 'smart post processing' is important to reduce the amount of data and, at the same time, increase the amount of information. This is tailored to the radiologist's needs. Interpretation is done at a separate workstation (Extended Brilliance workspace [EBW] Philips, Medical Imaging, Best, Netherlands) using interactive 2D viewing, i.e., viewing of axial, coronal and sagittal images with cross-referencing of abnormal or questionable findings. Selected significant reformatted images are sent to the picture archiving communication system (PACS) for the clinician to view. These are added to the reformatted axial images sent initially to the PACS station. This is also of value in conferences where direct retrieval of images are from PACS.

Clinical Indications

The clinical applications of the two modifications of CT enteroclysis overlap. In our early experience, we used CTE with positive enteral contrast for most small bowel investigations of possible small bowel obstruction (Fig. 3a, 3b). Since the introduction of multislice CT technology, we use CT enteroclysis with neutral enteral and iv contrast as our primary method of investigation when the small bowel is not distended, as determined by the scout radiograph, and when there is no contraindication to the use of iv iodinated contrast. This modification is faster, reproducible and allows a more global detailed evaluation

Table 3. CT Parameters

- Quad CT (MX 8000, Philips Medical Systems)
  3.2 mm slice width
  1.3 mm reconstruction interval
- Brilliance 16 channel CT (MX 8000 IDT, Philips Medical Systems)
  2.0 mm slice width
  1.0 mm reconstruction interval
- Brilliance 40 or 64 (Philips Medical Systems)
  Scan 40 × 0.625 mm
  *Recon 0.9 mm @ 0.45 mm
  AX
  Post process: COR 4@ 4 mm
  SAG

* Source raw images workstation for interpretation

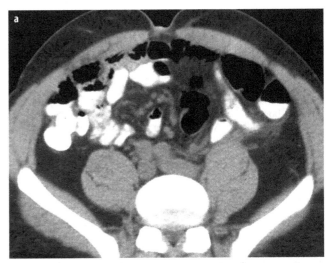

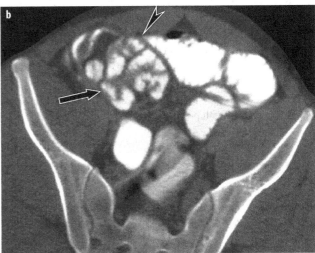

Fig. 3. A 38-year-old male with prior appendicectomy presenting with intermittent abdominal pain. **a** Conventional CT image showed no evidence of distended small bowel. **b** CTE with positive enteral contrast, performed three days later, showed distended proximal bowel loop with abrupt tapering of caliber (*arrowhead*) adjacent to anterior parietal peritoneum. Distal small bowel contains enteral contrast but was non-distended (*arrow*). Low-grade obstruction was diagnosed and surgically proven as being due to adhesions

not only of the small intestine, but also of the entire abdomen. It is well tolerated by patients if simple technical guidelines are observed and uses less radiation than positive enteral contrast.

Table 4 summarizes the current clinical indications of CTE with neutral enteral and iv contrast. Table 5 summarizes the current clinical indications of CTE with positive enteral contrast.

Miscellaneous Applications

CT enteroclysis has been of value in resolving the false positive and false negative interpretation of non-enteral volume-challenged small bowel studies that arise from the

Table 4. CTE with neutral enteral & iv contrast

CLINICAL INDICATIONS:
1. Unexplained GI bleeding - history of prior malignancy.
2. Unexplained anemia in elderly or younger patients without diarrhea. No heme positive stool.
3. Known Crohn's disease: Staging (Fig. 4).
4. Small bowel obstruction (SBO) - no evidence of significant small bowel distention on plain film.
5. ALTERNATE EXAM – Pre- or post capsule enteroscopy or when CO_2 double contrast barium enteroclysis is not technically possible (Fig. 5).

Table 5. CTE (positive contrast)

1. Suspected recurrent SBO or unexplained abdominal pain with negative conventional exams or iv contrast contraindicated (Fig. 6 a-c).
2. Suspected small bowel disease (unexplained lower GI bleeding, anemia, diarrhea, and history of NSAID intake) and iv contrast contraindicated or air (CO_2) Barium Enteroclysis not technically possible.
3. Subset of patients with SBO in whom general surgeons prefer conservative MX and SB distended on conventional exams.
4. SBO in the immediate post operative period.
5. History of prior abdominal surgery for malignant tumor.
6. History of prior radiation therapy.
7. Crohn's disease with prior surgery.

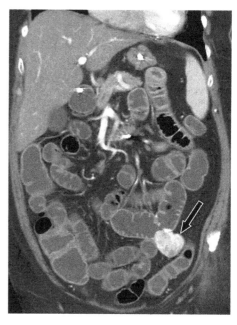

Fig. 5. Neutral enteral contrast CTE in a 63-year-old female with unexplained gastrointestinal (GI) bleeding. Wireless capsule endoscopy showed jejunal angioectasia (*not shown*). CTE showed a 3 cm hypervascular submucosal mass (*arrow*) arising from mid small bowel, proven to be a gastrointestinal stromal tumor at surgery

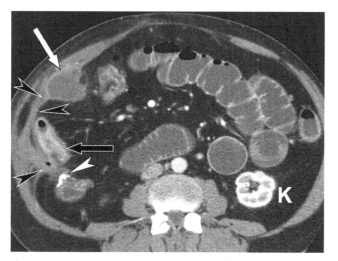

Fig. 4. Axial image of neutral enteral contrast CTE in a 62-year-old female with Crohn's disease showing a long fistulous track (*black arrowheads*) extending from the inflamed cecum (*black arrow*) to an abscess (*white arrow*). Prior terminal ileal resection is evidenced by surgical clips (*white arrowhead*). Note the late arterial phase of iv contrast bolus, indicated by enhancement of left renal cortex (*K*)

difficulties associated with small bowel non-filling, poor distention, peristalsis, or the simulation of wall thickening or pseudowaves caused by retained fluid that occurs with positive oral contrast [12]. In patients with symptoms of proximal small bowel obstruction, the performance of the CT enteroclysis with the catheter tip in the descending duodenum have resulted in more precise diagnosis.

We have observed abdominal pain and nausea in patients with irritable bowel syndrome due to the high infusion rates used with CT enteroclysis. This may be an important clinical observation once organic disease has been excluded [12]. Prompt adjustment of the infusion rate can diminish the discomfort without problems. Neutral enteral contrast is not seen fluoroscopically, so CT enteroclysis with this method is subject to difficulties that arise when evaluating non-distended bowel in patients that vomit or inadvertently lose small bowel contrast via the rectum. Experience and adherence to technical details alleviates this disadvantage.

Relevance of CTE for the Elective Investigation of Small Bowel Disease in the Era of Wireless Capsule Endoscopy

Pre-capsule Endoscopy

Except for emergent clinical investigation for possible small bowel diseases where abdominal CT will remain the primary method of investigation, the role of imaging is likely to undergo reassessment based on results of WCE in the elective work-up of patients [1]. In the patient without risk factors for a potentially obstructing small bowel lesion, radiology has a limited role. As stated earlier, where the indication raises the possibility of early Crohn's or NSAID enteropathy, air double-contrast enteroclysis is the most reliable method of imaging (Fig. 7). CTE should otherwise suffice for all pre-capsule radiologic investigations where there is a possibility of a potentially obstruct-

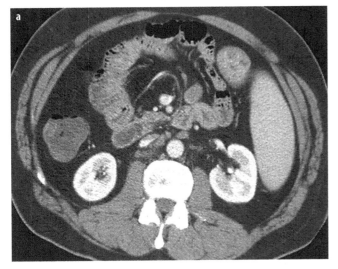

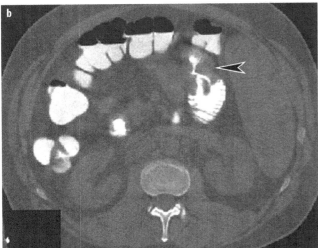

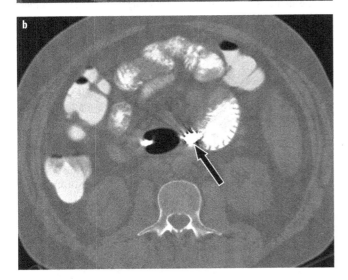

ing small bowel abnormality. How the introduction of the patency capsule will impact on utilization of radiologic investigation remains to be seen.

Post-capsule Endoscopy

As with all examinations where there is a human factor involved, perceptive errors are inevitable. The clinical significance of diminutive red spots without positive evidence of bleeding and the superficial mucosal 'scratches' shown by WCE are increasingly being questioned [1]. A mucosal 'scratch' is a nonspecific and will need fur-

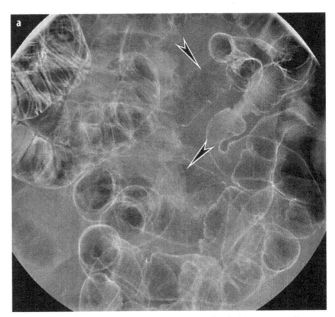

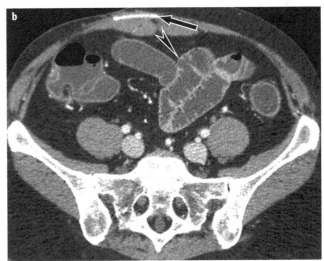

Fig. 6. Axial CT (**a**) and positive contrast CTE (**b, c**) in a 48-year-old male presenting with vomiting and weight loss. CT showed no obstruction or mass. Wireless capsule enteroscopy performed after CT was unsuccessful because the capsule was trapped in proximal small bowel. CTE showed annular mass (*arrowhead*, **b**) in proximal jejunum proven to be adenocarcinoma and capsule trapped in distal duodenum (*arrow*, **c**)

Fig. 7. A neutral enteral contrast CTEs (**a**) performed within two weeks of each other in a 54-year-old female with suspected Crohn's disease. Fluoroscopic study showed aphtae in small bowel loops (*arrowheads*). **b** Double contrast carbon dioxide-barium small bowel fluoroscopic enteroclysis. CTE of same loop (*arrowhead*) showed no abnormality. Note incidental abdominal wall mesh on image **b** (*arrow*)

ther characterization to make a precise diagnosis in some instances. We have unpublished data of an air double contrast barium enteroclysis carried out following WCE and interpreted by experienced endoscopists to assess the extent of, or to characterize Crohn's disease. This has shown the limitations of WCE in characterizing superficial ulcers and their precise location [22]. In one instance, radiologic examination showed a giant Meckel's diverticulum with ulcerations in the junction of the diverticulum to the ileum. In another patient, NSAID ulcers and diaphragm disease were shown by air enteroclysis and ascribed by WCE to Crohn's disease. Patients with persistent symptoms or bleeding with negative WCE require accurate radiologic investigations (Fig. 5). We have diagnosed a Meckel's diverticulum with a prior negative WCE. NSAID ulcers were shown by air double-contrast barium enteroclysis. Where the indication is a question of submucosal mass on WCE, CTE with neutral enteral and iv contrast is appropriate.

Disadvantages of CTE and Pitfalls

Nasoenteric tube placement is necessary for infusion, but its associated discomfort is alleviated by the use of conscious sedation and smaller tubes [16]. Conscious sedation requires dedicated personnel and makes the procedure longer and more expensive. In small institutions and non-tertiary care facilities this may not be practical. In patients who require nasogastric suction and potentially need a small bowel examination, the initial use of a decompression/enteroclysis catheter circumvents this disadvantage [23].

The logistics of performing CT when the fluoroscopic suite is far from the CT area is a deterrent. The addition of CT to enteroclysis increases the cost of the procedure and exposure of radiation to patients and radiologic personnel. The procedure therefore should be done only when clinically indicated.

Fluoroscopy should be limited when utilizing positive enteral contrast CTE. When feasible, CTE should be used with neutral enteral and iv contrast.

Radiation doses related to CT enteroclysis remain a significant issue. The use of a multidetector CT with 40 or more channels can reduce radiation by 10-66% [24]. This is because of a more efficient detector configuration, automatic exposure controls, improved filters and image post processing algorithms. MR enteroclysis has the advantage of lack of radiation exposure and safer contrast agents, but appears to be less accurate than CT enteroclysis. In a prospective comparison between MR enteroclysis and CT enteroclysis, the latter showed greater sensitivity and interobserver agreement for an array of pathological signs of small bowel diseases [25].

Conclusions

Small bowel imaging is a rapidly changing field. The early diagnosis of small bowel disease will remain a diagnostic challenge to radiologists [26]. CTE combines the advantages of CT and barium enteroclysis. Although it has disadvantages, international experience has shown that it has value for the investigation of small bowel diseases. The use of multislice technology and 2D reformatting have made organs that are more long than wide, such as the mesenteric small intestine, easier to examine with CTE. CTE in the non-emergent investigation of small bowel diseases utilizes a hybrid imaging technique with high negative predictive value, high sensitivity, and specificity. This method of investigation is needed when evaluating an organ with a low prevalence of disease, the clinical symptoms of which are non-specific and are mimicked by diseases of other abdominal organs.

References

1. Maglinte D (2005) Capsule imaging and the role of radiology in the investigation of diseases of the small bowel. Radiology 236:763-767
2. Maglinte DD, Lappas JC, Kelvin FM et al (1987) Small bowel radiography: how, when, and why? Radiology 163:197-305
3. Maglinte DD, Kelvin F, O'Connor K et al (1996) Current status of small bowel radiography. Abdom Imaging 2:247-257
4. Buckley JA, Jones B, Fishman EK (1997) Small bowel cancer: imaging features and staging. Radiol Clin North Am 35:381-402
5. Fishman EK, Wolf EJ, Jones B et al (1987) CT evaluation of Crohn's disease: effect on patient management. AJR Am J Roentgenol 148:537-540
6. Merine D, Fishman EK, Jones B (1989) CT of the small bowel and mesentery. Radiol Clin North Am 27:707-715
7. Maglinte DD, Hallett R, Rex D et al (2001) Imaging of small bowel Crohn's disease: can abdominal CT replace barium radiography? Emerg Radiol 8:127-133
8. Koppel R, Thiele J, Bosse J (1992) The Sellink CT method. [in German] Rofo Fortschr Geb Rontgenstr Neuen Bildgeb Verfahr 156:91-92
9. Bender GN, Timmons JH, Williard WC et al (1996) Computed tomographic enteroclysis: one methodology. Invest Radiol 31:43-49
10. Ros PR, Ji H (2002) CT: applications in the abdomen. Radiographics 22:697-700
11. Caoili EM, Paulson EK (2000) CT of small-bowel obstruction: another perspective using multiplanar reformations. Am J Roentgenol 174:993-998
12. Maglinte DD, Bender GN, Heitkamp DE et al (2003) Multidetector-row helical CT enteroclysis. Radiol Clin North Am 41:249-262
13. Horton KM, Fishman EK (2003) The current status of multidetector row CT and three-dimensional imaging of the small bowel. Radiol Clin North Am 41:199-212
14. Iddan GI, Swain CP (2004) History and development of capsule endoscopy. Gastrointest Endoscopy Clin N Am 14:1-9
15. Yamamoto H (2005) Double balloon endoscopy. Clin Gastroent Hepatol 3:S27-S29
16. Maglinte DD, Lappas JC, Heitkamp DE et al (2003) Technical refinements in enteroclysis. Radiol Clin N Am 41:213-229
17. Schober E, Turetschek K, Schima W et al (1997) Methylcellulose enteroclysis spiral CT in the preoperative assessment of Crohn's disease: radiologic pathologic correlation. Radiology 205:717 (abs)
18. Schoepf UJ, Holzknecht N, Matz C et al (2001) New developments in imaging the small bowel with multislice computed tomography and negative contrast medium. In: Reiser

MF (ed) Multislice CT. Springer, Berlin Heidelberg New York, pp 49-60

19. Rollandi GA, Curone PF, Conzi R et al (1999) Spiral CT of the abdomen after distention of small bowel loops with transparent enema in patients with Crohn's disease. Abdom Imaging 24:544-549

20. Romano S, De Lutio E, Rollandi GA et al (2005) Multidetector computed tomography enteroclysis (MDCT-E) with neutral enteral and IV contrast enhancement in tumor detection. Eur Radiol 15:1178-1183

21. Horton KM, Eng J, Fishman EK (2000) Normal enhancement of the small bowel: evaluation with spiral CT. J Comput Assist Tomogr 24:67-71

22. Maglinte DD (2005) Invited Commentary to: Hara AK, Leighton JA, Virender K et al. Imaging of small bowel disease:

comparison of capsule endoscopy, standard endoscopy, barium examination, and CT. Radiographics 25:697-718

23. Maglinte D, Kelvin F, Rowe M et al (2001) Small-bowel obstruction: optimizing radiologic investigation and nonsurgical management. Radiology 218:39-46

24. Mannudeep K, Rizzo SMR, Novelline RA (2005) Technologic innovations in computer tomography dose reduction: implications in emergency settings. Emerg Radiol 11:127-128

25. Duvoisin B, Meuli R, Michetti P et al (2003) Prospective comparison of MR enteroclysis with multidetector spiral-CT enteroclysis: interobserver agreement and sensitivity by means of 'sign-by-sign' correlation. Eur Radiol 13:1303-1311

26. Maglinte D (2006) Small bowel imaging: a rapidly changing field and a challenge to radiology. Eur Radiol Jan 5:1-5

Imaging of the Colon and Rectum: Inflammatory and Neoplastic Diseases

R.M. Gore[1], J. Stoker[2]

[1] Department of Radiology, Evanston Northwestern Healthcare, Northwestern University, Evanston, IL, USA
[2] Department of Radiology, Academic Medical Center, University of Amsterdam, The Netherlands

Introduction

Inflammatory and neoplastic diseases of the colon and rectum are relatively common. Cross-sectional imaging plays an important part in the work-up of patients with these disorders. Diverticulitis, appendicitis, and the inflammatory and infectious colitides are among the commonest causes of acute abdominal pain. Affected patients frequently present with non-specific symptoms and often the first radiologic test that they undergo is computed tomography (CT). By virtue of its ability to directly image pathologic changes in the colon wall, serosa, surrounding mesentery and peritoneum, CT can provide crucial information for accurate diagnosis and prompt management. In patients with perianal fistulas, magnetic resonance imaging (MRI) is the preferred imaging technique, as the combination of high intrinsic contrast resolution and large field of view provides detailed information on the presence and extent of the disease. CT-colonography (CTC) is valuable for the detection of colorectal cancer and adenomatous polyps. For the work-up of patients with rectal cancer, endosonography (EUS) and especially MRI are crucial for management.

This presentation describes the features of these disorders, provides differential diagnostic guidelines and indicates the role of imaging in disease management.

Inflammatory Disorders

Ulcerative Colitis

Ulcerative colitis is characterized pathologically by extensive ulceration and diffuse inflammation of the mucosa. The disease characteristically begins in the rectum and extends proximally to involve part or all of the colon. The pathological changes found in the very early stages of ulcerative colitis are below the spatial resolution of CT. With progressive disease, submucosal edema may be seen, producing a target sign. Severe mucosal ulceration can denude certain portions of the colonic wall, leading to inflammatory pseudopolyps (Fig. 1). When sufficiently large, these pseudopolyps can be visualized on CT.

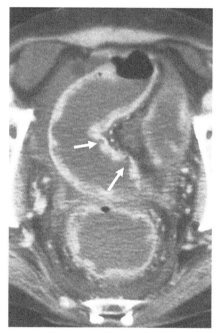

Fig. 1. Acute ulcerative colitis. CT demonstrates deep ulcerations (*arrows*) of the fluid-filled rectosigmoid. Inflammatory pseudopolyps appear as residual islands of inflamed mucosa, which protrude above the denuded colonic surface

Mural thickening and lumen narrowing are the CT hallmarks of subacute and chronic ulcerative colitides. Mural thinning, unsuspected perforations, and pneumatosis can be detected on CT in patients with toxic megacolon. In this regard, CT can be quite helpful in determining the urgency of surgery for patients with stable abdominal radiographs yet a deteriorating clinical course [1-3].

In chronic ulcerative colitis, the muscularis mucosae becomes markedly hypertrophied, often by up to a factor of 40. Forceful contraction of this hypertrophied longitudinal muscle may pull the mucosa away from the submucosa, producing diffuse or segmental narrowing of the lumen. The contraction also causes shortening of the colon. The submucosa becomes thickened due to the deposition of fat or, in acute and subacute cases, edema. Submucosal thickening further contributes to lumen narrowing. Additionally, the lamina propria is thickened due to round cell infiltration in both acute and chronic ulcerative colitides.

On CT, these mural changes produce a target or halo appearance when axially imaged: the lumen is surrounded by a ring of soft tissue density (mucosa, lamina propria, hypertrophied muscularis mucosae). This is surrounded by a low-density ring (fatty infiltration of the submucosa), which in turn is surrounded by a ring of soft tissue density (muscularis propria). This mural stratification is not specific and can also be seen in Crohn's disease, infectious enterocolitis, pseudomembranous colitis, ischemic and radiation enterocolitides, mesenteric venous thrombosis, bowel edema and graft-versus-host disease [1-3].

There are certain CT findings that can help differentiate granulomatous and ulcerative colitis. Mural stratification, that is, the ability to visualize individual layers of bowel wall, is seen in 61% of patients with chronic ulcerative colitis but only in 8% of patients with chronic granulomatous colitis. In addition, mean colon wall thickness in chronic ulcerative colitis is 7.8 mm, significantly smaller than that observed in Crohn's colitis (11 mm). Finally, the outer contour of the thickened colonic wall is smooth and regular in 95% of ulcerative colitis cases, while serosal and outer mural irregularities are present in 80% of patients with granulomatous colitis [1-3].

Rectal narrowing and widening of the presacral space are hallmarks of chronic ulcerative colitis. CT depicts the anatomic alterations that underlie these rather dramatic morphologic changes. The rectal lumen is narrowed due to the previously described mural thickening that attends chronic ulcerative colitis. As a result, the rectum has a target appearance on axial scans, which should not be mistaken for the external anal sphincter, mucosal prolapse, or the levator ani muscles. The increase in the presacral space is caused by proliferation of the perirectal fat. On CT, this fat is characterized by an increased number of nodular and streaky soft tissue densities and an abnormal attenuation value 10-20 HU higher than the normal extraperitoneal or mesenteric fat. These fatty changes relate to a number of factors, including *ex vacuo* replacement by fat of the void produced by rectal lumen narrowing and lipodystrophy resulting from an influx of inflammatory cells and edema. Edematous adipose tissue and enlarged lymph nodes are often observed in the perirectal region in patients with chronic ulcerative colitis upon abdominoperineal resection [1-3].

Crohn's Disease

Crohn's disease most commonly affects the terminal ileum and proximal colon. The acute, active phase of Crohn's disease is characterized by focal inflammation, aphthoid ulceration with adjacent cobblestoning, an often transmural inflammatory reaction with lymphoid aggregates and granuloma formation, fissures, fistula and sinus tracts. The chronic and resolving phase of this disorder is associated with fibrosis and stricture formation. When Crohn's disease is limited to the mucosa, the CT scan is often normal. Although inflammatory and post-in-flammatory pseudopolyps may be identified on CT, the assessment of the mucosa is best reserved for barium studies and colonoscopy, which are more direct and sensitive. Crohn's disease causes mural thickening of the gut in the range of 1-2 cm. This thickening, which occurs in up to 83% of patients, is most frequently observed in the terminal ileum, but other portions of the small bowel, colon, duodenum, stomach, and esophagus may be similarly affected [1-3].

During the acute, non-cicatrizing phase of Crohn's disease, the small bowel and colon maintain mural stratification and often have a target or double-halo appearance. As in ulcerative colitis, there is a soft tissue density ring (corresponding to mucosa), which is surrounded by a low-density ring. This ring has an attenuation near that of water or fat (corresponding to submucosal edema or fat infiltration, respectively), which in turn is surrounded by a higher density ring (muscularis propria). Inflamed mucosa and serosa may show significant contrast enhancement following bolus intravenous contrast administration, and the intensity of enhancement correlates with the clinical activity of disease [1-3].

The CT demonstration of mural stratification, that is, the ability to visualize distinct mucosal, submucosal, and muscularis propria layers, indicates that transmural fibrosis has not occurred and that medical therapy may be successful in ameliorating lumen compromise. Additionally, prior to the onset of fibrosis, the edema and inflammation of the bowel wall that cause mural thickening and lumen obstruction are reversible to some extent. A modest decrease in wall thickness often produces a dramatic increase in the cross-sectional area of the lumen and resolution of the patient's obstructive symptoms. Loss of mural stratification is indicative of transmural fibrosis [1-3].

In patients with long-standing Crohn's disease and transmural fibrosis, mural stratification is lost so that the affected bowel wall typically has homogeneous attenuation on CT. Homogeneous attenuation of the thickened bowel wall in the presence of good intravascular contrast medium levels and thin-section scanning suggests irreversible fibrosis so that anti-inflammatory agents may not provide significant reduction in bowel wall thickness. If these segments become sufficiently narrow, surgery or stricturoplasty will be necessary to relieve the patient's obstruction.

The palpation of an abdominal mass or separation of bowel loops on a barium study in a patient with Crohn's disease evokes an extensive differential diagnosis: abscess, phlegmon, 'creeping fat' or fibrofatty proliferation of the mesentery, bowel wall thickening, and enlarged mesenteric lymph nodes. Each of these disorders has significantly different prognostic and therapeutic implications. This diagnostic dilemma is further complicated by the fact that many patients are receiving immunosuppressive therapy that can mask signs and symptoms. CT can readily differentiate the extraluminal manifestations of Crohn's disease.

Fibrofatty proliferation, also known as 'creeping fat' of the mesentery, is the most common cause of separation of bowel loops seen on barium studies in patients with Crohn's disease. On CT, the sharp interface between bowel and mesentery is lost and the attenuation value of the fat is elevated by 20-60 HU due to the influx of inflammatory cells and fluid. Mesenteric adenopathy with lymph nodes ranging in size between 3 and 8 mm may also be present. If these lymph nodes are larger than 1 cm, the presence of lymphoma or carcinoma, both of which occur with greater frequency in Crohn's disease, can be excluded [1-3].

Contrast-enhanced CT scans often show hypervascularity of the involved mesentery, manifesting as vascular dilatation, tortuosity, prominence, and wide spacing of the vasa recta. These distinctive vascular changes have been termed the 'comb sign'. Identification of this hypervascularity suggests active disease and may be useful in differentiating Crohn's disease from lymphoma or metastases, which tend to be hypovascular lesions.

Pseudomembranous Colitis

Pseudomembranous colitis is being encountered with increasing frequency as a nosocomial infection complicating antibiotic therapy. This potentially life-threatening disorder is caused by overgrowth of *Clostridium difficile* and the subsequent release of a cytotoxic enterotoxin, which causes ulceration of the colonic mucosa and the formation of 2-3 mm pseudomembranes consisting of fibrin, mucus, sloughed epithelial cells, and leukocytes. Mild cases may demonstrate only mucosal irregularity and nodularity, with small plaque formation that cannot be detected radiologically. In advanced cases, there is thickening of haustral folds, a shaggy wall contour, and mucosal plaques.

CT shows a pancolitis with mural thickening that may be irregular or polypoid and have a shaggy endoluminal contour. The wall thickening (Fig. 2), usually 1.6-1.8 cm, is a result of submucosal edema. Mucosal and serosal enhancement are seen following intravenous contrast administration. The haustra are also thickened and edematous producing an 'accordion pattern', which is highly suggestive of pseudomembranous colitis. This pattern consists of contrast material trapped between thickened haustral folds that are aligned in a parallel fashion. This appearance can sometimes simulate deep ulcerations or fissures. Pericolic stranding, ascites, pleural effusions, and subcutaneous edema are other ancillary CT findings. Complications of untreated pseudomembranous colitis include toxic megacolon and intestinal perforation with subsequent peritonitis. CT is also useful for monitoring the response to medical therapy with oral vancomycin and metronidazole [4, 5].

AIDS-related Colitis

Cytomegalovirus and cryptosporidiosis are becoming relatively common pathogens, due to acquired immunodeficiency syndrome (AIDS). Patients with CD4 lymphocyte counts of 200 mm^3 or less are at greatest risk for these infections. Typically, the cecum and proximal ascending colon are affected by these organisms, however, a pancolitis with continuous lesions may occur. CT shows mural thickening of the involved segments of colon, with low attenuation in the region of the submucosa due to edema as well as pericolonic fluid and standing of the adjacent fat. Pneumatosis and ascites have also been described [5].

Typhlitis

Typhlitis (neutropenic colitis) is a potentially fatal infection of the cecum and ascending colon caused by enteric pathogens in patients with severe immunosuppression. It is most frequently seen in patients with acute leukemia receiving chemotherapy, but also occurs in the setting of AIDS, aplastic anemia, multiple myeloma, or bone marrow transplantation. Bacteria, viruses, and fungi penetrate the damaged cecal mucosa and proliferate due to the profound neutropenia. There is edema and inflammation of the cecum, ascending colon, and occasionally ileum. Fever, abdominal pain, nausea and diarrhea are presenting symptoms. Prompt diagnosis and supportive therapy with intensive antibiotics and fluids are required to prevent transmural necrosis and perforation. Surgical resection is indicated in patients with transmural necrosis, intramural perforation, abscess, or uncontrolled sepsis and gastrointestinal hemorrhage.

The inherent risks of bowel perforation caused by barium enemas and colonoscopies in these critically ill patients mean that CT is the study of choice in typhlitis. CT demonstrates circumferential mural thickening (1-3 cm) of the cecum, low density areas within the colonic wall secondary to edema, pericolonic inflammation and fluid, and in severe cases, pneumatosis. Clinically, CT is used to monitor decreases in mural thickness after therapy and to detect subtle pneumoperitoneum in cases of silent perforation or necrosis [6, 7].

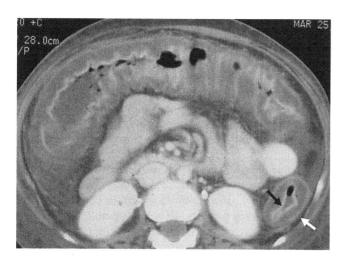

Fig. 2. Pseudomembranous colitis. There is mural and haustral thickening of the colon associated with submucosal edema (*white arrow*, enhancing muscularis propria; *black arrow*, enhancing mucosa)

Graft-Versus-Host Disease

Colonic complications of graft-versus-host (GVH) disease are common. In this disorder, mature donor lymphocytes attack recipient tissue in bone marrow transplantation patients. Acute GVH disease may manifest with profuse diarrhea, nausea, vomiting, intestinal hemorrhage, and cramping abdominal pain. Transmural inflammation is common but frank perforation is unusual.

Initially, CT shows diffuse mural thickening of the colon with submucosal edema and increased intraluminal secretions. In chronic GVH disease, submucosal fat may deposit rapidly and be readily identified on CT [4].

Differential Diagnosis of the Colitides

The differentiation of granulomatous colitis and ulcerative colitis is important in terms of medical management, surgical options, and prognosis. This distinction can usually be made on the basis of colonoscopy with biopsy histology, double-contrast barium enema, disease distribution, and clinical course. CT can occasionally help distinguish these disorders by demonstrating differences in mural thickness, wall density and distribution of colonic involvement, as well as the presence or absence of small bowel disease, abscess, fistula, and fibrofatty mesenteric proliferation.

Idiopathic inflammatory bowel disease must also be differentiated from infectious colitides. Although there is considerable overlap in the CT findings of these disorders, there are certain differentiating features. The presence of ascites is more suggestive of an acute, rather than chronic, cause of colonic inflammation. Peritoneal fluid is commonly found in the acute colitides, particularly pseudomembranous, infectious, and ischemic colitis, and not in chronic inflammatory bowel disease. Ascites is only infrequently seen in patients with acute inflammatory bowel disease. Submucosal fat deposition detected by CT is primarily found in subacute and chronic colitides, usually ulcerative colitis, and not in acute disease.

Appendicitis

Acute appendicitis is the most common abdominal surgical emergency, affecting 250,000 individuals in the United States annually. The lifetime risk of developing acute appendicitis is 8.6% for men and 6.7% for women. Radiologists play a critical role in evaluating patients with suspected appendicitis and minimizing complications by confirming or excluding the diagnosis in atypical cases. They also reduce the number of misdiagnoses and negative laparotomies, provide a correct alternate diagnosis, and manage appendiceal abscesses and post-operative complications. Contrast-enhanced helical CT has a sensitivity, specificity, and accuracy over 95% for the diagnosis of acute appendicitis [8-10].

On CT, the abnormal appendix presents as a slightly distended, fluid-filled, or collapsed structure, approxi-mately 0.5-2 cm in diameter. Inflammatory hyperemia causes the wall of the diseased appendix to show homogenous enhancement during the arterial phase of contrast administration. The wall is circumferentially and asymmetrically thickened (usually 1-3 mm). Periappendiceal inflammation, the hallmark of appendicitis, is characterized by increased hazy density or linear stranding of adjacent mesenteric fat, by fluid-containing abscesses, and by ill-defined, heterogeneous soft-tissue densities representing a phlegmon [8-10]. There may be secondary inflammatory and edematous changes, with thickening of the wall of the adjacent ileum and cecum, which may mimic primary ileocolic inflammatory disease (Fig. 3).

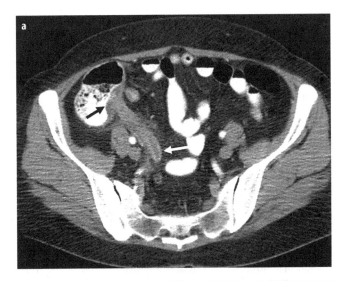

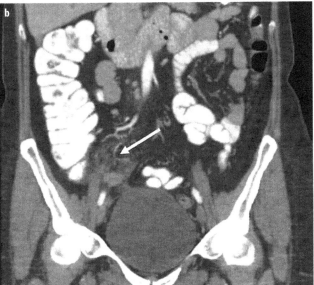

Fig. 3. Acute appendicitis. **a** Axial image demonstrates a dilated appendiceal lumen and abnormal mural enhancement (*white arrow*). Note the thickening of the adjacent cecum (*black arrow*). **b** Coronal reformatted image shows inflammatory changes (*arrow*) in the mesoappendix

On non-contrast CT scans, the diagnosis of acute appendicitis requires the detection of a thickened appendix (diameter exceeding 6 mm) with associated inflammatory changes in the periappendiceal fat, or abnormal thickening of the right lateroconal fascia, with or without a calcified appendicolith. The detection of an appendicolith confirms a specific diagnosis of appendicitis in the appropriate clinical setting. An appendicolith can be visualized on CT in approximately 28% of adult patients (compared with 10% for plain films), reflecting the higher sensitivity of CT in detecting small intra-abdominal calcifications [8-10].

The combination of right lower quadrant inflammation, a phlegmon, and an abscess adjacent to the cecum is suggestive but not diagnostic of appendicitis. Indeed, if an abnormal appendix or an appendicolith is not shown, the differential diagnosis must also include Crohn's disease, cecal diverticulitis, ileal diverticulitis, perforated cecal carcinoma, and pelvic inflammatory disease. A barium enema is required to visualize the appendix and evaluate the colon and terminal ileum for primary intestinal disease. Abscesses may be found in locations distant from the cecum because of the length and position of the appendix and the patterns of fluid migration in the peritoneal cavity.

The majority (60-70%) of patients referred for cross-sectional imaging with suspected appendicitis do not have this disease. Although most patients have benign, self-limited gastrointestinal disorders such as viral gastroenteritis, CT and ultrasound (US) can often suggest a specific alternate diagnosis [8-10].

Adnexal cysts, masses, salpingitis, and tubo-ovarian abscesses can be readily shown on US. Ureteral calculi and pyelonephritis can be detected on CT and US. Enlarged lymph nodes in the right lower quadrant suggest mesenteric adenitis or infectious ileitis; mural thickening of the terminal ileum can be seen in Crohn's disease or infectious ileitis.

Diverticulitis

It is estimated that 10-25% of individuals with diverticulosis will suffer from episodes of peridiverticular inflammation during their lifetime. In the United States, this complication accounts for approximately 200,000 hospitalizations and a health care expenditure of four billion dollars annually. Among patients who are hospitalized, 10-20% require emergency operations.

Inflammatory change in the pericolic fat (Fig. 4) is the hallmark of diverticulitis on CT, and is seen in 98% of cases. The extent of the inflammatory reaction is related to the size of the perforation, bacterial contamination, and the host response. Mild cases may manifest as areas of slightly increased density of fat adjacent to the involved colon or as fine linear strands with small fluid collections or bubbles of extraluminal air. In sigmoid diverticulitis, the fluid is typically decompressed into the inferior interfascial plane. Due to hypervascularity of the inflamed area, contrast-enhanced CT scans often reveal engorged mesenteric vessels in the involved pericolic fat.

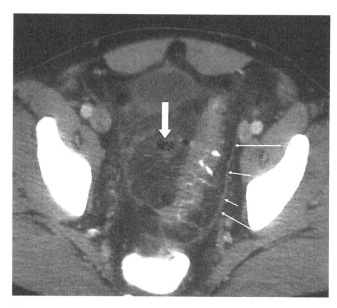

Fig. 4. Acute diverticulitis. There are diverticula and mural thickening of the sigmoid colon with inflammatory change and gas collection (*large arrow*) in the sigmoid mesocolon. Fluid is also present in the combined interfascial plane (*small arrows*)

Pericolic heterogeneous soft tissue densities representing phlegmons and partially loculated fluid collections indicating abscess are seen in more severe cases. The abscess cavities usually contain air bubbles or air-fluid levels. They develop within the sigmoid mesocolon or are sealed off by the sigmoid colon and adjacent small bowel loops. Less commonly they may form in the groin, flank, thigh, psoas muscle, subphrenic space or liver [11].

Using CT, diverticula are seen at the site of perforation or adjacent to it in about 80% of cases. They appear as small out-pouchings of air, contrast, or fecal material projecting through the colonic wall. Symmetric mural thickening of the involved colon by approximately 4-10 mm is seen in about 70% of cases, however if there is marked muscular hypertrophy, the wall of the colon can measure up to 2-3 cm in thickness.

CT can also demonstrate intramural abscesses and fistula, and is helpful in patients with suspected colovesical fistulas. In the latter case, a pericolic inflammatory mass is seen involving the bladder wall and intraluminal gas confirms the diagnosis.

CT has a reported sensitivity of up to 98% in the diagnosis of diverticulitis [11]. Additionally, CT can demonstrate extension of the disease, such as abscess and peritonitis remote from the colon and can guide percutaneous abscess drainage. CT can diagnose other pathological conditions that can clinically simulate diverticulitis.

Epiploic Appendagitis

Primary epiploic appendagitis is a relatively uncommon condition that results from an acute inflammation of the appendices epiploicae. This disorder is often associated

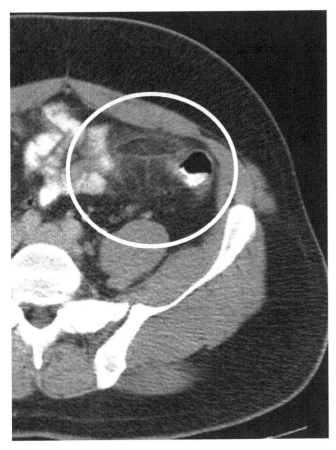

Fig. 5. Epiploic appendagitis. Inflammatory changes are present in the pericolic fat (*circle*). The central portion of the inflammatory change is fat density, indicating an inflamed epiploic appendage

with torsion and infarction of these appendices and can simulate diverticulitis if they occur in the sigmoid colon, and appendicitis if they are located in the proximal colon. CT reveals a characteristic small, round, or oval fat-containing mass with associated inflammatory reaction of the pericolic fat (Fig. 5) [12].

Epiploic appendagitis is a self-limited process with clinical resolution seen within a few days. Follow-up CT examination may show total resolution in shrinkage with eventual calcification of the inflamed and infarcted epiploic appendix.

Perianal Fistulas

Perianal fistulas primarily occur as the result of fistulous disease originating in the anal glands near the anal crypts (cryptoglandular hypothesis), or in patients with Crohn's disease [13]. Infection of the anal glands may result in abscess formation. It is a relatively common condition with a prevalence of approximately 0.01%, predominantly affecting young adults.

The tracks may have a simple superficial course, or may have a complicated course. The complicated tracks may be intersphincteric (through the internal anal sphincter and then downward through the intersphincteric space), transsphincteric (transversing not only the internal sphincter but also the external sphincter or puborectis muscle), supralevator, or extrasphincteric (extension to the rectum without involvement of the anal sphincter). These complicated tracks require detailed imaging for proper therapy, as inadequate treatment may lead to recurrent disease. The surgeon must be aware of the presence and number of tracks and their extent, the location of internal opening, and presence of abscesses.

Preoperative evaluation of these fistulas may include physical examination, examination under anesthesia (EUA), EUS, or MRI. Physical examination has significant shortcomings, especially in patients with recurrent disease. EUA can be used to determinine the extent of the disease, immediately followed by treatment. However, EUA has limitations and disadvantages, mostly related to probing. Firstly, not all fistulas have an external opening that can be probed, and probing may miss secondary tracks. It is well-recognized that missed extensions are the commonest cause of recurrence, which reaches 25% in some series. Forceful probing may lead to perforation of the levator plate, worsening the extent of the disease. Patients with recurrent disease are likely to harbor missed disease, but are also most difficult to assess. Digital palpation frequently cannot distinguish between scarring due to repeated surgery and induration due to an underlying extension.

EUS, which can be enhanced by hydrogen peroxide installation in the track, may be used to determine disease extent. Initial reports were encouraging, but later studies have been less sanguine, especially when comparison is made to MRI. This discrepancy probably relates to operator expertise, since EUS is highly operator dependent. Insufficient penetration beyond the external sphincter, especially with high-frequency transducers, limits the ability to resolve ischioanal and supralevator sepsis, with the result that EUS may miss extensions from the primary tract. EUS is useful for demonstrating the internal opening. However, it is often difficult to differentiate infection from postoperative fibrosis by EUS.

MRI has been proven to provide the most comprehensive assessment of patients with perianal fistulas, facilitating accurate identification of tracks and extensions as well as abscesses. An MRI examination for perianal fistulas should include T2-weighted sequences in multiple planes, a fat-saturation sequence, and preferably a contrast-enhanced (fat-saturation) T1-weighted sequence [14].

Tracks (Fig. 6) are identified at T2 as hyperintense longitudinal structures, often with a hypointense, fibrous wall. Some collateral inflammation is often appreciated at fat saturation sequences. After intravenous contrast medium administration the lining of the wall enhances. Non-enhancing fluid can be identified in the center of the track or the track can be completely obliterated by granulation tissue. In the latter case, there is complete en-

Fig. 6. A male patient with Crohn's disease and perianal fistulas. **a** Axial T2-weighted turbo spin-echo demonstrates multiple tracks (*arrowheads*), both intersphincteric as well as outside the anal sphincter. At the right an abscess (*A*) is seen in the ischioanal space. **b** Coronal oblique T2-weighted TSE demonstrates the abscess with supralevator extension (*arrow*)

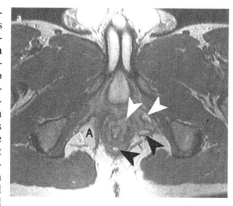

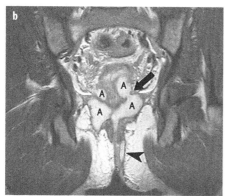

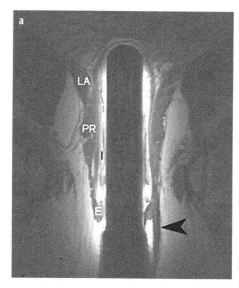

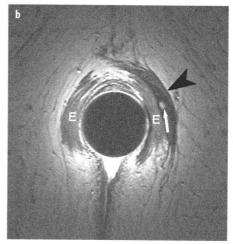

Fig. 7. a Coronal T2-weighted turbo spin-echo with endoanal coil shows a fibrous track (*arrowhead*) extending through the left external sphincter. Normal sphincter anatomy at the right side: external sphincter (*E*), internal sphincter (*I*), puborectal muscle (*PR*) as well as the levator ani plate (*LA*). **b** Axial T2-weighted turbo spin-echo demonstrates the hyperintense track (*arrow*) surrounded by fibrous tissue (*arrowhead*), along the left external sphincter (*E*)

hancement of the part of the track that is hyperintense at T2 (Fig. 7). Abscesses are readily appreciated on fat saturation sequences, although some small fluid collections can be more difficult to identify. External phased array coils are used, which may have limitations for the detection of superficial extensions and difficulty in locating the precise level on the internal opening. Endoluminal MRI may provide more information on these findings.

Results of a prospective triple-blinded comparison of the accuracy of AES, pelvic MRI, and surgical EUA in perianal Crohn's disease showed that AES correctly classified fistulas in 91% of cases, compared with 87% for pelvic MRI, and 91% for surgical evaluation [15]. Combination of any two of the three modalities increased accuracy to 100%. Another study, in which MRI and AES were compared with surgical findings, showed MRI to be superior to AES for classification of fistulas, with sensitivities of 84% versus 60% for the two modalities, and specificities of 68% and 21%, respectively.

Several studies have indicated the positive effect of preoperative MRI on patient outcome. In one study, the therapeutic effect of MRI before EUA was 21.1% [16]. Additionally, it was shown that recurrence of disease after surgery could be reduced by about 75% if surgery was guided by MRI.

The differential diagnoses of perianal fistulas primarily concern fistulas originating from skin appendages (acne conglobata, suppurative hidradenitis and pilonidal sinus). The first of these are commonly easy to recognize

clinically, but diagnosis of pilonidal sinus is more difficult. Imaging can be used to differentiate between perianal fistula and pilonidal sinus. A study in seven patients with pilonidal sinus, and in 14 sex- and age-matched individuals with perianal fistulas has demonstrated that these conditions can be discriminated, due to the fact that the former condition has an absence of intersphincteric sepsis or enteric opening. Osteomyelitis of the pelvis or femur may give rise to abscesses and tracks that extend to the anorectal region, while osteomyelitis is a rare finding in perianal fistulas due to Crohn's disease. Differentiating these two conditions is usually not difficult, as the predominant disease localization (either extensive bone marrow edema or extensive tracks with intersphincteric extension and internal opening) establishes the diagnosis.

Neoplastic Diseases

Colorectal cancer is a common disease and is one of the leading causes of cancer-related death in many Western countries. Imaging plays an important role in the detection of colorectal cancer and of their precursor polyps, and in staging of rectal cancer.

The vast majority of colorectal cancers are adenocarcinoma and there is a well-established adenoma-carcinoma sequence. Cancer can present as a mass that may cause lumen obstruction. Some cancers may have a carpet-like presentation. Polyps are mostly sessile, but may be pedunculated or flat. Currently, it is not fully established whether flat adenomas are more aggressive.

Other malignancies of the colon and rectum are rare, and include soft tissue cancers, gastrointestinal stromal tumors and extension of tumor from adjacent organs and peritoneal metastases. The differentiation between diverticulitis and cancer may be difficult, particularly in the sigmoid colon. The presence of fluid in the root of the sigmoid mesentery, engorgement of adjacent sigmoid mesenteric vasculature and a tethered or sawtooth luminal configuration favors the diagnosis of diverticulitis. Conversely, the presence of enlarged pericolic lymph nodes, mural thickness greater than 1.5 cm, and an abrupt transition zone raises the possibility of colon cancer. Ischemic colitis may also lead to bowel wall thickening, but the clinical history (e.g. extensive atherosclerosis) and imaging findings (no enlarged lymph nodes, more gradual transition) help to differentiate. At the rectosigmoid, endometriosis may simulate colorectal cancer, but the location (often anterior, adjacent to the pouch of Douglas or rectovaginal septum) and morphology help to differentiate between these two conditions. At MRI endometriosis has typical findings: fibrosis with small hyperintense foci on T1-weighted sequences representing blood, or cystic masses that are often hyperintense on T1-weighted sequences and intermediate signal intensity on T2-weighted sequences (so-called shading) due to the presence of blood in a cyst.

Colorectal Cancer: CT Colonography (Virtual Colonoscopy)

CTC is used for the detection of polyps and colorectal cancer in symptomatic patients, patients with failed colonoscopy (pain, sharp bowel curvatures or bowel stenosis) and in screening. CT of the air- or carbon dioxide-distended colon is performed in supine and prone positions, as some bowel segments may be collapsed in one position. This dual positioning also assists movement of residual fluid and stool that may obscure the bowel surface. The use of oral iodine contrast media (e.g. Gastrografin) has facilitated identification of submerged lesions as well as tagging of residual stool. The use of intravenous contrast medium has no clear advantage for polyp detection and may even be counterproductive with the use of oral fluid tagging.

The main purpose of CTC is to detect clinically significant lesions such as colorectal carcinomas and large adenomatous polyps, which are its precursors. As adenomatous and nonadenomatous lesions cannot be discriminated with CTC, the primary focus of most studies is polyps ≥ 10 mm, as the likelihood of adenomas and malignancy is size-related. Although the primary interest is in polyps ≥ 10 mm, polyps ranging in size from 5-9 mm are also considered relevant.

In symptomatic populations CTC is an accurate technique with a detection sensitivity for colorectal cancer of 95.9% and a specificity of > 99% [17]. For patients with polyps ≥ 10 mm, sensitivity is 85-92.5% and specificity 95-97.4%, while for patients with polyps ≥ 6 mm, sensitivity is 70-86.4% and specificity 86.1-93% [17, 18]. Intravenous contrast medium can be used for the detection of lymphadenopathy and liver metastases in symptomatic patients in one position.

In colorectal cancer, extension outside the colon, such as infiltration of pericolic fat and loss of fat planes between the colon and adjacent organs, can be readily evaluated. Pathways of lymph node metastases can be predicted based on the site of the primary tumor. Complications of primary colonic malignancies, such as obstruction, perforation, and fistula can be visualized with CT.

The liver, the primary site for distant metastases, needs to be examined for the presence of colorectal liver metastases. CT and MRI are the principal diagnostic techniques for detection of liver metastases, with an increasing role of fluorine-18-fluorodeoxyglucose (FDG) positron emission tomography (PET). FDG PET has significantly higher sensitivity on a per-patient basis, compared with that of CT and MRI, but not on a per-lesion basis [19]. Sensitivity estimates for enhanced MR imaging (superparamagnetic iron oxide [SPIO] or gadolinium) are significantly superior to those for helical CT with 45 g of iodine or less.

Data on CTC in surveillance/screening of populations are still limited. The sensitivity in patients with polyps ≥ 10 mm varies considerably (55-94%), while specificity is high (92-96%) [20]. The studies differ considerably in methodology, including prior reading experience, review methods (two-dimensional [2D] or three-dimensional [3D]), bowel preparation and reference standards. All these factors may have contributed to the differences seen.

CTC examinations have traditionally been performed after extensive bowel cleansing, a major deterrent for full structural colon examinations. Several studies have demonstrated the feasibility of CTC after limited bowel preparation. A low-fiber diet and the use of oral contrast medium has been shown to be sufficient for good CTC results for the detection of colorectal cancer and polyps.

Pitfalls include untagged stool (inhomogeneous, moves in position), complex folds (3D is helpful), extrinsic compression (2D is helpful), ileocecal valve (combined 2D and 3D evaluation), while flat lesions can be difficult to detect. Evaluation of the sigmoid can be difficult in patients with extensive diverticulosis and muscular hypertrophy. Collapsed bowel segments should be scrutinized in the other position. It is important to report the quality of the examination (distension, tagging) and whether a colonoscopy is indicated.

For screening purposes, radiation exposure is a drawback of CT. MRI can be used as an alternative to CT, although this is less common. MR-colonography can be performed after limited bowel preparation, however the optimal MR protocol has not been determined.

Rectal Cancer: Diagnostic Work-up

Adenocarcinoma is the most common rectal malignancy. The diagnosis is usually histologically established prior to imaging. Cross-sectional imaging is used to stage the tumor. The treatment of rectal cancer depends on the extent of disease and has changed substantially over the last decade. EUS and MRI are important in the management of these patients. T2-weighted sequences are pivotal in MRI of rectal cancer. These provide optimal contrast between the rectal wall and surrounding fat and organs. T1-weighted sequences after intravenous contrast medium administration do not provide much additional information. No bowel preparation is necessary.

Rectal tumors are identified as lesions with intermediate signal intensity, while stool often has an inhomogeneous low signal intensity at T2-weighted sequences. Tumors present as a mass, but may also have a more superficial extent. Mucinous tumors have a high signal intensity.

Tumor limited to (sub)mucosa (T1 disease) is often treated by transanal endoscopic microsurgery. EUS is preferable for local staging of these tumors. The higher spatial resolution of EUS as compared to MRI results in a more detailed demonstration of the rectal wall layers. EUS depicts five interfaces, while MRI shows a maximum of two interfaces. This leads to a significantly higher ($p = 0.02$) specificity of EUS (86%) as compared to MR imaging (69%), indicating overstaging of T1 (or lower) tumors with MR imaging [21]. Endoluminal US and MR imaging have similar sensitivity estimates of 94% for these tumors.

The tumor often invades deeper than the (sub)mucosa and may extend into the lamina propria (T2), beyond the muscularis propria (T3) (Fig. 8) or even involve surrounding structures (T4). For muscularis propria invasion, EUS and MR imaging have similar sensitivities; specificity of EUS (86%) is significantly higher than that of MR imaging (69%) [21]. For perirectal tissue invasion, sensitivity of EUS (90%) is significantly higher than that of CT (79%) and MR imaging (82%); specificities are comparable (75%, 78%, and 76%). For adjacent organ invasion and lymph node involvement (Fig. 9), estimates for EUS, CT, and MR imaging are comparable (70%, 72%, 74%, respectively). Specificity estimates are also comparable (97%, 96%, 96%). Stenotic tumors may hamper endosonography.

The importance of T-staging has decreased with the widespread use of total mesorectal excision (TME). In this procedure, the rectal cancer and the surrounding envelope of mesorectal fat bordered by the mesorectal fascia is removed *en bloc*. This operation has been shown to

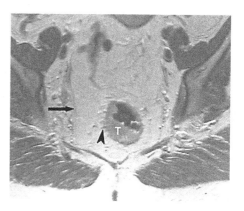

Fig. 8. Coronal oblique T2-weighted turbo spin-echo of a rectal tumor (*T*) extending through the rectal wall into the mesorectal fat. A spiculated margin (*arrowhead*) is seen, where imaging cannot differentiate between desmoplastic tumor reaction without or with tumor. There is several centimeters distance between the tumor margin (including spiculations) and the mesorectal fascia (*arrow*) and therefore total mesorectal excision is possible. There are not any enlarged lymph nodes

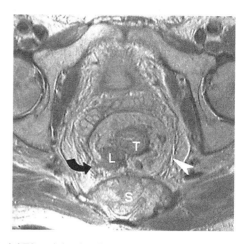

Fig. 9. Axial T2-weighted turbo spin-echo of a rectal tumor (*T*) with multiple mesorectal lymph nodes. In general, imaging is not an accurate technique for differentiating between malignant and benign lymph nodes. However, in this patient one lymph node (*L*) extends through the mesorectal fascia (*curved arrow*) and one presacral lymph node (*S*) has invaded the sacrum, indicating malignancy loaded lymph nodes. Normal mesorectal fascia at the left (*arrowhead*)

reduce significantly tumor recurrence rate. For this treatment, determining the distance between tumor and mesorectal fascia (circumferential resection margin; CRM) has become crucial. TME was introduced due to the high initial local tumor recurrence (approximately 28%). With TME the recurrence rate has decreased to 10-15%. In Europe, mobile rectal cancers are treated with preoperative radiotherapy before TME and this has led to a further decrease of recurrence, especially for cancers in the mid-rectum (3.9% vs 14.9%; $p = < 0.001$).

MRI can accurately determine the distance between tumor and mesorectal fascia and differentiate between patients with a wide circumferential resection margin, close margin and involved margin, with accuracy rates of 92-100% and high reproducibility (Fig. 8 and 9) [22, 23]. Low rectal cancers and anterior cancers are more difficult to assess than other rectal cancers, as the mesorectal fascia is less readily identified.

Detection of nodal disease is important since it is a predictor for distant metastases and local recurrence. In rectal cancer, lymph drainage is upward along the superior rectal vessels to the inferior mesenteric vessels, while the lower rectum drains along the middle rectal vessels to the internal iliac vessels. In patients treated with TME, perirectal nodes are removed, but lateral nodes may lead to recurrent disease. Lateral lymphatic spread is more prevalent in low rectal cancer. To reduce the local recurrence rate, radiotherapy and dissection of the lateral nodes is used, although there has been little interest shown in the latter treatment. Nevertheless, improved preoperative identification of lymphatic spread is a major step forward in the treatment of rectal cancer.

The accuracy of MRI, EUS, and CT with respect to lymph node staging is disappointing. The size criterion used to differentiate between benign and malignant nodes has serious limitations [24]. In a systematic review, sensitivity estimates for EUS, CT, and MR imaging were comparably low: 67%, 55%, and 66%, respectively [19]. Specificity values were also comparable: 78% for EUS, 74% for CT, and 76% for MR imaging. Improved lymph node criteria, such as presence of a spiculated border, indistinct border and mottled heterogenic pattern strongly correlate with tumor invasion ($p < 0.001$), but still have limitations [25]. The use of ultra small iron oxide particles (USPIO) has shown promising results in differentiating normal sized nodes that contain tumors [26].

References

1. Schreyer AG, Seitz J, Feuerbach S et al (2004) Modern imaging using computer tomography and magnetic resonance imaging for inflammatory bowel disease (IBD). Inflamm Bowel Dis 10:45-54
2. Markose G, Ng CS, Freeman AH (2003) The impact of helical computed tomography on the diagnosis of unsuspected inflammatory bowel disease in the large bowel. Eur Radiol 13:107-113
3. Furukawa A, Saotome T, Yamasaki M et al (2004) Cross-sectional imaging in Crohn disease. Radiographics 24:689-702
4. Horton KM, Corl FM, Fishman EK (2000) CT evaluation of the colon: inflammatory disease. Radiographics 20:399-418
5. Turner DR, Markose G, Arends MJ et al (2003) Unusual causes of colonic wall thickening on computed tomography. Clin Radiol 58:191-200
6. Gluecker TM, Williamson EE, Fletcher JG et al (2003) Diseases of the cecum: a CT pictorial review. Eur Radiol 13(Suppl 4):L51-L61
7. Kirkpatrick ID, Greenberg HM (2003) Gastrointestinal complications in the neutropenic patient: characterization and differentiation with abdominal CT. Radiology 226:668-674
8. Pinto Leite N, Pereira JM, Cunha R et al (2005) CT evaluation of appendicitis and its complications: imaging techniques and key diagnostic findings. AJR Am J Roentgenol 185:406-417
9. Daly CP, Cohan RH, Francis IR et al (2005) Incidence of acute appendicitis in patients with equivocal CT findings. AJR Am J Roentgenol 184:1813-1820
10. Paulson EK, Harris JP, Jaffe TA et al (2005) Acute appendicitis: added diagnostic value of coronal reformations from isotropic voxels at multi-detector row CT. Radiology 235:879-885
11. Kircher MF, Rhea JT, Kihiczak D, Novelline RA (2002) Frequency, sensitivity, and specificity of individual signs of diverticulitis on thin-section helical CT with colonic contrast material: experience with 312 cases. AJR Am J Roentgenol 178:1313-1318
12. Singh AK, Gervais DA, Hahn PF et al (2005) Acute epiploic appendagitis and its mimics. Radiographics 25:1521-1534
13. Halligan S, Stoker J (2006) Imaging fistula-in-ano. Radiology (in press)
14. Horsthuis K, Stoker J (2004) MRI of perianal Crohn's disease. AJR Am J Roentgenol 183:1309-1315
15. Schwartz DA, Wiersema MJ, Dudiak KM et al (2001) A comparison of endoscopic ultrasound, magnetic resonance imaging, and exam under anesthesia for evaluation of Crohn's perianal fistulas. Gastroenterology 121:1064-1072
16. Buchanan G, Halligan S, Williams A et al (2002) Effect of MRI on clinical outcome of recurrent fistula-in-ano. Lancet 360:1661-1662
17. Halligan S, Altman DG, Taylor SA et al (2005) CT colonography in the detection of colorectal polyps and cancer: systematic review, meta-analysis, and proposed minimum data set for study level reporting. Radiology 237:893-904
18. Mulhall BP, Veerappan GR, Jackson JL (2005) Meta-analysis: computed tomographic colonography. Ann Intern Med 142:635-650
19. Bipat S, van Leeuwen MS, Comans EF et al (2005) Colorectal liver metastases: CT, MR imaging, and PET for diagnosis-meta-analysis. Radiology 237:123-131
20. Pickhardt PJ, Choi JR, Hwang I et al (2003) Computed tomographic virtual colonoscopy to screen for colorectal neoplasia in asymptomatic adults. N Engl J Med 349:2191-2200
21. Bipat S, Glas AS, Slors FJ et al (2004) Rectal cancer: local staging and assessment of lymph node involvement with endoluminal US, CT, and MR imaging. A meta-analysis. Radiology 232:773-783
22. Beets-Tan RG, Beets GL, Vliegen RF et al (2001) Accuracy of magnetic resonance imaging in prediction of tumour-free resection margin in rectal cancer surgery. Lancet 357:497-504
23. Brown G, Radcliffe AG, Newcombe RG et al (2003) Preoperative assessment of prognostic factors in rectal cancer using high-resolution magnetic resonance imaging. Br J Surg 90:355-364
24. Brown G, Richards CJ, Bourne MW et al (2003) Morphologic predictors of lymph node status in rectal cancer with use of high-spatial-resolution MR imaging with histopathologic comparison. Radiology 227:371-377
25. Kim JH, Beets GL, Kim MJ et al (2004) High resolution MR imaging for nodal staging in rectal cancer: are there criteria in addition to the size? Eur J Radiol 52:78-83
26. Koh DM, Brown G, Temple L et al (2004) Rectal cancer: mesorectal lymph nodes at MR imaging with USPIO versus histopathologic findings. Initial observations. Radiology 231:91-99

CT Colonography

M. Macari[1], C.D. Johnson[2]

[1] Department of Radiology, NYU School of Medicine, New York, NY, USA
[2] Department of Radiology, Mayo Clinic, Rochester, MN, USA

Introduction

Computed tomography colonography (CTC, also known as virtual colonoscopy) has been used for over a decade to investigate the colon for colorectal neoplasia. Numerous clinical and technical advances have allowed CTC to advance from a research tool to a viable option for colorectal cancer screening. Slowly the clinical community is beginning to realize its promise. However, controversy remains among radiologists, gastroenterologists, and other clinicians, regarding its utilization in clinical practice.

On the one hand there is tremendous excitement about a noninvasive imaging examination that can reliably detect clinically significant colorectal lesions. However, this is tempered by several recent studies that show the sensitivity of CTC may not be as great when performed and interpreted by radiologists without expertise and training. The potential to miss significant lesions exists even among experts, and moreover, if polyps are unable to be differentiated from folds and residual fecal matter, it will result in unnecessary colonoscopies.

A recent meta-analysis of published CTC studies has determined that several factors may be important for increasing the sensitivity of CTC. These include the use of a multi-detector CT (MDCT) scanner, the use of thin CT sections, and possibly the utilization of a three dimensional (3D) fly-through data interpretation technique [1].

Currently, there are not enough trained endoscopists to screen the U.S. population at average risk for colorectal cancer. There are certainly not enough trained radiologists to make a substantial impact on colon caner screening with CTC. Radiologists need to understand the issues related to colon cancer screening, how CTC may impact on colon cancer evaluation, and importantly, learn the techniques of patient preparation, data acquisition, and data interpretation. If radiologists do not embrace CTC, ultimately gastroenterologists will.

The Problem: Colon Cancer

Colon cancer is the second leading cause of cancer death in the United States, and it accounts for approximately 10% of all cancer deaths in both men and women combined [2, 3]. 150,000 new cases and 50,000 deaths result from colon cancer every year in the United States [2]. This translates into 137 deaths per day or six deaths per hour. This is unfortunate, since most cases of colon cancer are preventable if detected as precancerous adenomas. It is estimated that up to 80-90% of all cases of colon cancer develop from small adenomas that undergo mutations and slowly advance over time [4].

However, it should be noted that most adenomas do not progress to colon cancer, and the vast majority of diminutive lesions ($\leq$ 5 mm) in the colon are non-adenomas [5, 6]. This has led to debate in the medical community about the size at which a colon lesion should be considered clinically important [7]. Most gastroenterologists feel that the small lesions are probably not important if routine screening is performed. Larger lesions (those over 5 mm) should be removed unless there are contraindications to endoscopy and polypectomy, or if the patient is of an advanced age. Unfortunately, some colon cancers develop very rapidly and would not be detected even with the current screening techniques.

A number of screening options are available for the detection of precursor adenomas in the colon. These include fecal occult blood test (FOBT), sigmoidoscopy, double contrast barium enema (DCBE), and colonoscopy [2, 8]. Both FOBT and sigmoidoscopy have been shown to decrease the morbidity and mortality of colon cancer [9, 10]. However, there is a growing consensus that a full structural examination of the colon is warranted in order to optimize colon cancer screening. This can be performed by DCBE, colonoscopy, or CTC.

Complete colonoscopy allows the most thorough evaluation of the colon with the added benefit of the possibility of biopsy or excision of suspicious lesions. Colonoscopy is considered the reference standard for colonic evaluation [2]. However, there are several important limitations to the widespread use of screening colonoscopy, including need for sedation, the potential risk of perforation and bleeding (0.1-0.3%), costs of the procedure including the need for sedation, failure to complete the examination in 5-10% of patients, and an insufficient workforce of trained endoscopists to meet increased demand. Moreover, in an optimized study, the sensitivity of CTC was superior to colonoscopy for detecting adenomas over 10 mm [6]. Other studies have also shown that CTC can detect larger lesions that were missed at colonoscopy [5]. For these reasons, CTC is being further investigated and is being used clinically to evaluate the colon for polyps and cancers.

CTC Technique

The technical aspects of CTC continue to evolve. What is essential is that the colon needs to be cleansed, distended, and scanned with a low dose technique in both the supine and prone positions.

Bowel Preparation

There are several techniques that may be used for bowel preparation, and there remains controversy as to how to optimize patient preparation. The goal is to have a well-prepared, well-distended colon that will facilitate polyp detection and minimize false positive findings. A clean, well-distended colon facilitates detection of colorectal abnormalities whether two dimensional (2D) or 3D techniques are used for data interpretation. More importantly, it often maximizes our ability to differentiate polyps, folds, and residual fecal matter within the colon.

There are three commercially available bowel preparations in the U.S, which include cathartics such as magnesium citrate and phospho-soda, and colonic lavage solutions such as polyethylene glycol. In our experience, the polyethylene glycol preparation frequently leaves a large amount of residual fluid in the colon. While this preparation is adequate for colonoscopy, large amounts of residual fluid will limit the effectiveness of CTC. With conventional colonoscopy, residual fluid can be endoscopically aspirated from the colon. With CTC, the examination is typically limited to only two acquisitions, supine and prone. While supine and prone imaging allows for fluid redistribution, this does not ensure full mucosal evaluation if large amounts of fluid are present. Regarding bowel preparation, polyethylene glycol should be utilized in all patients with substantial cardiac or renal insufficiencies. The polyethylene-glycol preparation results in no fluid shifts and no electrolyte imbalances. Therefore, it is safe to use in these patients.

Some investigators have found that the use of intravenous (IV) contrast material may facilitate colorectal polyp detection when large amounts of fluid are present. Occasionally polyps are obscured by residual fluid. After IV contrast administration, a polyp will enhance, and it may become visible despite being submerged in the fluid. The downsides of the routine administration of contrast are the costs, the need for IV access, and the risk of allergy from the iodinated contrast material.

Given the limitations of bowel preparation, including poor patient compliance and reluctance, as well as residual fecal material that can make interpretation difficult, the possibility of fecal and fluid tagging for CTC is being investigated. Fecal tagging is obtained by having the patient ingest small amounts of barium or iodine with their meals prior to imaging. The high attenuation contrast material will be incorporated within residual fecal matter, facilitating differentiation from polyps. Some researchers have advocated fecal tagging, since tagged fecal matter should allow the improved differentiation of residual stool from colorectal polyps.

Colonic Distension

After colonic preparation, the examination is ready to be performed. Colonic distension should be performed entirely by a trained technologist or a nurse. A radiologist does not need to be present for high quality data acquisition to proceed. An experienced technologist or nurse is required, thus minimizing radiologist time needed for data acquisition.

Immediately prior to data acquisition, the patient should evacuate any residual fluid from the rectum. Therefore, easy access to a nearby bathroom is essential. For colonic insufflation, either room air or carbon dioxide (CO_2) can be used. Room air is easy, clean, and inexpensive to use. Proponents of CO_2 argue that because it is readily absorbed from the colon it causes less cramping following the procedure than room air insufflation. While initial discomfort is usually present with either CO_2 or room air, delayed cramping appears to be a lesser problem with CO_2.

The use of a bowel relaxant is controversial. Previous data have shown minimal benefit to the routine use of IV or intramuscular (IM) glucagon. We do not routinely use a bowel relaxant. This minimizes cost and patient anxiety since it does not necessitate the use of needles. Excellent results have been achieved distending the colon without the use of a bowel relaxant. A report from England showed that hyoscine butylbromide improved colonic insufflation and suggested that it should be routinely administered when available [11]. However, this product has not been approved by the FDA and is not available for use in the United States.

Data Acquisition

Over the past decade, there have been three important advances in CTC data acquisition, including reduction in radiation exposure, improved CT slice profile, and shorter acquisition times. These advances have been facilitated by the development and installation of multi-detector row CT scanners. The scanners allow four to 64 slices to be obtained in a single rotation of the X-ray tube. Moreover, gantry rotation times have decreased so that now most CT scanners allow tube rotation in 0.5 seconds or less. Multidetector row CT scanners allow large volumes of near isotropic data to be acquired in a single breath-hold.

Utilizing a 16 slice multidetector row CT scanner with 0.75 mm thick collimation and a pitch of 1.5, the same Z-axis coverage can be obtained in 15-20 seconds. Data can be reconstructed as 1 mm thick sections overlapped every 0.75 mm. Using a 64-row multidetector CT scanner, acquisition times are routinely less than 10 seconds.

The optimal slice profile for CTC has not been determined, but it is likely that data acquired with thin sections, approximately 1 mm, will improve sensitivity for small polyps and specificity. Using a four-row scanner, a 1-1.25 mm detector configuration is recommended. Others have advocated a 4×2.5 mm detector configuration [12]. There are two benefits of the 2.5 mm detector configuration. First, the mAs can be lowered and there is an inherent decrease in radiation exposure at 2.5 mm, when compared to 1 mm collimation on a four-row detector system. In addition, there are fewer images that need to be acquired.

Radiation Dose

When considering an imaging examination that utilizes ionizing radiation for screening, exposure is a serious concern. Radiation dose can be decreased at CT by increasing pitch and slice collimation or by decreasing the kVp or mAs. Absorbed dose and mAs values are directly proportional. Since there is extremely high tissue contrast between insufflated gas and the colonic wall, substantial reductions in mAs can be obtained without sacrificing polyp detection. The increased noise resulting from acquisitions acquired with low mAs techniques does not appear to affect polyp detection. In 2002, a study comparing CTC to colonoscopy in 105 patients showed that the sensitivity of CTC in detecting 10 mm polyps was less than 90% using an effective mAs value of 50 [13]. The resultant effective dose for the patient in both supine and prone imaging was 5.0 mSv for men and 7.8 mSv for women. The effective dose utilizing this technique is similar to the dose reported for a DCBE. Since that publication, several studies have shown that mAs values can be decreased even further [12].

Data Interpretation

Once the colon has been cleaned, distended and scanned, the data need to be interpreted. There are two primary techniques for data interpretation: a primary 2D or a 3D approach. In either case, the alternative viewing technique needs to be available for problem solving and to aid in differentiating folds, fecal matter, and polyps. Moreover, the interpreter needs to be familiar with a given workstation in order to optimize data interpretation.

Performance

Four large recently published studies have shown that there continues to be variability in the reported sensitivity of CTC in detecting clinically significant colorectal polyps [6, 14-16]. Moreover, as stated earlier, a meta-analysis of published studies suggests that slice collimation and a primary 3D technique may be important variables for sensitivity improvement (Table 1). Reader experience is also a factor, but cannot account for all the variability [15]. We need to continue to study the reasons for the variability in CTC sensitivity. In the future, as computer-aided detection (CAD) improves, this may lead to an improvement in overall sensitivity.

Indications for CTC

The indications for CTC continue to grow [17]. Indications with scientific validation include incomplete colonoscopy and evaluating the proximal colon in patients with colonic obstruction. Other indications that have received acceptance from the medical community include patients who require a colon examination and cannot have colonoscopy safely. These patient groups include patients on anticoagulants and with a prior adverse event related to sedation. Data from the Pickhardt study [6] supports a screening indication for CTC, but this remains controversial. The use of CTC in symptomatic patients is also controversial, as many experts would recommend colonoscopy in these patients. As most colon neoplasms are not associated with symptoms, it seems reasonable to select symptoms as indications for a CTC examination (anemia, change in bowel habits, abdominal pain).

CTC is not appropriate in certain situations. There is no clear data that CTC can successfully image patients with inflammatory bowel disease. Further, patients with acute gastrointestinal blood loss (most commonly due to angiodysplasia and diverticular bleeding) are better imaged by colonoscopy. Patients with suspected diverticulitis are well-served with a CT examination, but do not require the laxative preparation or colonic insufflation required with CTC.

Table 1. Summary, CTC sensitivity

Author	# of Pts	Sens < 6	6-9 mm	> 9 mm
Rockey (2005)	614	–	60	64
Cotton (2004)	600	7.6	22.7	51.9
Macari (2004)	186	14.7	46.2	90.9
Van Gelder (2004)	249	40.6	76.7	77.8
Iannaccone (2004)	203	87.1		100
Pickhardt (2003)	1233		83.6	92.2
Iannaccone (2003)	158	51.4	83.3	100
Johnson (2003)	703		47.1	46.3
Yee (2001)	300	66.9	81.8	92.7
Hara (1997)		25.9	57.1	70

Pitfalls

Errors at CTC can be due to a multitude of factors. The most common causes of error are related to technique, experience/training, and lack of recognition of uncommon but important presentations of polyps. Technical inaccuracies are probably the most important cause of error, especially for larger lesions (1 cm or larger in diameter) [18]. Every technical step must be carefully followed in order to achieve a high-quality and accurate examination. The commonest problems are suboptimal distention and inadequate preparation of the colon. Distention can be reliably achieved with the use of a mechanical insufflator, and a warning to and acceptance by patients of a brief episode of discomfort during image acquisition. The use of the spasmolytic butyl scopolamine has also been shown to be effective in improving distention. In patients with a colon segment that is poorly distended in both the prone and supine position, a decubitus view (usually right lateral decubitus) can be very helpful [19]. Inadequate preparation of the colon can be minimized by providing easily understood instructions, and if possible an educational encounter with the patient is recommended to ensure understanding about the timing and amounts of the various required preparatory agents.

Experience and training are the keys to high-quality interpretations [20]. Spinzi et al. has shown that interpreting at least 75 examinations is required for competent interpretation [21]. Our experience has shown that most individuals are not adequately trained after a weekend course of lectures, including a 40-50 case hands-on experience. In testing readers for the National CT Colonography Trial (ACRIN 6664), only one third of readers were deemed expert at the end of a weekend course. Most readers were able to perform at 60%-80% sensitivity for large lesions after this amount of training. Expertise requires additional experience, and review of positive cases with emphasis on detecting the most difficult lesions.

Familiarity with the appearance of the most difficult lesions [22], especially flat adenomas, is important in order to achieve the highest performance rating [23, 24]. The most common errors that the novice reader makes are misinterpreting a cancer as a segmental region of collapse. In addition, reporting polyps less than 5 mm in diameter is associated with an unacceptably high false positive rate. We encourage our staff not to report these biologically unimportant bumps of less than 5 mm. The expert reader most commonly makes mistakes by not recognizing a lesion that is seen in only a single position (either prone or supine). Experts also tend to discount lesions as stool in segments of the colon with suboptimal preparation. Both expert and novice readers find flat lesions difficult to detect. Lesions that have an irregular surface are also often falsely considered as stool. Recognition that some adenomas, especially villous adenomas, have an irregular surface is important.

Tagging of stool should prevent many of these types of errors in the future. Tagging, however, can induce other errors. Tagging that is too dense can cause streak artifacts. In addition, barium tagging agents can adhere to the wall of the colon and even cover polyps. It is important to carefully inspect the wall beneath the barium (whether in pools or as a circumferential coating). In many instances a bone window setting is helpful to assess the colon wall adjacent to high attenuation contrast material. Pedunculated polyps can move within the colon lumen and resemble moving stool at first glance. It is important to search for the fixed attachment of the pedunculated polyp stalk to the colon wall.

Large lesions, especially those within the right and transverse colon, can cause the colon to rotate as the patient is turned from supine to prone position [25]. The sheer weight of the lesion and a loose colon mesentery probably account for this occurrence. Therefore, if a large lesion is seen in the dependent location of the colon on both the supine and prone views, the filling defect is not necessarily stool. First, a search should ensue to confirm that the colon has rotated. This is straightforward in the right colon, as the ileocecal valve can be easily identified, and its position confirmed on both views. In other parts of the colon this can be difficult. Second, the cleanliness of the colon should be assessed. A filling defect in an otherwise clean colon should be regarded as a real lesion. Finally, if necessary, intravenous contrast material can be administered [26]. All polyps 5 mm or larger will enhance at least two-fold following intravenous contrast material. Untagged stool does not enhance. This can be very helpful in selected patients with a confusing filling defect. Intravenous contrast material can also be helpful in patients with a large amount of residual colonic fluid that cannot be moved between imaging positions if the patient did not receive a tagging agent. If stool and fluid tagging is utilized, IV contrast material could actually obscure a lesion.

The Unprepared Colon

Nearly all of the work on CTC to date has revolved around the laxative-prepared colon. As the promise of this technique is being realized, it is possible that compliance with colorectal screening guidelines will not improve appreciably even if CTC becomes widely accepted and available. The single biggest obstacle to guideline compliance is the inconvenience and discomfort associated with laxative purgation. If the laxatives could be excluded from the preparation, this would most likely result in improved compliance. Preliminary work in this field is encouraging. The basis for a laxative-free examination is the ability to adequately tag the stool in the colon. Theoretically, if the attenuation of the stool is changed significantly from soft tissue, a computer could electronically remove the tagged stool, leaving a dataset similar to the cathartic-cleansed colon. Ideally, this would be done without dietary modification or disruption of lifestyle. Callstrom and colleagues [27] demonstrated that stool can be adequately tagged without dietary modification using barium liquid in divided doses (administered at meals and at bedtime) over 48 hours. Other investigators have confirmed these findings with some modifications. Lefere [28] has worked on dietary restrictions using a low fiber diet combined with barium to create low volume well-tagged stool. In these cases, the colon can be examined without electronic cleansing. Zalis [29] has utilized iodinated contrast material to create uniform stool labeling and effective stool subtraction. Iannaccone [30] demonstrated that large doses of oral iodinated contrast material without subtraction can result in polyp detection similar to the cleansed colon. One issue that needs to be better understood is the common association of diarrhea with iodinated contrast material and its effect on patient compliance for colorectal screening. Clearly, the feasibility of examining the non-cathartic prepared colon has been proven. Once the technical issues are agreed upon, a new wave of CTC will occur with the promise of a full structural examination without the burden of the laxative preparation.

Quality Improvement

Radiologists must take an active role in monitoring and improving their individual practice. Regular assessment of the adequacy of patient preparation, distention and tagging should be performed. Further, a log of all cases that are referred to colonoscopy should be performed to assess true and false positives. A simple quality assessment form to be completed after each examination and collated by an assistant can be easily implemented without disruption of clinical workflow. Regular review of all data should be required. Sharing of problems and insights among colleagues can lead to improvements throughout the practice.

In summary, CTC is an exciting technique for the detection of colorectal neoplasia. Careful attention to the technical requirements of the examination (patient preparation, insufflation, data acquisition, reader training and interpretation methodology) is required for a high-quality examination. Performance data indicates that CTC has the potential to detect colorectal polyps with the same sensitivity and specificity as colonoscopy. The indications for the examination are growing, but patients with inflammatory bowel disease and active gastrointestinal hemorrhage should be examined with colonoscopy. Common pitfalls include the lack of attention to the technical aspects of the exam, adequate training and experience, and familiarity with the appearance of flat adenomas. CTC without laxative purgation will likely occur rapidly after the technical requirements of this examination are confirmed. Radiologists must commit themselves to a vigilant CTC quality assessment program to maintain high standards of care.

References

1. Mullhall BP, Veerappan GR, Jackson JL (2005) Meta-analysis: computed tomographic colonography. Am Intern Med 142:635-650
2. Ransohoff DF, Sandler RS (2002) Clinical practice: screening for colorectal cancer. NEJM 346:40-44
3. Jemal A, Tiwari RC, Murray T et al (2004) Cancer statistics 2004. CA Cancer J Clin 54:8-29
4. Muto T, Bussey HJR, Morson BC (1975) The evolution of cancer of the colon and rectum. Cancer 36:2251-2270
5. Macari M, Bini EJ, Jacobs SL et al (2004) Significance of missed polyps at CT colonography. AJR Am J Roentgenol 183:127-134
6. Pickhardt PJ, Choi JR, Hwang I et al (2003) Computed tomographic virtual colonoscopy to screen for colorectal neoplasia in asymptomatic adults. NEJM 349:2191-2200
7. Zalis ME, Barish MA, Choi JR et al (2005) CT colonography reporting and data system: a consensus proposal. Radiology 236:3-9 (review)
8. Podolsky DK (2000) Going the distance - the case for true colorectal-cancer screening. NEJM 343:207-208
9. Mandel JS, Bond JH, Church TR et al (1993) Reducing mortality from colorectal cancer by screening for fecal occult blood. NEJM 328:1365-1371
10. Selby JV, Friedman GD, Quesenberry PC, Weiss NS (1992) A case control study of screening sigmoidoscopy and mortality from colorectal cancer. NEJM 326:653-657
11. Taylor SA, Halligan S, Goh V et al (2003) Optimizing colonic distention for multi-detector row CT colonography: effect of hyoscine butylbromide and rectal balloon catheter. Radiology 229:99-108
12. Iannaccone R, Laghi A, Catalano C et al (2003) Detection of colorectal lesions: lower-dose multi-detector row helical CT colonography compared with conventional colonoscopy. Radiology 229:775-781
13. Macari M, Bini EJ, Xue X et al (2002) Colorectal neoplasms: prospective comparison of thin-section low-dose multi-detector row CT colonography and conventional colonoscopy for detection. Radiology 224:383-392
14. Cotton PB, Durkalski VL, Pineau BC et al (2004) Computed tomographic colonography (virtual colonoscopy): a multicenter comparison with standard colonoscopy for detection of colorectal neoplasia. JAMA 291:1713-1719
15. Johnson CD, Harmsen WS, Wilson LA et al (2003) Prospective blinded evaluation of computed tomographic colonography for screen detection of colorectal polyps. Gastroenterology 125:311-319
16. Rockey DC, Paulson E, Niedzwiecki D et al (2005) Analysis of air contrast barium enema, computed tomographic colonography, and colonoscopy: prospective comparison. Lancet 365:305-311
17. Fletcher JG, Booya F, Johnson CD, Ahlquist DA (2005) CT colonography: unraveling the twists and turns. Curr Opin Gastroenterol 21:90-98
18. Gluecker T, Fletcher JG, Welch TJ et al (2004) Characterization of lesions missed on interpretation of CT colonography using 2D search method. AJR Am J Roentgenol 182:881-889
19. Rogalla P, Lembcke A, Ruckert JC et al (2005) Spasmolysis at CT colonography: butyl scopolamine versus glucagon. Radiology 236:184-188
20. Taylor SA, Halligan S, Burling D et al (2004) CT colonography: effect of experience and training on reader performance. Eur Radiol 14:1025-1033
21. Spinzi G, Belloni G, Martegani A et al (2001) Computed tomographic colonography and conventional colonoscopy for colon diseases: a prospective, blinded study. Am J Gastroenterology 96:394-400
22. Pickhardt PJ (2004) Differential diagnosis of polypoid lesions seen at CT colonography (virtual colonoscopy). Radiographics 24:1535-1559

23. Fidler JL, Johnson CD, MacCarty RL et al (2002) Detection of flat lesions in the colon with CT colonography. Abdom Imaging 27:292-300

24. Pickhardt PJ, Nugent PA, Choi JR, Schindler WR (2004) Flat colorectal lesions in asymptomatic adults: implications for screening with CT virtual colonoscopy. AJR Am J Roentgenol 183:1343-1347

25. Laks S, Macari M, Bini EJ (2004) Positional change in colon polyps at CT colonography. Radiology 231:761-766

26. Sosna J, Morrin MM, Kruskal JB et al (2003) Colorectal neoplasms: role of intravenous contrast-enhanced CT colonography. Radiology 228:152-156

27. Callstrom MR, Johnson CD, Fletcher JG et al (2001) CT colonography without cathartic preparation: feasibility study. Radiology 219:693-698

28. Lefere PA, Gryspeerdt SS, Baekelandt M, Van Holsbeeck BG (2004) Laxative-free CT Colonography. AJR Am J Roentgenol 183:945-948

29. Zalis ME, Perumpillichira J, Del Frate C, Hahn PF (2003) CT colonography: digital subtraction bowel cleansing with mucosal reconstruction initial observations. Radiology 226:911-917

30. Iannaccone R, Laghi A, Catalano C et al (2004) Computed tomographic colonography without cathartic preparation for the detection of colorectal polyps. Gastroenterology 127:1300-1311

Imaging of Liver Diseases

E. Rummeny[1], R. Baron[2]

[1] Department of Diagnostic Radiology, Technische Universität Muenchen, Munich, Germany
[2] Department of Radiology, University of Chicago, Chicago, IL, USA

Introduction

Modern imaging technology has allowed imaging of the liver to excel in ways not dreamed possible just ten or 15 years ago. It is imperative for radiologists to be aware of new capabilities and opportunities for evaluating liver disease by imaging. Imaging of the liver, similar to other organs, runs the gamut from the detection of anatomic variations and congenital anomalies, visualization of vascular disease, detection, characterization and staging of liver tumors and infections, and evaluation of trauma and post-surgical changes. Differing modalities and the understanding of different imaging techniques, including contrast utilization, is essential to optimize patient diagnoses.

In the current environment of cost containment, the most appropriate modality should be chosen to answer the clinical question. Ultrasonography (US) is widely available and is the most inexpensive modality for imaging the liver parenchyma. However, it is limited by low sensitivity and specificity. Contrast-enhanced computed tomography (CT) has emerged as the modality of choice for routine liver imaging. Magnetic resonance (MR) imaging is used primarily as a problem solving technique for liver evaluation when CT or US are equivocal. The present chapter highlights imaging of hepatic parenchymal diseases focusing on CT and MR, but including US and scintigraphy in selected cases. Course participants should gain an understanding of how these liver diseases appear at CT and MR and learn how to optimize contrast enhancement techniques and diagnoses by learning the impact of timing in the different phases of contrast enhancement after intravenous (iv) injection of contrast agents. The relative performance of different imaging modalities in diagnosing liver diseases will be compared.

Imaging Techniques

The advent of multidetector CT resulted in the concept of organ imaging in multiple planes, rather than single sequential slices. Thus, with multi-detector systems of more than 40 channels, one can image the entire abdomen in less than ten seconds, and the liver in five seconds or less, using the thinnest detector configuration of less than a millimeter, maximizing multiplanar reconstruction capabilities. When viewed electronically, reconstructed sections of 3-5 mm are preferred in order to realistically view these images. Timing of image acquisition in relation to contrast material administration depends on whether one needs to image during early arterial phase (for arterial anatomy), late arterial phase (for hypervascular tumor detection/characterization) or portal venous phase (for most routine imaging and hypovascular tumor detection). Typically, 42-45 g of iodine should be administered, which can be accomplished with 120-150 ml of contrast, depending on concentration. We administer contrast at 3 cc/sec when only portal phase imaging is to be done, and at 5 cc/sec for arterial phase imaging, with timing at 20 sec for early arterial phase (arterial mapping) and 30-35 sec for late arterial (tumor visualization). Timing of portal phase imaging varies depends on the rate of infusion and patient's fluid volume status and vascular circulation time (approximately 70 sec for 3 cc/sec, and 60 sec for 5 cc/sec). The choice of combinations of these phases of imaging depends on the individual indication [1, 2].

MR examination of liver includes sequences providing T1, T2, and with contrast enhancement. Specific pulse sequences depend on the make of the scanner, patient compliance and the clinical question being addressed [3]. In-and out-of-phase T1 imaging is recommended to allow for maximal tumor detection and characterization of fat. In general, dynamic imaging with extracellular gadolinium-based contrast agents is used for lesion characterization and detection of tumors in a setting of cirrhosis, and tissue-specific agents are also used to maximize detection of metastases in a non-cirrhotic liver [4, 5].

US can be performed with and without the use of contrast agents, which otherwise improve lesion detection and characterization, while scintigraphy may be used in selected cases for differentiation of benign and malignant tumors. However, new MR hepatocyte specific agents can perform this function as well, avoiding additional imaging tests.

Benign Hepatic Tumors

Hemangioma is the most common benign liver tumor. It is composed of multiple vascular channels lined by a single layer of endothelial cells. The size may vary from a few millimeters to more than 10 cm. If they are larger than 10 cm in diameter, hemangiomas are designated giant hemangiomas. In over 50% of cases, more than one hemangiomas is present.

US of a typical hemangioma shows a sharply circumscribed, well-defined hyperechoic lesion with distal acoustic enhancement (Fig. 1). However, about 20% of hemangiomas lack this typical appearance.

On CT, hemangiomas are sharply defined, hypodense masses compared to the adjacent hepatic parenchyma on unenhanced images. They have a distinctive enhancement pattern characterized by sequential contrast opacification beginning at the periphery as one or more nodular or globular areas of enhancement, and proceeding toward the center. The key factor is that all areas of lesion enhancement should appear with the same enhancement as blood pool elsewhere (Fig. 2). MRI is useful in differentiating hemangiomas from malignant hepatic neoplasms, based on very long T2 relaxation of the hemangioma compared with other hepatic masses. Other characteristic MRI features include a sharp margin and internal homogeneity. Similar to CT, key to diagnosis is typically early enhancing peripheral nodular enhancement on dynamic T1 images, with progressive fill-in on delayed images on dynamic gadolinium-enhanced MRI. However, in some cases, hemangiomas may be atypical. With both CT and MRI it is important to remember that central fibrous scarring prevents some large lesions from completely enhancing in this dynamic process. Furthermore, on MR images some giant hemangiomas of the liver may show a rim of low signal corresponding to a rim of high density on CT related to hemosiderin deposits. Other atypical hemangiomas may have high blood flow due to arteriovenous shunting [6-9].

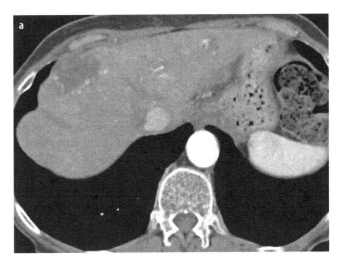
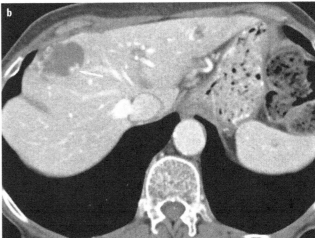
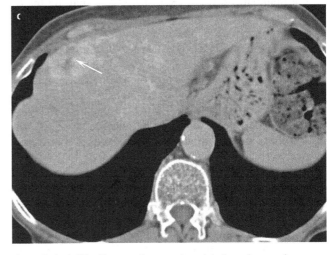

Fig. 2. Spiral CT of hemangioma. **a** Arterial phase image shows peripheral enhancement. **b** Note peripheral nodular enhancement during portal venous phase (*arrow*). **c** Delayed phase shows contrast enhancement of the whole lesion, except for central scar (*arrow*)

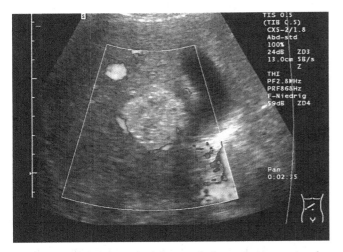

Fig. 1. Hemangioma, typical hyperechoic appearance at color Doppler sonography. Note central hypoechoic structures due to scar formation

Focal Nodular Hyperplasia (FNH) is a benign tumor of the liver, most likely caused by a hyperplastic response to a localized vascular abnormality. FNH reveals the nonspecific findings of an ill-defined lesion on US. The central scar may be detected as a hyperechoic area, but often cannot be differentiated from other areas of hyperechoic or isoechoic appearance. The use of color flow Doppler US demonstrates blood vessels within the scar. Due to the prominent arterial vascular supply, FNH undergoes marked homogenous enhancement during the arterial phase of contrast-enhanced CT [10], except for the scar, which often enhances on delayed scans. On unenhanced MR images, FNH often has signal intensity characteristics close to hepatic parenchyma, but usually slightly different on either T1 or T2 images. The central scar is most often hypointense on T1-weighted images and hyperintense on T2-weighted images. Gadolinium-enhanced MRI reveals enhancement similar to that observed with contrast-enhanced CT. One key feature is that, other than the scar, these lesions tend to be very homogeneous in appearance. Additionally, FNH shows enhancement on delayed images after administration of hepatobiliary contrast agents such as Gd-EOB-DTPA or mangafodipir trisodium (Primovist®, Teslascan®) and signal loss after administration of RES agents such as superparamagnetic iron oxide (SPIO) [4, 11]. This uptake parallels uptake of Tc-99m sulfur-colloid in scintigraphy and is a useful tool for characterization.

Hepatocellular Adenoma (HA) is an uncommon benign, but pre-malignant neoplasm with non-specific US findings. Pathologically, most HAs are large (usually > 10 cm), solitary lesions with a smooth, thin tumor capsule, often rich in fat and void of portal tracts but containing RES cells. Intratumoral hemorrhage can produce areas of infarction and fibrosis.

CT and MRI appearances of HA are also non-specific. On unenhanced CT images, the lesion may be hypodense due to the presence of fat, old necrosis or hemorrhage, or it may be hyperdense owing to recent hemorrhage or large amounts of glycogen. Substantial enhancement during the arterial and early portal venous phases of contrast enhancement may be noted. On MRI, most lesions are heterogeneous in signal intensity, with a majority being hyperintense on T1-weighted images and isointense or hyperintense on T2-weighted images [12]. On out-of-phase or fat-suppressed MR images, hepatic adenomas may appear hypointense compared to the liver (Fig. 3). On dynamic contrast-enhanced gradient echo imaging, adenomas usually appear hyperintense compared to hepatic parenchyma. Like focal nodular hyperplasia, HAs may show delayed enhancement with hepatobiliary contrast agents but opposite to FNH wash-out effects on very late images taken 1-3 hours after the injection of, for example, Gadobenate Dimeglumine (MultiHance) [19]. After administration of SPIO, HA may show uptake within the lesion and therefore signal loss on T2-weighted MR images [13].

Hepatic cysts are common liver lesions, with an incidence between 5 and 14% in the population, with a higher prevalence in women. At US, hepatic cysts are anechoic. On CT scans, hepatic cysts appear as well-circumscribed, homogeneous masses of near-water attenuation

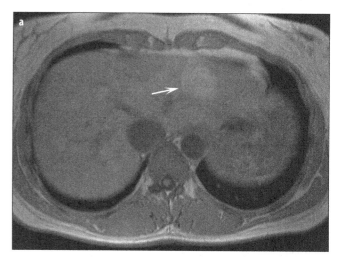

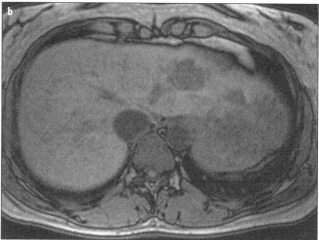

Fig. 3. MRI of hepatic adenoma. **a** On T1-weighted image the lesion is iso- to slightly hyperintense (*arrow*). **b** T1-weighted out-of-phase image shows the lesion as hypointense area due to fat content within the adenoma

value (< 20 Hounsfield Units [HU]), that shows no contrast enhancement after iv contrast material administration. Small lesions may appear to have higher density because of partial volume averaging. An US evaluation is usually helpful in demonstrating the cystic character of the mass. On MRI, they are well-defined, homogeneous lesions that are hypointense on T1-weighted images and on US they are anechoic and markedly hyperintense on heavily T2-weighted images. Abscess, hydatid cyst, intrahepatic biloma, and cystic neoplasms may be distinguished from simple cysts by virtue of features such as a thick, irregular wall, mural nodules, internal septations, or density greater than 20 HU [14].

Other Benign Tumors

Rare benign liver tumors which contain fat, include lipoma, angiomyolipoma, myelolipoma, and angiomyelolipoma. The imaging diagnosis of these uncommon benign tumors is based on the identification of fat within the mass [15], although caution is advised, since hepatic adenoma and hepatocellular carcinoma can also contain fat. More commonly, focal fatty infiltration, while not a neoplasm, can simulate a mass lesion, and this can be categorized by in- and out-of-phase T1 MR imaging. Small biliary hamartomas can be seen in the liver, and can appear cystic. These are usually less than 5 mm in diameter, but occasionally can simulate small neoplasms.

Malignant Primary Tumors

Hepatocellular Carcinoma (HCC) is the most common abdominal tumor worldwide, primarily found in Asian and Mediterranean populations. In European countries, HCC is found mostly in patients with liver cirrhosis or hemochromatosis. HCC consists of abnormal hepatocytes arranged in a typical trabecular, sinusoidal pattern. It may be solitary, multifocal, or diffusely infiltrating. US may show HCC as an iso-, hypo- or hyperintense lesion. The capsule appears as a hypoechoic rim surrounding the lesion. Using new contrast agents for US, such as Echovist® and others, the degree of vascularity within the tumor can be demonstrated.

Most HCCs are hypodense when visualized on plain CT images. Due to their predominant arterial supply, HCC are seen as transiently hyperdense masses in the arterial phase of hepatic enhancement (Fig. 4). They become isodense with hepatic parenchyma or hypodense in the portal venous phase of enhancement. On delayed images, the capsule and septa demonstrate prolonged enhancement, whereas contrast wash-out from the tumor

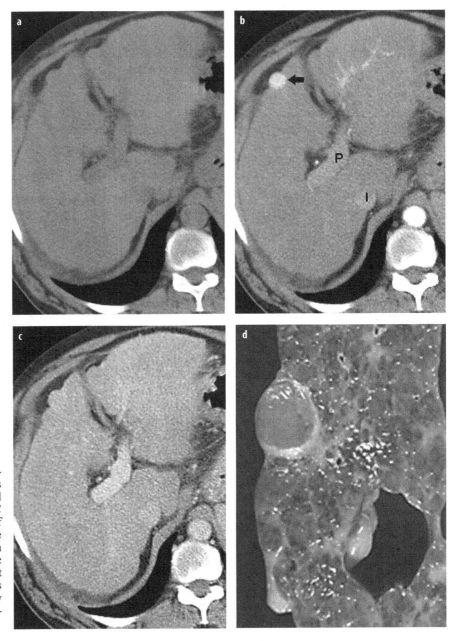

Fig. 4. Spiral CT of small HCC. **a** Unenhanced CT shows only changes of cirrhosis with nodular contour to liver. **b** Arterial phase image shows small enhancing HCC nodule (*arrow*) seen only on this phase of imaging. Note that this is a late arterial phase image, as evidenced by early enhancement in portal vein (*P*) and inferior vena cava (*I*). **c** Portal venous phase image shows wash-out of contrast in tumor such that the lesion is again isointense with liver. **d** Pathology specimen confirming small HCC with surrounding fibrous capsule

makes the lesion again appear hypodense. Contrast-enhanced CT is capable of showing the vascular invasion and arterioportal shunting associated with HCC. Diffusely infiltrating and small HCCs in cirrhosis may be difficult to detect with CT. Since HCC lesions are typically hypervascular with a primarily arterial blood supply, 'tumor seeking agents' such as lipiodol can be injected angiographically via hepatic arteries for improved detection of small nodules on lipiodol-enhanced CT performed 4-7 days after application of the contrast medium. Furthermore, in combination with cytostatic drugs, lipiodol can be used for chemo-embolization of HCC. Larger HCC lesions typically have a mosaic appearance due to hemorrhage and fibrosis [16]. Also, about 10% of small HCC can appear hypodense compared to liver, and are thus thought to be well-differentiated lesions.

Typical MRI findings of HCC include a capsule, central scar, intratumoral septa, daughter nodules, and tumor thrombus. While most large HCC are hyperintense on T2-weighted images, small lesions less than 2 cm are often isointense, with the spectrum including a hypointense appearance. On T1-weighted images, HCC has variable signal intensity relative to hepatic parenchyma. A tumor capsule may be seen on T1-weighted images (Fig. 5). HCCs characteristically show early peak contrast enhancement, and absent or minimal delayed enhancement [17], and delayed images most often exhibit a tumoral wash-out on T1 images appearing hypointense. These enhancement features are useful in differentiating HCC from hemangioma, which generally shows early peripheral enhancement, marked peak enhancement more than 2 minutes after injection, and marked delayed enhancement at 10-12 minutes. HCC may show enhancement on delayed images after mangafodipir administration. However, such enhancement is not specific for HCC and can be seen with other primary hepatocellular tumors, such as FNH and adenoma, and also with hepatic metastases from hypervascular tumors.

Fibrolamellar hepatocellular carcinoma is a less aggressive tumor with a better prognosis than HCC. It consists of malignant hepatocytes separated into cords by fibrous strands. On CT, fibrolamellar HCC appears as a large, well-defined vascular mass with a lobulated surface and often a central scar. On MRI, fibrolamellar HCC appears hypointense on T1-weighted images and hyperintense on T2-weighted images, with the central scar being hypointense on both sequences. The scar in FNH is hyperintense on T2-weighted images and shows delayed enhancement, whereas that in fibrolamellar HCC has been reported to be hypointense on T2-weighted images with less often delayed enhancement [18]. In contrast to the homogeneous appearance of FNH, these lesions are more often characterized as heterogeneous in appearance following contrast administration.

Other uncommon malignant primary tumors of the liver include intrahepatic cholangiocarcinoma, biliary cystadenocarcinoma, hepatoblastoma, primary lymphoma of liver, epithelioid hemangioendothelioma, angiosarcoma,

connective tissue sarcoma and undifferentiated embryonal sarcoma. Cholangiocarcinoma can be suggested when marked delay retention of iodinated or gadolinium based contrast is seen at 8-10 minutes post administration, and is due to the fibrous content of tumors [19]. Angio-

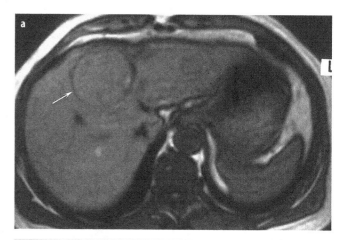

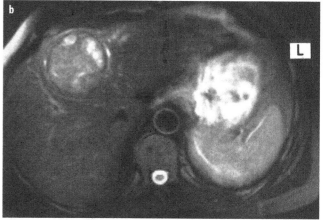

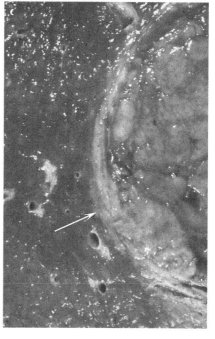

Fig. 5. MRI of HCC. **a** T1-weighted GRE scan shows the tumor isointense to liver and delineates a hypointense capsule (*arrow*). **b** T2-weighted images with signs of necrosis within the tumor. **c** Pathology specimen confirming a surrounding fibrous capsule (*arrow*)

sarcoma can have a variety of appearances, and may rarely simulate hemangioma, although usually either its diffuse nature or contrast characteristics do not match blood pool, allowing for a proper diagnosis [19].

Hepatic Metastases

At US, metastases may appear hypoechoic, isoechoic or hyperechoic in echogenicity. On a dynamic contrast-enhanced CT study, most metastases appear hypovascular and hypodense relative to liver parenchyma on portal venous phase. Hypervascular metastases, most commonly seen in renal cell, pancreatic islet cell tumors, sarcomas and breast tumor patients, may become isodense and may be difficult to detect during the redistribution phase of enhancement. These hypervascular metastases are more easily identified during the hepatic arterial phase of enhancement. At MRI, metastases are usually hypointense on T1-weighted images and hyperintense on T2-weighted images [20]. Peritumoral edema makes lesions appear larger on T2-weighted images and is very suggestive of a malignant mass [21]. High signal intensity (SI) on T1-weighted sequences has also been described and is presumably related to the internal content of a paramagnetic substance (Table 1). Some lesions may have a central area of hyperintensity ('target sign') on T2-weighted images, which corresponds to central necrosis. Metastases from colorectal carcinoma may reveal low signal intensity central areas relative to the higher intensity tumor edge on T2-weighted images ('halo sign'). On dynamic contrast-enhanced MRI, metastases demonstrate enhancement characteristics similar to those described for CT. Metastases may demonstrate a hypointense rim compared with the center of the lesion on delayed images ('peripheral wash-out' sign). Most recent studies have shown MRI to be more sensitive than contrast-enhanced CT (Fig. 6) for the detection of hepatic metastases [22].

Hepatic Abscesses

Abscess appearances can vary depending on etiology (peribiliary abscesses tend to be small and scattered adjacent to the biliary tree; portal distribution of infection from appendicitis or diverticulitis tends to lead to larger cystic lesions).

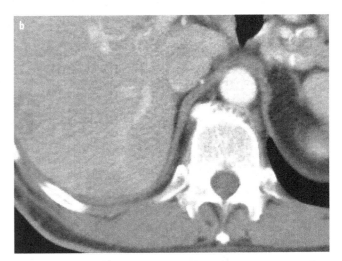

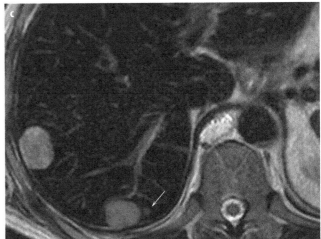

Fig. 6. Liver metastases from breast cancer. **a** Contrast enhanced Spiral CT. **b** SPIO-enhanced T2-weighted MR image, note the improved detection and delineation of the metastases (*arrow*)

US reveals a cystic lesion with internal echoes. On CT, hepatic abscess appears as a hypodense lesion with a capsule that may show enhancement. 'Cluster sign' may be noted as focal clusters of lesions when multiple abscesses are present [23]. The CT appearance of hepatic abscess is non-specific and can be mimicked by cystic or necrotic metastases. Though present in only a small minority of cases, presence of central gas is highly specific for abscess. On MRI, hepatic abscesses are hypointense relative to liver parenchyma on T1-weighted images and markedly hyperintense on T2-weighted images, often surrounded by a local area of slight T2 hyperintensity representing perilesional edema.

The CT appearance of *amebic liver abscess* is non-specific. It usually appears as a solitary, hypodense lesion with an enhancing wall that may be smooth or nodular, often associated with an incomplete rim of edema. With MRI, the lesions are hypointense on T1-weighted images and heterogeneously hyperintense on T2-weighted images [24].

Table 1. MR features

T1-weighted hyperintense lesions	Probable cause of hypertensity
Melanoma metastases	Melanin, extracellular methemoglobin
Colonic adenocarcinoma	Hemorrhage or coagulative necrosis
Ovarian adenocarcinoma	Protein
Multiple myeloma	Protein
Pancreatic mucinous cystic tumor	Protein

Table 2. Classification of common hepatic neoplasms

Cell Type	Benign	Malignant
Cholangiocellular	Hepatic cysts Biliary cystadenoma Bile duct adenoma	Biliary cystadenocarcinoma Cholangiocarcinoma
Hepatocellular	Hepatocellular adenoma Focal nodular hyperplasia Nodular regenerative hyperplasia Adenomatous hyperplasia	Hepatocellular carcinoma Fibrolamellar hepatocellular carcinoma
Mesenchymal	Mesenchymal hamartoma Hemangioma Infantile hemangioendothelioma Lymphangioma Lipoma, angiomyolipoma Leiomyoma Fibroma	Angiosarcoma Connective tissue sarcoma Undifferentiated embryonal sarcoma
Miscellaneous	–	Metastasis Lymphoma Hepatoblastoma

On CT scan, involvement of liver by *Echinococcus granulosus (hydatid cyst)* appears as unilocular or multilocular cysts with thin or thick walls, usually with the daughter cysts seen as smaller cysts with septations at the margin of mother cyst. On MRI, the presence of a hypointense rim on T1- and T2-weighted images and a multiloculated appearance are considered to be important diagnostic features [25].

Diffuse Liver Disease

Fatty liver (hepatic steatosis) may be associated with a variety of clinical disorders. US shows a diffuse or focal increase in the echogenicity of the liver. Increased fat content produces a decrease in mean hepatic CT attenuation value [26]. Milder degrees of diffuse fatty change can be diagnosed when the attenuation value of the liver is less than that of the spleen on plain study. Fatty liver may be more difficult to diagnose on scans obtained after administration of iv contrast material. Focal fatty infiltration frequently has a segmental or wedge-shaped configuration and characteristically produces no mass effect or bulging of the hepatic contour. In addition, it is simpler to diagnose when it occurs in typical locations such as adjacent to the gallbladder fossa. Normal coursing of hepatic vessels can often be seen in the affected area. MRI is extremely useful in providing definite diagnosis when the CT scan is equivocal. Proton chemical shift imaging techniques (in- and out-of-phase imaging) can readily diagnose focal and diffuse fatty infiltration [27].

The role of imaging in *cirrhosis* is to identify effects of portal hypertension and to detect HCC. The liver in early cirrhosis often has a normal appearance on CT. Early CT features include hepatomegaly and heterogeneity of hepatic parenchymal attenuation. Advanced cirrhosis is characterized by decreased hepatic volume with prominence of the porta hepatis and intrahepatic fissures, decreased size of the right hepatic lobe and medial segment of the left lobe, with a corresponding relative increase in the size of the caudate lobe and left lateral segment [28]. *Regenerative nodules* are seen on CT in those patients with siderotic nodules (dense on unenhanced CT, and signal void on MRI) and are better appreciated on MRI than on CT due to greater MR susceptibility to iron [29]. *Dysplastic nodules* (DN) represent a continuum and transition between regenerative nodules and HCC, and therefore is an important imaging diagnosis. When large, they are characteristically hyperintense on T1-weighted images and hypointense on T2-weighted images. On the contrary, HCCs generally appear iso- or hyperintense on T2-weighted images. Unfortunately, all small DNs and many large DNs have no characteristic appearance and are often not visualized. Although early enhancement on dynamic enhanced MRI may help in reliably distinguishing HCC from DN, some DN will exhibit marked contrast enhancement.

In patients being screened for cirrhosis and possible transplantation, 10-20% of patients harbor a HCC (higher rates for patients with hepatitis B and C), and arterial phase imaging is the only methodology that with high sensitivity (70-80%) can detect these patients [30]. Caution is recommended, however, as it is now known that many small benign lesions can enhance and simulate HCC, most prominently in patients with hepatic vascular disorders, particularly Budd-Chiari [31, 32]. Probably the best approach to a patient with just one or a few small enhancing nodules is to take the same approach as upon visualizing a lung nodule in a cancer patient - suspicious but not definitive.

Of the myriad of lesions simulating HCC in cirrhosis (arteriovenous [AV] malformation, small hemangiomas, infracted regenerative nodules among the less common), the most common and problematic lesions, that can enhance are enhancing benign or dysplastic regenerating nodules (usually small, but not always) and focal confluent fibrosis [32]. Key to the latter diagnosis is the characteristic finding of associated overlying capsular retraction, and characteristic locations and shape (wedge shaped, radiating to porta hepatic).

Extrahepatic imaging features of cirrhosis are ascites, splenomegaly and portosystemic collateral vessels.

Differential Diagnosis

The approach to characterizing a focal liver lesion seen on CT begins with the determination of its density. If the lesion is of near water density, homogenous in character and has sharp margins, then a cyst should be considered and can be confirmed with an equilibrium phase CT, US or MRI (T2 bright and non-enhancing post gadolinium).

If the lesion has some enhancement, then the next analysis requires a determination of whether the enhancement is peripheral and nodular, with the density of the lesions appearing similar to density of blood vessels. In this case, a hemangioma may be diagnosed with confidence. On the other hand, thick irregular, heterogeneous enhancement suggests a malignant mass.

Arterially enhancing lesions include FNH, hepatocellular adenoma, HCC and metastases from carcinoid, melanoma, renal cell carcinoma, breast, sarcoma and islet cell tumor. In general, HCC is considered when there is a setting of cirrhosis, while FNH is considered in young women and hepatic adenoma in patients on oral contraceptives, anabolic steroids or with history of glycogen storage disease.

References

1. Gazelle GS, Haaga JR (1992) Hepatic neoplasms: surgically relevant segmental anatomy and imaging techniques. AJR Am J Roentgenol 158:1015-1018
2. Laghi A, Iannaccone R, Rossi P et al (2003) Hepatocellular Carcinoma: detection with triple-phase multi-detector row helical CT in patients with chronic hepatitis. Radiology 226:543-549
3. Sharma R, Saini S (1999) Role and limitations of magnetic resonance imaging in the diagnostic work-up of patients with liver cancer. J Comput Assist Tomogr 23(Suppl 1):S39-S44
4. Semelka RC, Helmberger TKG (2001) Contrast agents for MR imaging of the liver. Radiology 218:27-38
5. Grimm J, Muller-Hulsbeck S, Blume J et al (2001) Comparison of biphasic spiral CT and MnDPDP-enhanced MRI in the detection and characterization of liver lesions. Rofo Fortschr Geb Rontgenstr Neuen Bildgeb Verfahr 173:266-272
6. Clement O, Siauve N, Lewin M et al (1998) Contrast agents in magnetic resonance imaging of the liver: present and future. Biomed Pharmacother 52:51-58
7. Coumbaras M, Wendum D, Monnier-Cholley L et al (2002) CT and MR imaging features of pathologically proven atypical giant hemangiomas. AJR Am J Roentgenol 179:1457-1463
8. Jang HJ, Kim TK, Lim HK et al (2003) Hepatic hemangioma: atypical appearance on CT, MR imaging, and sonography. AJR Am J Roentgenol 180:135-141
9. Vilgrain V, Boulos L, Vullierme MP et al (2000) Imaging of atypical hemangiomas of the liver with pathologic correlation. Radiographics 20:379-397
10. Brancatelli G, Federle M, Grazoli L et al (2001) Focal nodular hyperplasia: CT findings with emphasis on multiphasic helical CT in 78 patients. Radiology 219:61-68
11. Grandin C, Van Beers BE, Robert A et al (1995) Benign hepatocellular tumors: MRI after superparamagnetic iron oxide administration. J Comput Assist Tomogr 19:412-418
12. Arrive L, Flejou J-F, Vilgrain V et al (1994) Hepatic adenoma: MR findings in 51 pathologically proved lesions. Radiology 193:507-512
13. Bartolotta TV, Midiri M, Galia M et al (2001) Benign hepatic tumors: MRI features before and after administration of superparamagnetic contrast media. Radiol Med (Torino) 101:219-229
14. Baron RL, Ferris JV (2004) Primary tumors of the liver and biliary tract. In: Husband JE, Reznek RH (eds) Imaging in oncology, 2nd edn. Taylor & Francis, London, pp 245-272
15. Sung KF, Chen TC, Hung CF et al (2001) Angiomyolipoma of the liver: case report. Chang Gung Med J 24:318-323
16. Steven WR, Gulino SP, Batts KP et al (1996) Mosaic pattern of hepatocellular carcinoma: histologic basis for a characteristic CT appearance. J Comput Assist Tomogr 20:337-342
17. Peterson MS, Baron RL (2001) Radiologic diagnosis of hepatocellular carcinoma. Clin Liver Dis 5:123-144
18. Ichikawa T, Federle MP, Grazioli L et al (1999) Fibrolamellar hepatocellular carcinoma: imaging and pathologic findings in 31 recent cases. Radiology 213:352-361
19. Grazioli L, Morana G, Kirchin MA, Schneider G (2005) Accurate differentiation of focal nodular hyperplasia from hepatic adenoma at gadobenate dimeglumine-enhanced MR imaging: prospective study. Radiology 236:166-177
20. Imam K, Bluemke DA (2000) MR imaging in the evaluation of hepatic metastases. Magn Reson Imaging Clin N Am 8:741-756
21. Lee MJ, Saini S, Compton CC et al (1991) MR demonstration of edema adjacent to a liver metastasis: pathologic correlation. AJR Am J Roentgenol 157:499-501
22. Semelka RC, Cance WG, Marcos HB et al (1999) Liver metastases: comparison of current MR techniques and spiral CT during arterial portography for detection in 20 surgically staged cases. Radiology 213:86-91
23. Jeffrey RB, Tolentino CS, Chang FC et al (1998) CT of small pyogenic hepatic abscesses: the cluster sign. AJR Am J Roentgenol 151:487-489
24. Barreda R, Ros PR (1992) Diagnostic imaging of liver abscess. Crit Rev Diagn Imaging 33:29-58
25. Taourel P, Marty-Ane B, Charasset S et al (1993) Hydatid cyst of the liver: comparison of CT and MRI. J Comput Assist Tomogr 17:80-85
26. Jacobs JE, Birnbaum BA, Shapiro MA et al (1998) Diagnostic criteria for fatty infiltration of the liver on contrast-enhanced helical CT. AJR Am J Roentgenol 171:659-664
27. Levenson H, Greensite F, Hoefs J et al (1991) Fatty infiltration of the liver: quantification with phase-contrast MR imaging at 1.5 T vs biopsy. AJR Am J Roentgenol 156:307-312
28. Mortele KJ, Ros PR (2001) Imaging of diffuse liver disease. Semin Liver Dis 21:195-212
29. Rode A, Bancel B, Douek P et al (2001) Small nodule detection in cirrhotic livers: evaluation with US, spiral CT, and MRI and correlation with pathologic examination of explanted liver. J Comput Assist Tomogr 25:327-336
30. Peterson MS, Baron RL, Marsh JW et al (2000) Pretransplantation surveillance for possible hepatocellular carcinoma in patients with cirrhosis: epidemiology and CT-based tumor detection rate in 430 cases with surgical pathological correlation. Radiology 217:743-749
31. Viligrain V, Lewin M, Vons C et al (1999) Hepatic nodules in Budd Chiari Syndrome: imaging features. Radiology 210:443-449
32. Baron RL, Peterson MS (2001) Screening the cirrhotic liver for hepatocellular carcinoma with CT and MR: opportunities and pitfalls. Radiographics 21:S117-S132

Diseases of the Pancreas, Part I: Pancreatitis

T. Helmberger

Clinic for Radiology and Nuclear Medicine, University Hospitals of Schleswig – Holstein, Campus Luebeck, Luebeck, Germany

Introduction

The incidence of pancreatic inflammation in the western world ranges from 110-240 cases/million. In about 80% of these cases the reason for the disease is an undetected gall stone or alcohol abuse. While in men 30-50 years of age alcohol is the main reason, gall stones are predominantly responsible for the onset of the disease in women. Nevertheless, there are many other factors that cause pancreatitis (Table 1).

The manifestations of pancreatitis range widely, from forms that are mild and self-limiting, to severe, lethal forms in acute pancreatitis, to forms with permanent loss of exocrine and/or endocrine function, as seen in chronic pancreatitis [1-5].

In clinical reality, it can be difficult to differentiate cystic changes of the pancreas from cystic tumors, and chronic pancreatitis (CP) from pancreatic cancer, due to their similarity in imaging presentation. The differential diagnosis is of utmost importance as these conditions have significantly different management and prognoses. The differential diagnoses in terms of solid and cystic tumors will be discussed in 'Diseases of the Pancreas, Part II: Tumors', by Ruedi Thoeni.

Acute Pancreatitis

Acute pancreatitis (AP) is defined as an inflammatory process involving a gland that is normal prior to the attack, and which returns to normal once the derangements that precipitated the attack have been corrected.

AP is a common problem with a rising incidence in the western world – in the US there are about 200,000 admissions/year and about 10,000 deaths/year.

Table 1. Potential factors causing pancreatitis

Metabolic	Alcohol
	Drugs (e.g. glucocorticosteroids, azathioprine, hydrochlorothiazide, furosemide, sulfonamides, estrogens, pentamidine, didanosine (DDI), valproic acid)
	Hypertriglyceridemia
	Hyperalimentation with lipids
	Hypercalcemia
	Hyperparathyroidism
Mechanical/obstructive	Gall stones
	Tumours (pancreas CA, common bile duct CA, TU of the ampulla and duodenum, metastases)
	Sphincter of Oddi Dysfunction
	Post upper gastorintestinal surgery
	Post endoscopy
	Post abdominal trauma
	Duodenal obstruction/scar (e.g. after ulcer disease)
Infectious	Mumps
	Coxsackie virus infection
	Ascaris infection with mechanical component
Vascular	Panarteriitis nodosa
	Post cardiac and pulmonary surgery
	Severe arteriosclerosis
Other	Hereditary, idiopathic
	Anomalies (pancreas divisum, anulare)
	Autoimmune
	Scorpion sting/gila monster bite

AP is more often seen in the elderly population (50-60 years of age). The most common causes of AP are cholelithiasis (75%) and alcohol abuse (15%). Other causes are metabolic disorders (e.g., hypercalcemia, hyperlipidemia Type I and V), infections (e.g., parasites, hepatitis, HIV), trauma (e.g., penetrating ulcer, abdominal surgery, endoscopic retrograde cholangiopancreatography [ERCP]), drugs (e.g., azathioprine, furosemide, sulfonamides, steroids), and structural abnormalities (e.g., pancreas divisum, choldeochocele). In 10-15% of patients no obvious cause can be found, however, biliary microlithiasis might be the most likely cause in these cases (Table 1).

From a pathophysiological point of view, the most likely factors for the sudden onset of AP are: (1) pancreatic hypersecretion, (2) intra- and extravasation of pancreatic secretions, and (3) premature activation of pancreatic enzymes followed by autodigestion and necrosis of the pancreatic gland and peripancreatic tissues.

From the clinical point of view, AP can be divided into a mild and severe form almost paralleled by the pathophysiological finding of an interstitial (edematous) and necrotizing form [6, 7].

The mild form of AP (approximately 50% of the cases) is characterized by mild symptoms and transitory elevation of amylase levels that recover rapidly without complications. In general, the gland may be enlarged due to a moderate edema, and peripancreatic fluid collections can be present; however, in 30% of the cases no morphological changes can be appreciated. In cholelithiasis, a segmental pancreatitis – mainly of the pancreatic head – is found in up to 20% of cases (Fig. 1).

While ultrasound (US) may reveal a normal to mildly enlarged gland with homogeneous (hypoechoic) echogenicity, sufficient visualization by US is possible in only 60-70% of cases. In contrast-enhanced computed tomography (CT) as well as in magnetic resonance imaging (MRI) (which is, in general, not necessary), the gland is diffusely enlarged and a small amount of fluid can be seen outlining the gland. Moreover, imaging is needed to rule out other underlying conditions that can be accompanied by hyperamylasemia, such as bowel obstruction, bowel infarction, gangrenous cholecystitis or perforated ulcers.

In the progressive mild to moderate forms of AP the contour of the gland becomes shaggy. On CT and MRI, the appearance of the parenchyma may get heterogeneous and small intraglandular and/or retroperitoneal fluid collections adjacent to the organ may develop (Fig. 2).

The severe forms of pancreatitis are determined by a delayed or no response to conservative therapy or even deterioration under therapy. The mortality rate at the latter stage is almost 100%.

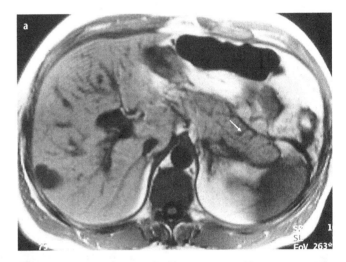

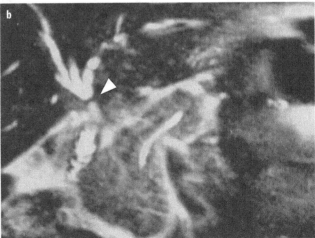

Fig. 2. MRI in acute pancreatitis after cholecystectomy and reconstruction of the extrahepatic common bile duct. The side branches of the pancreatic duct are slightly dilated (*arrows*). **a** A small fluid rim on the anterior renal fascia can be appreciated on the T1-weighted gradient-echo image. **b** The heavily T2-weighted image reveals fluid outlining the pancreatic gland and the slightly dilated pancreatic duct. Note the moderate stenosis (*arrowhead*) of the common bile duct (CBD) after surgical reconstruction

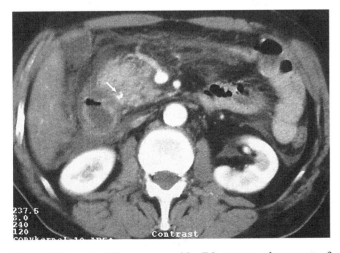

Fig. 1. CT in acute biliary pancreatitis. Edematous enlargement of the pancreatic head, exudation surrounding the duodenum and along the pararenal fascia. The reason for the acute panceatitis is a biliary stone 'trapped' in the ampullary region (*arrow*)

Typical findings in severe (necrotizing) AP are varying degrees of parenchymal necrosis accompanied by progressive exudation, superinfection of necrotic tissue, hemorrhage, abscess formation, phlegmon (~ inflammatory pannus), and vascular erosion (Fig. 3b).

According to these pathomorphological conditions, the pancreas and its surroundings present a rather wide spectrum of imaging findings. In severe cases, US imaging is often compromised by overlying gas, peripancreatic exudation and phlegmoneous changes. After necrosis, the pancreatic appearance becomes increasingly hypoechoic without differentiation of vital from necrotic tissue. Therefore, US is generally used for second line, complementary imaging in follow-up to detect fluid formations such as pseudocysts.

Parenchymal necrosis is best displayed on contrast-enhanced CT during at least the portal venous phase. Characteristic findings are patchy areas of lack of enhancement, (pseudo) fragmentation, and liquid necroses. Additionally, increasing peripancreatic exudations dis-

secting along retroperitoneal fascial planes into the mesocolon and the small bowel mesentery are frequently seen, as well as peripancreatic inflammatory tissue (phlegmon) and infected areas. In less than 10% of cases, small amounts of intraperitoneal fluid (ascites) are seen, whereas large volumes of intraperitoneal fluids are very rare.

With respect to the literature, there is no significant superiority of MRI over CT in the diagnosis of AP and related complications. The superior tissue resolution and the higher sensitivity to slight edematous or necrotic changes, hemorrhage or fluid dissection of fat planes favor MRI. However, these advantages are often hampered by the impaired study conditions in severely ill patients that may degrade the image quality. In severe AP, pancreatic flow can be reduced by iodinated contrast agents, which is followed by an increased rate of necrosis and mortality. This may make MRI the favorable staging tool in AP, however, this potential complication has never been proven for the non-ionic contrast agents that are used nowadays almost exclusively in CT [8-10].

The local inflammatory conditions are often complicated by regional and systemic involvement induced by autodigestion and activation of systemic inflammatory mediators [11-17].

The rapid change of the local pancreatic and overall abdominal situation demands an adequate diagnostic and therapeutic regime in order to avoid a disastrous outcome. Several clinical and laboratory scoring systems were established to stage and predict the clinical course of severe AP (Ranson's score, APACHE II, Glasgow criteria (also known as Imrie criteria), MOSS score, serum-methemalbumin, trypsin-activated peptide, C-reactive protein; see Table 2). However, these scoring systems are mainly dependent on systemic alterations and are quite non-specific in that they do not address the local pancreatic situation [18-25]. Balthazar et al. [26, 27] proved that contrast-enhanced CT is the most helpful diagnostic modality for detecting complications that may necessitate medical, surgical or interventional management, and can predict the patient's outcome depending on the local pancreatic situation. The proposed 5-grade scoring system

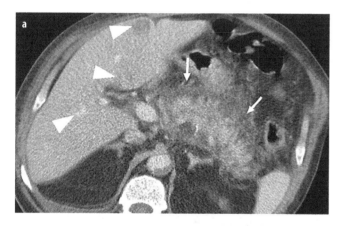

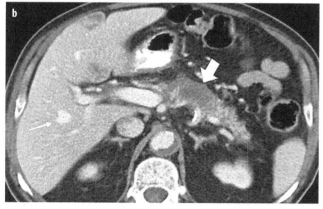

Fig. 3. Acute severe pancreatitis. **a** At the patient's admission, contrast-enhanced CT during the venous phase displayed a fuzzy contour of the pancreatic gland together with peripancreatic exudation (*arrow*). Note the hypo- and hyperdense hepatic lesions (*arrowheads*). **b** A control scan 10 days later revealed an almost normal gland with resorption of the peripancreatic fluid. However, there was an area with a lack of enhancement representing focal necrosis (*large arrow*). In the liver, one lesion turned out to be a hemangioma (*arrow*) while the other two lesions were small abscesses

Table 2. Ranson score based on present clinical and laboratory signs at admission and 48 hour follow-up (each sign = 1 point)

At admission	48-hour follow-up
Age > 55	Hematocrit fall > 10%
WBC > 16.000	Blood urea nitrogen rise > 5 mg/dL
Blood Glucose > 200 mg/dL	Ca (serum) < 8 mg/dL
Serum LDH > 350 IU/L	PO2 < 60 mm Hg
SGOT (AST) > 250 U/L	Base deficit > 4 meq/L
	Estimated fluid sequestration > 600 ml

Score	Mortality
0 - 2	< 10%
3 - 5	10 - 20%
> 5	> 50%

(Table 3, 4), by estimating the presence and degree of pancreatic and peripancreatic inflammation and fluid accumulation and by detecting the presence and extent of pancreatic necrosis together with the estimation of the lack of enhancement of the gland (< 30%, 30-50%, > 50%, respectively), can be translated into a CT-severity index (Table 4) that allows the estimation of complications (morbidity) and mortality (Fig. 4). If more than 50% of the volume of the pancreas is necrotic, the morbidity rate rises up to almost 100%. However, recently a modified and simplified CT severity index was proposed by Mortele et al. [28], correlating more closely with patient outcome measures than the currently accepted CT severity index (Table 4).

About a fifth of the patients without necrotic changes of the pancreatic gland also develop local complications. Fluid collections are seen in up to 50% of patients with AP. In about half of these patients these collections resolve spontaneously within several weeks. In the rest however, the fluid collections will persist, eventually followed by encapsulation, superinfection (abscess), or formation of a pseudocyst.

Complications in AP

Pseudocysts are fluid collections with a noticeable capsule. They typically develop 4-5 weeks after the onset of AP. On US, CT and MRI, they present a typical cyst-like

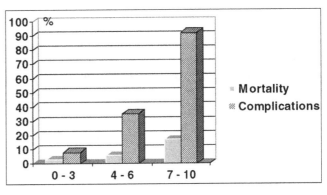

Fig. 4. CT severity index related to the degree of necrosis of the pancreatic parenchyma (according to Balthazar). Grad A = 0, B = 1, C = 2, D = 3, E = 4; no necrosis = 0, 30% of necrosis = 2, < 50% = 4, > 50% = 6 (data from [29])

appearance, in general without septations. Since large cysts are prone to complications (such as rupture, infection, hemorrhage, biliary obstruction or fistulization to the GI tract), cysts greater than 5-7 cm should be treated by percutaneous drainage or operative marsupilization.

In a septic patient, fluid collections that are not water-like, and rim enhancement in contrast enhanced CT or MRI studies, imply the presence of abscesses until proven otherwise. Gas is detected as a characteristic sign of an infected fluid collection in only 20% of cases with pancreatic abscesses. Percutaneous aspiration or drain-placement is the proper treatment.

In contrast to abscess formations, superinfected necrotic areas of the pancreas are much more difficult to handle. Percutaneous drainage therapy is mostly frustrating due to the more solid consistency of the infected necrosis, however, a biopsy is often needed to prove the diagnosis. In most cases, a percutaneous, endoscopy-guided necrosectomy or a surgical intervention has to be considered.

Table 3. CT grading in acute pancreatitis (according to Balthazar)

Grade	CT findings
A	Normal
B	Focal (~ 20%), diffuse enlargement of the gland, irregular contour, inhomogeneous density
C	Grade B + inflammation in peripancreatic fat
D	Small, mostly occasionally fluid collections or phlegmon
E	Two or more fluid collections, gas within the pancreas or retroperitoneum

Table 4. 'Classic' and modified CT severity index

CT Severity Index	Points	Modified CT Severity Index	Points
Pancreatic inflammation		Pancreatic inflammation	
- Normal pancreas	0	- Normal pancreas	0
- Focal or diffuse enlargement of the pancreas	1	- Intrinsic pancreatic abnormalities with or without inflammatory changes in peripancreatic fat	2
- Intrinsic pancreatic abnormalities with inflammatory changes in peripancreatic fat	2	- Pancreatic or peripancreatic fluid collection or peripancreatic fat necrosis	4
- Single, ill-defined fluid collection or phlegmon	3		
- Two or more poorly defined collections or presence of gas in or adjacent to the pancreas	4		
Pancreatic necrosis		Pancreatic necrosis	
- None	0	- None	0
- ≤ 30%	2	- ≤ 30%	2
- > 30-50%	4	- > 30%	4
- > 50%	6	- Extrapancreatic complications (one or more of pleural effusion, ascites, vascular complications, parenchymal complications, or gastrointestinal tract involvement)	2

Pseudoaneurysm formation and hemorrhage may result from the extravasated pancreatic enzymes that cause vascular injury, and are typically late complications that occur after several episodes of severe AP. While pseudoaneurysms are generally easily detected by any kind of imaging modality, retroperitoneal hemorrhage is best depicted by contrast-enhanced CT or unenhanced MRI. Angiography with arterial embolization is the treatment of choice and is generally superior to the surgical therapy.

Groove Pancreatitis

The so-called 'groove pancreatitis', first described by Becker [30], is a rare, 'late' complication occurring after several AP attacks, and is defined as an inflammatory reaction and fluid collection located in the groove between the head of the pancreas, the duodenum and the common bile duct. The anterior anlage of the pancreas seems to be mainly affected, with duodenal stenosis and/or strictures of the common duct in about 50% of the cases. Therefore, this disease may mimic pancreatic head cancer, necessitating surgical exploration. Dynamic CT and MR imaging with delayed enhancement of collagen fibrous tissue during the late post-equilibrium phase can characterize a potential soft tissue mass as fibrosis and may, in the absence of complications, allow surgical exploration to be avoided [31, 32].

Autoimmune Pancreatitis

Autoimmune pancreatitis (AIP) is a relatively new syndrome of clinical and histologic findings and has also been described as 'lymphoplasmocytic sclerosing pancreatitis with cholangitis', 'nonalcoholic duct-destructive chronic pancreatitis' and 'chronic sclerosing pancreatitis'. A number of features can be found, including hypergammaglobulinemia, elevation of serum IgG4, IgG4-containing immune complexes and a number of antibodies, such as antinuclear antibodies, antibodies against lactoferrin, carbonic anhydrase type II, and rheumatoid factors. Histological features include fibrosis with lymphoplasmacytic infiltration of interlobular ducts. The majority of lymphocytes are CD8+ and CD4+ T-lymphocytes, while B-lymphocytes are less frequent. In general, diagnosis of AIP is established by clinical signs and laboratory and morphological findings. An association with other autoimmune disease such as Sjögren-syndrome, primary biliary cirrhosis, primary sclerosing cholangitis, Crohn's disease or ulcerating colitis, systemic lupus erythematosus, and retroperitoneal fibrosis is found in a third of the cases.

At imaging, a focal ('mass-forming') or diffuse ('sausage-like') enlargement of the pancreas may be present. In contrast-enhanced studies, peripancreatic nodular or rim-like enhancement can be appreciated. Focal AIP of the head that involves the pancreatic and distal common bile duct needs to be differentiated from pancreatic carcinoma, necessitating biopsy proof.

Most patients appear to respond to steroid treatment according to their symptoms, and laboratory and morphological findings [33-38].

Chronic Pancreatitis

CP is determined by a continuing (aseptic) inflammation of the gland, characterized by irreversible morphological and functional damage. The most common reasons are chronic alcohol abuse (70%) and cholelithiasis (20%), rare cases are caused by cystic fibrosis or are idiopathic, without any apparent cause. Typically, patients 30-40 years of age present with a history of epigastric pain (95%), weight loss (95%) and signs of endo-/exocrine deficiency (diabetes mellitus 58%, malabsorption syndrome and steatorrhea 80%). Acute exacerbations of CP are accompanied by episodes of pain that may mimic an acute abdomen. With progressive destruction of the gland, CP can become painless after several years. In about 1.5-12% of cases, CP can be complicated by pancreatic cancer.

Tumor markers such as CA 19-9 and CA-50 may also be elevated transiently and are unspecific. Laboratory tests for secretin-creozyme and secretin-cerulein have a high diagnostic accuracy, except in the early stages, but are invasive and cumbersome for the patient. These tests are of particular importance for the diagnostically challenging, newly defined small duct CP, where chronic inflammation occurs without duct abnormalities.

In CP, the most characteristic findings are dilatations of the pancreatic main duct and of ductal side branches (70-90%) together with small cystic changes, scattered glandular and ductal calcifications (40-50%), and ductal protein plugs. The grade and shape of ductal dilatation may help to differentiate chronic (benign) obstructions from malignant occlusions. In CP the contour of the pancreatic duct and its side branches is commonly irregular (73%), while this is true only in 15% of the cases in pancreatic malignancies. Additionally, the duct commonly forms less than 50% of the pancreatic anterior-posterior diameter in CP, while the opposite is true in pancreatic cancers (due to obstructive atrophy) (Fig. 5).

In CP, the gland may present a normal appearance in 15-20% of cases, however, a diffuse (50%) or focal (25%) enlargement is more common, and may raise the suspicion of a neoplasm. With time, atrophy of the organ will occur in 10-50%. The varying appearance of CP explains the shortcomings in establishing diagnosis: without gross morphologic changes it is very difficult to diagnose incipient forms of CP. Moreover, morphologic changes correlate very poorly with the functional exocrine and endocrine deficit, therefore endoscopically-guided (endoscopical US) or percutaneous biopsy may be necessary for differentiation.

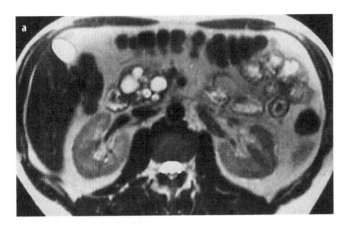

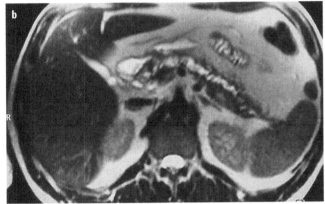

Fig. 5. CP by MRI. Cystic degeneration of the pancreatic head (**a**), together with irregular dilatation of the pancreatic main duct (**b**) in MRI (fast spin echo T2)

Complications in CP

Beside consolidated cystic degeneration in terms of cystic branch and side branch dilatation of the pancreatic duct and peripancreatic pseudocyst formation, complications may occur, such as common bile duct obstruction secondary to fibrosis, splenic vein thrombosis (note: upper GI bleeding is possible due to gastric varices in the absence of esophageal varices!), pancreatic fistulae, and communication between the pancreatic duct and abdominal organs or the skin.

Diagnostic Challenges in CP

In general, diagnostics of inflammatory and tumorous pancreatic conditions rely on imaging such as US, CT, MRI and – more invasively – ERCP). Imaging findings are ruled by the macro-structural changes of the organ and its surrounding.

Calcifications in CP can easily be depicted using plain films and US. Additionally, US is able to display ductal dilatation, micro- and macrocystic changes, and the gland itself.

Contrast-enhanced multidetector CT (MDCT) is well-established to assess ductal changes, calcifications, the

form and shape of the pancreatic gland, and potential concomitant conditions such as pseudocysts. This also enables multiplanar, curved reconstructions for a high-resolution display of the total gland and the run of the duct. Depending on the fibrotic changes in CP, contrast enhancement can be variable by CT, whereas most ductal carcinomas present no or only minor enhancement during arterial-dominant- and parenchymal-phase imaging. However, late enhancement can be seen on delayed imaging without substantial additional information.

Beside the superior tissue resolution for the differentiation of varying 'qualities' of pancreatic parenchyma, using unenhanced and Gd-DTPA-enhanced T1-weighted sequences (± fat suppression) and heavily T2-weighted sequences, MRI is capable of best displaying the pancreatic gland and the pancreatic duct, including first-generation side arms and small stones. Nevertheless, ERCP does show initial ductal changes (Table 4) superior to all other imaging modalities, but the clinical significance of these minor changes remains contentious, compromised by the fact of potentially 'unphysiological' distension of the ducts by contrast medium injection.

Pancreatic cancer (PCa) is the most crucial complication in CP and is the major challenge for diagnostics because focal enlargement of the gland induced by a fibrotic inflammatory pseudotumor may be indistinguishable from pancreatic carcinoma. According to the recent literature, a comparison of state-of-the-art MDCT and MRI reveals no difference in the detection rate of PCa. Nevertheless, CP is still the major factor for a missed diagnosis due to its potential tumor-like appearance. However, if local or regional lymph node enlargement, vascular encasement, or remote metastases are displayed, the differential is ruled by these secondary signs of malignancy. Then, it is most important to stage the tumor correctly to allow for further treatment stratification (Table 2, 3). In ambiguous cases, biopsy or even surgical exploration may still be necessary.

CP can cause a focal pancreatic mass indicative of a neoplasm. Moreover, CP represents a major risk factor for PCa with a 26-fold increased risk of developing cancer, according to an international, multicenter cohort study [39].

Therefore, the differential between CP and PCa is still challenging, stressing a variety of methods. The sensitivities and specificities of US, CT, and MRI for PCa were reported as 76-83% and 91-93%, respectively. Nevertheless, the rate of incorrect diagnoses is still up to 25%. Using various differential criteria (Table 5) may help to improve the overall diagnostic accuracy beyond pure image interpretation.

Recently, new methods and techniques for discriminating between CP and PCa have been described, these include the oxygen insensitivity test, FDG-PET or in vivo proton MR spectroscopy, in addition to conventional pathologic studies of brush cytology. Nevertheless, in general, these new methods are not yet well established [40, 41].

Table 5. Differential criteria for CP versus PCa

	CP	PCa
History	+++	–
Duct	irregular	smooth
Duct/parenchyma	< 0.5	> 0.5
Calcification	+++	–
Enhancement	diffuse	focal
Cysts	+++	(+)
Lymphnodes	(+)	++
Metastases	–	+++

Nevertheless, up to now biopsy is the most reliable diagnostic tool to establish diagnosis in ambiguous cases of pancreatic masses. There is no significant difference for endoscopial compared to percutaneous procedures, but laparoscopical procedures are compromised by an increased chance of adverse events, such as potential tumor seeding.

Pancreatitis in Children

Fortunately, pancreatitis in childhood is rare. The best known causes of pancreatitis are trauma to the pancreas (typically bicycle accident), genetically transmitted hereditary pancreatitis, and cystic fibrosis. Nevertheless, in most cases the reason for pancreatitis is unknown (idiopathic pancreatitis), although microcalculi and protein plugs are discussed as potential reasons. In general, diagnosis can be established based on the history, the clinical findings, and imaging findings that are not different from that seen in adults [42-44].

References

1. Mitchell RM, Byrne MF, Baillie J (2003) Pancreatitis. Lancet 361:1447-1455
2. Glasbrenner B, Kahl S, Malfertheiner P (2002) Modern diagnostics of chronic pancreatitis. Eur J Gastroenterol Hepatol 14:935-941
3. Etemad B, Whitcomb DC (2001) Chronic pancreatitis: diagnosis, classification, and new genetic developments. Gastroenterology 120:682-707
4. Halonen KI, Leppaniemi AK, Puolakkainen PA et al (2000) Severe acute pancreatitis: prognostic factors in 270 consecutive patients. Pancreas 21:266-271
5. Bank S, Indaram A (1999) Causes of acute and recurrent pancreatitis. Clinical considerations and clues to diagnosis. Gastroenterol Clin North Am 28:571-589, viii
6. Cavallini G, Frulloni L, Bassi C et al (2004) Prospective multicentre survey on acute pancreatitis in Italy (ProInf-AISP): results on 1005 patients. Dig Liver Dis 36:205-211
7. Losanoff JE, Asparouhov OK, Jones JW (2001) Multiple factor scoring system for risk assessment of acute pancreatitis. J Surg Res 101:73-78
8. Plock JA, Schmidt J, Anderson SE et al (2005) Contrast-enhanced computed tomography in acute pancreatitis: does contrast medium worsen its course due to impaired microcirculation? Langenbecks Arch Surg 390:156-163
9. Werner J, Schmidt J, Warshaw AL et al (1998) The relative safety of MRI contrast agent in acute necrotizing pancreatitis. Ann Surg 227:105-111
10. Robinson PJ, Sheridan MB (2000) Pancreatitis: computed tomography and magnetic resonance imaging. Eur Radiol 10:401-408
11. Pamuklar E, Semelka RC (2005) MR imaging of the pancreas. Magn Reson Imaging Clin N Am 13:313-330
12. Laurens B, Leroy C, Andre A et al (2005) [Imaging of acute pancreatitis]. J Radiol 86(6 Pt 2):733-746
13. Vaishali MD, Agarwal AK, Upadhyaya DN et al (2004) Magnetic resonance cholangiopancreatography in obstructive jaundice. J Clin Gastroenterol 38:887-890
14. Arvanitakis M, Delhaye M, De Maertelaere V et al (2004) Computed tomography and magnetic resonance imaging in the assessment of acute pancreatitis. Gastroenterology 126:715-723
15. Akahane T, Kuriyama S, Matsumoto M et al (2003) Pancreatic pleural effusion with a pancreaticopleural fistula diagnosed by magnetic resonance cholangiopancreatography and cured by somatostatin analogue treatment. Abdom Imaging 28:92-95
16. Sica GT, Miller FH, Rodriguez G et al (2002) Magnetic resonance imaging in patients with pancreatitis: evaluation of signal intensity and enhancement changes. J Magn Reson Imaging 15:275-284
17. Okai T, Fujii T, Ida M et al (2002) EUS and ERCP features of nonalcoholic duct-destructive, mass-forming pancreatitis before and after treatment with prednisolone. Abdom Imaging 27:74-76
18. Taylor SL, Morgan DL, Denson KD et al (2005) A comparison of the Ranson, Glasgow, and APACHE II scoring systems to a multiple organ system score in predicting patient outcome in pancreatitis. Am J Surg 189:219-222
19. Mentula P, Kylanpaa ML, Kemppainen E et al (2005) Early prediction of organ failure by combined markers in patients with acute pancreatitis. Br J Surg 92:68-75
20. Leung TK, Lee CM, Lin SY et al (2005) Balthazar computed tomography severity index is superior to Ranson criteria and APACHE II scoring system in predicting acute pancreatitis outcome. World J Gastroenterol 11:6049-6052
21. Johnson CD, Toh SK, Campbell MJ (2004) Combination of APACHE-II score and an obesity score (APACHE-O) for the prediction of severe acute pancreatitis. Pancreatology 4:1-6
22. Gerlach H (2004) Risk management in patients with severe acute pancreatitis. Crit Care 8:430-432
23. King NK, Powell JJ, Redhead D et al (2003) A simplified method for computed tomographic estimation of prognosis in acute pancreatitis. Scand J Gastroenterol 38:433-436
24. Triester SL, Kowdley KV (2002) Prognostic factors in acute pancreatitis. J Clin Gastroenterol 34:167-176
25. Sandberg AA, Borgstrom A (2002) Early prediction of severity in acute pancreatitis. Is this possible? Jop 3:116-125
26. Balthazar EJ (2002) Staging of acute pancreatitis. Radiol Clin North Am 40:1199-1209
27. Balthazar EJ (2002) Acute pancreatitis: assessment of severity with clinical and CT evaluation. Radiology 223:603-613
28. Mortele KJ, Wiesner W, Intriere L et al (2004) A modified CT severity index for evaluating acute pancreatitis: improved correlation with patient outcome. AJR Am J Roentgenol 183:1261-1265
29. Balthazar EJ, Robinson DL, Megibow AJ, Ranson JH (1990) Acute pancreatitis: value of CT in establishing prognosis. Radiology 174:331-336
30. Becker V (1973) Proceedings: Fundamental morphological aspects of acute and chronic pancreatitis [author's transl]. Langenbecks Arch Chir 334:317-322
31. Irie H, Honda H, Kuroiwa T et al (1998) MRI of groove pancreatitis. J Comput Assist Tomogr 22:651-655
32. Gabata T, Kadoya M, Terayama N et al (2003) Groove pancreatic carcinomas: radiological and pathological findings. Eur Radiol 13:1679-1684
33. Okazaki K (2005) Autoimmune pancreatitis: etiology, pathogenesis, clinical findings and treatment. The Japanese experience. Jop 6:89-96

34. Sahani DV, Kalva SP, Farrell J et al (2004) Autoimmune pancreatitis: imaging features. Radiology 233:345-352
35. Farrell JJ, Garber J, Sahani D et al (2004) EUS findings in patients with autoimmune pancreatitis. Gastrointest Endosc 60:927-936
36. Wakabayashi T, Kawaura Y, Satomura Y et al (2003) Clinical and imaging features of autoimmune pancreatitis with focal pancreatic swelling or mass formation: comparison with so-called tumor-forming pancreatitis and pancreatic carcinoma. Am J Gastroenterol 98:2679-2687
37. Ito K, Koike S, Matsunaga N (2001) MR imaging of pancreatic diseases. Eur J Radiol 38:78-93
38. Irie H, Honda H, Baba S et al (1998) Autoimmune pancreatitis: CT and MR characteristics. AJR Am J Roentgenol 170:1323-1327
39. Lowenfels AB, Maisonneuve P, Cavallini G et al (1994) Prognosis of chronic pancreatitis: an international multicenter study. International Pancreatitis Study Group. Am J Gastroenterol 89:1467-1471
40. Cho SG, Lee DH, Lee KY et al (2005) Differentiation of chronic focal pancreatitis from pancreatic carcinoma by in vivo proton magnetic resonance spectroscopy. J Comput Assist Tomogr 29:163-169
41. van Kouwen MC, Laverman P, van Krieken JH et al (2005) FDG-PET is able to detect pancreatic carcinoma in chronic pancreatitis. Eur J Nucl Med Mol Imaging 32:399-404
42. Manfredi R, Lucidi V, Gui B et al (2002) Idiopathic chronic pancreatitis in children: MR cholangiopancreatography after secretin administration. Radiology 224:675-682
43. DeBanto JR, Goday PS, Pedroso MR et al (2002) Acute pancreatitis in children. Am J Gastroenterol 97:1726-1731
44. Levy MJ, Geenen JE (2001) Idiopathic acute recurrent pancreatitis. Am J Gastroenterol 96:2540-2555

Diseases of the Pancreas, Part II: Tumors

R.F. Thoeni

Department of Radiology, University of California, San Francisco, CA, USA

Introduction

Ultrasonography may be used as the initial screening method in patients with jaundice and upper abdominal pain and might determine that a pancreatic tumor causes the symptoms, but helical computed tomography (CT), especially multi detector-row helical CT (MDCT), with its superb spatial resolution, is considered the imaging method of choice for detecting neoplastic changes in the pancreas [1-5]. Generally, magnetic resonance imaging (MRI) is used in patients with suspected small pancreatic tumors and as a problem-solving modality that may help to clarify internal architecture, particularly in patients with cystic lesions when CT is equivocal [6-8]. Nevertheless, improved MR sequence design has led to higher tissue contrast and faster scanning that has resulted in more accurate detection and staging of pancreatic neoplasms, particularly of small adenocarcinomas, small islet cell tumors and cystic neoplasms [9]. Endoscopic ultrasonography (EUS) also can detect small pancreatic tumors [10-12] and characterize pancreatic lesions, especially for patients with cystic masses [13]. EUS has shown excellent results in cyst aspiration and biopsies of the pancreas, but is not universally accepted [14, 15]. The role of MRI and CT vis-a-vis EUS needs further definition through exploration of a large series of small pancreatic tumors. Furthermore, it is expected that new EUS instruments with increased resolution and deeper penetration will be developed. A wider acceptance of EUS for the pancreas will depend on training a large number of operators that can provide reproducible results based on standard techniques and possibly, on the use of an intravenous contrast material [16]. In recent years, positron emission tomography (PET), particularly PET/CT, has been increasingly used for assessing patients with suspected pancreatic tumors. However, its ultimate role still needs further definition, as the published results are somewhat conflicting [17-20]. Also, somatostatin receptor scintigraphy has gained popularity in recent years for neuroendocrine tumor detection [21]. This discussion will focus on diagnosing and staging the various pancreatic neoplasms with CT and MRI and will also mention EUS, PET/CT and somatostatin receptor scintigraphy where appropriate.

Ductal Adenocarcinoma of the Pancreas

About 90% of all neoplasm of the pancreas are ductal adenocarcinomas. It is a common neoplastic disease with a poor prognosis. It is estimated that approximately 32,000 Americans will die of this disease in 2005 [22]. Pancreas carcinoma is the fourth leading cause of death in the USA and its five-year survival rate remains dismal, at less than 5%. This poor outcome is largely related to the aggressiveness of the tumor and in most cases, to late diagnosis. The initial diagnosis of pancreatic tumor, particularly if the patient presents with jaundice and the tumor is located in the head, may be made by ultrasound. Ultrasonographic signs of pancreatic carcinoma include focal or diffuse pancreatic mass, which is hypoechoic relative to normal gland parenchyma, and dilatation of the pancreatic and/or biliary ducts. The accuracy of ultrasound for detecting the level of bile duct obstruction varies greatly, and its staging of pancreatic carcinoma is inferior to that of CT. Ultrasonography often fails to provide an adequate examination of the entire gland, resulting in an overall decrease in sensitivity. Some of these limitations are overcome by endosonography, but even for EUS, tumors in the tail of the pancreas are not always accessible.

For optimal evaluation of pancreatic adenocarcinomas by MDCT, a dual- or triple-phase pancreas protocol should be used that includes thin sections (1.25-2.5 mm) and a rapidly delivered bolus of contrast material (we use 150 ml at 4-5 ml/sec). Water as oral contrast material is best for better assessing extension of the tumor to the stomach and/or duodenum. We recommend a scan delay of 20 sec for the arterial phase, a scan delay of 40-45 sec for the pancreatic phase and a scan delay of 80 sec for the hepatic phase. The arterial phase permits evaluation of vascular involvement by tumor and is best for 3D angiography, if requested by surgery. Vascular involvement and tumor mass are best detected in the late arterial or pancreatic phase, whereas the hepatic phase serves for visualizing the liver and entire abdomen to detect liver metastases and peritoneal seeding [23]. Some authors have shown that the early arterial phase may not be needed [23], and in at least one recent publication, a single-phase thin-slice MDCT technique was recommended for best results in assessing resectability of pancreatic adenocarcinoma [24].

On CT, pancreatic adenocarcinoma arises from the pancreatic duct and usually appears as a low-density mass often associated with poorly defined margins and pancreatic and/or bile duct dilatation (Fig. 1). The low-density central zone represents the hypovascular, scirrhous tumor surrounded by normal parenchyma or inflammatory tissue caused by obstructive pancreatitis. Cystic degeneration is occasionally seen [13]. Frequently, pancreatic duct obstruction causes atrophy of the pancreatic parenchyma and only a thin rim of parenchyma may be seen accompanying a dilated duct. Tumor obstruction of the main pancreatic duct can lead to rupture of side branches, resulting in formation of pseudocysts. Occasionally, no low-density mass is identified, but a dilated duct is seen proximal to a small imperceptible tumor mass. Ancillary findings are local tumor extension including direct invasion of neighboring organs and vessels (loss of fat planes surrounding the celiac axis, SMA, etc., so-called vascular 'cuffing') and metastatic disease to local lymph nodes, as well as spread to liver, peritoneum (often associated with ascites) and more distant sites. The so-called 'double-duct sign' (dilatation of the biliary and pancreatic ducts) occurs in less than 5% of patients with pancreatic carcinoma. Biductal obstruction also may be seen in bile duct or ampullary carcinoma, pancreatitis and ampullary stenosis.

If MRI is used, T1-weighted fat-suppressed sequences and dynamic gadolinium-enhanced spoiled gradient echo (SPGR) sequences appear to be superior to T2-weighted sequences due to the fact that most pancreatic carcinomas have a significant desmoplastic reaction that renders the tumor less conspicuous on T2-weighted images. T1-weighted fat-suppressed images using an early (arterial) gadolinium-enhanced SPGR sequence provide the best delineation of the tumor, particularly if it is small.

CT imaging results for pancreatic carcinoma vary widely, but with current generation scanners and state-of-the-art scanning techniques, a sensitivity of more than 90% for detecting pancreatic carcinoma can be achieved [1, 24]. Small metastatic implants on liver and peritoneum are the most likely lesions to be missed by CT. CT generally provides accurate information on vascular involvement as long as a pancreatic protocol is observed and for resectability, sensitivities of more than 80% have been obtained [1]. Presently, most studies show a slight advantage of helical CT over MR for detecting and staging pancreatic adenocarcinomas. A recent meta-analysis that compared CT, MRI and US, demonstrated a sensitivity and specificity of 91% and 85% for helical CT and a sensitivity and specificity of 84% and 82%, respectively for MRI [1]. In the same analysis for determining resectability, the sensitivity and specificity of helical CT was 81% and 82% and for MRI it was 82% and 78%. For US, the sensitivity for diagnosing pancreas carcinoma was much lower, as was the specificity for determining

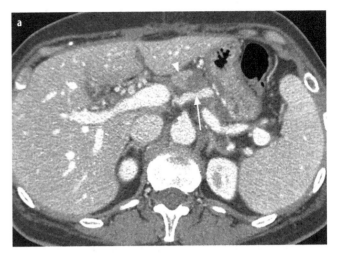

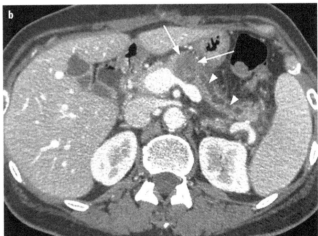

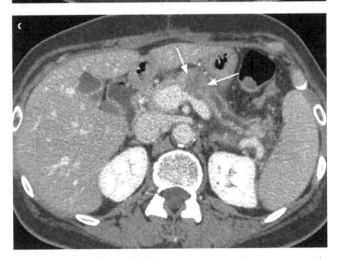

Fig. 1. a Thin-section MDCT of pancreas carcinoma, pancreatic phase. A low-attenuation mass is apparent in the distal body of pancreas with slight indentation of the splenic artery (*arrow*). This appearance does not necessarily constitute adherence or invasion, and a graft or stent can be placed due to the short segment involved. The mass is easily distinguished from adjacent normal pancreas (*arrowhead*). **b** Thin-section MDCT of pancreas carcinoma, pancreatic phase, 1 cm below 1a. Note the oval-shaped mass of low attenuation (*arrows*) and the dilated pancreatic duct (*arrowheads*) abruptly ending at the mass. **c** Thin-section MDCT of pancreas carcinoma, hepatic phase, same level as 1b. While the mass (*arrows*) is still evident, it is less conspicuous in the hepatic phase

resectability. Only one MR study using gadolinium and MR angiography revealed superiority over CT. The advantage of MRI is thought to be in the area of small tumors, which do not alter the contour of the gland [25]. At present, CT is the modality of choice in the work-up of suspected pancreatic disease and MRI appears to be a problem solving modality. MRI may be helpful in cases where clinical suspicion of disease is very high but results with MDCT are negative or equivocal. In addition, when choosing an imaging modality, one has to take into account the fact that with MDCT, imaging of the pancreas, including preparation, takes a small fraction of the time needed for a complete MRI of the pancreas. Overall, MR of the pancreas should be considered in patients (1) with elevated serum creatinine, allergy to iodine contrast, or other contraindications for iodine contrast administration; (2) with prior CT imaging who have focal enlargement of the pancreas with no definable mass; (3) whose clinical history suggests malignancy and in whom CT imaging is equivocal or difficult to interpret; and (4) whose case requires distinction between chronic pancreatitis with focal enlargement and pancreatic cancer [6].

False positive diagnoses of pancreatic cancer occur, especially in patients with chronic pancreatitis, and, therefore, percutaneous aspiration biopsies are needed if nonoperative treatment is planned. Fine-needle aspiration biopsy of pancreatic cancer under CT-guidance is a frequently performed procedure and is associated with severe pancreatitis in less than 3% of cases. Pancreatitis is more likely to occur if normal parenchyma is biopsied. Therefore, biopsies should be carefully planned by placing the needle into the mass itself and by avoiding puncture of the pancreatic duct. The sensitivity of percutaneous CT biopsies reaches 79%, with a positive predictive value of 100% and a negative predictive value of 47% [14]. Because of possible tumor seeding in the needle tract, patients with potentially resectable tumors (only 10% of all cases) who are acceptable candidates for surgery should undergo exploratory surgery [10]. Today, percutaneous CT biopsies of the pancreas are often replaced by endoscopic biopsies that have a sensitivity of 80% with a positive predictive value of 99% and a negative predictive value of 73%, particularly if CT is equivocal or negative with a strong clinical suspicion of tumor and when the lesion is less than 3 cm in size [14].

While EUS excels at detecting even small pancreatic adenocarcinomas, reaching sensitivities as high as 97% [16] and can be used in the differential diagnosis of pancreatic tumors, it demonstrates poor sensitivity and specificity for diagnosing vascular involvement by tumor [26]. EUS suffers from limited depth penetration and cannot always distinguish between an inflammatory and neoplastic process in the pancreas.

PET, and particularly PET/CT, has emerged as an important modality for effectively managing patients with suspected pancreatic cancer. Nevertheless, more studies are needed to demonstrate its true value and cost-effectiveness, since some of the studies found no benefit over

CT alone [17]. In one PET study, if helical CT was positive for pancreas carcinoma, PET was found to have a sensitivity of 92% and a specificity of 68% and if CT was negative, the sensitivity of PET was 73% and the specificity 86% [20]. PET/CT allows a more precise localization of hot tracer spots and has been shown to improve patient management before possible resection. In one PET/CT study, management was changed in 16% of patients with pancreatic cancer that were initially staged as being resectable [18]. In suspected tumor recurrence, PET reliably detected local recurrence and was advantageous in diagnosing distant disease [19].

Neuroendocrine Tumors of the Pancreas

Functioning Neuroendocrine Tumors

Among functioning neuroendocrine tumors (NET, formerly called islet cell tumors) of the pancreas, insulinoma is the most common tumor, followed by gastrinoma, glucagonoma, VIPoma and other secretory neoplasms, which are more rarely encountered. In functioning pancreatic adenomas, the clinical diagnosis is based on clinical data and laboratory tests that usually permit an accurate diagnosis. Cross-sectional imaging is used only for localizing the pancreatic neoplasm.

NETs represent a challenge to the radiologist. Extrapancreatic NETs that are small and located in the duodenal or gastric wall are the least likely to be detected preoperatively by any of the radiographic techniques, and even intraoperative ultrasonography fails to detect these lesions. These ectopic lesions are more likely to occur in patients with multiple endocrine adenomatosis (MEA) or multiple endocrine neoplasia (MEN). For insulinomas, angiography is reported to reach sensitivities between 59 and 80%, while venous sampling reaches sensitivities between 77 and 94%, with results slightly better for gastrinomas [27]. A combination of intraoperative palpation and intraoperative ultrasonography was found to achieve best results during surgery. Intraoperative ultrasound is particularly important in patients with multiple lesions and MEN, as under these conditions, ectopic tumors are quite frequent and often difficult to find with CT or MRI.

On CT and MRI, functioning NETs show intense enhancement in the arterial phase with rapid wash-out in the portal venous phase (Fig. 2). The most common NET, the insulinoma, is usually small ($\leq$ 2 cm in diameter). Metastases occur in only 5-10% of cases. All other NETs tend to be large and have metastases in 60-65% of cases. The appearance of liver metastases in patients with functioning NET is similar to that of the primary tumor.

The reported sensitivity of conventional CT for detecting an insulinoma ranges from 28-79% with a mean of 38% and is slightly higher for gastrinomas, primarily due to their larger size. The dual-phase MDCT protocol with thin sections improved the detection rate to 94% and reached 100% if combined with EUS [28]. Endoscopic

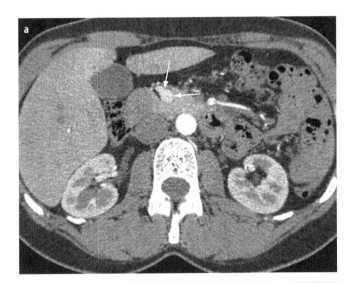

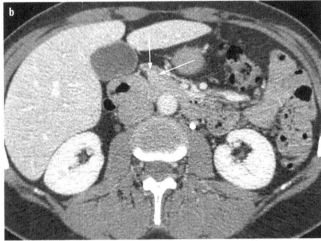

Fig. 2. a Thin-section MDCT of a neuroendocrine tumor of the pancreas (insulinoma), early arterial phase. A small hypervascular mass (*arrows*) is seen in the neck of the pancreas. **b** Thin-section MDCT of a neuroendocrine tumor of the pancreas (insulinoma), hepatic phase. In this phase the mass in the neck of the pancreas (*arrows*) is barely seen

ultrasound provides excellent results in the head of the pancreas, but results are less convincing for the tail of the pancreas because of its distance from the stomach. EUS usually allows detection of even small NETs and their precise location. Ectopic gastrinomas may be missed by EUS, but combination with somatostatin receptor scintigraphy increases the combined overall sensitivity to 93% for gastrinomas [10]. The sensitivity of transabdominal ultrasound for detecting insulinomas ranges from 19-60% with a mean of 46%, and therefore should not be used for this purpose.

Functioning NETs of the pancreas are of low signal intensity on T1-weighted and of high signal intensity on T2-weighted images [8]. Occasionally, an insulinoma can be of dark signal intensity on T2-weighted sequences due to a fibrous stroma. In our study, we reached a MRI sensitivity of 85% for detecting functioning NETs of 2 cm

or less in diameter, which is similar to the sensitivity achieved by invasive procedures and is superior to most of the MRI results reported in the literature [8]. Previous MR series reported a sensitivity of 100% [29], but the number of patients examined was small. For gastrinomas, some reports have shown MRI sensitivities of 25-62% [30, 31]. With present techniques, MRI should detect lesions greater than 2 cm, with a sensitivity of greater than 85%. Therefore, MRI appears to be a useful technique for diagnosing small pancreatic NETs, but optimal MRI techniques and state-of-the-art equipment need to be used. Overall, MRI results are presently surpassed by contrast-enhanced MDCT because of volume imaging and very thin sections.

Somatostatin receptor scintigraphy using various derivatives of long-acting somatostatin analogues [21] can be used for small gastrinomas, somatostatinoma, glucagonoma, carcinoid and VIPoma, but insulinomas may be missed due to reduced receptor expression [32]. Somatostatin receptor scintigraphy with ^{111}In-octreotide can often diagnose small lesions only suspected on CT or MRI [33] and detect metastases not diagnosed with other modalities.

Non-functioning Neuroendocrine Tumors

The non-functioning endocrine tumor is the third most common NET and represents 15-25% of all these tumors. It arises from alpha or beta cells. The neoplasm is hormonally quiescent (probably with very minimal secretion) and often presents as a mass with or without jaundice or gastric outlet obstruction. The tumor is usually located in the pancreatic head and can measure up to 20 cm in diameter. There may be solid and necrotic components and coarse calcifications are present in up to 25%. The mass is hypervascular, with a late capillary stain. The tumor does not encase vessels but in 80-100% of cases shows malignant transformation with liver metastases and adenopathy. The five-year survival is 44%. The key features of non-functioning NETs are large size, hypervascularity and absence of vascular encasement. Results with CT and MRI are similar.

Cystic Neoplasms of the Pancreas

Serous and Mucinous Cystic Neoplasms of the Pancreas

Cystic neoplasms of the pancreas are uncommon tumors and are seen in less than 5% of pancreatic neoplasms. Pancreatic cystic neoplasms are classified into two categories, serous cystic (usually microcystic, occasionally unilocular) neoplasms that are benign, and mucinous cystic (macrocystic) neoplasms that are potentially malignant or already malignant at the time of diagnosis. There is a rare macrocystic variant, which is benign and exhibits radiological features similar to those of mucinous cystadenoma. Serous and mucinous cystic neoplasms, except for intraductal papillary mucinous tumors (IPMT) do not communicate with the pancreatic duct.

Serous cystic neoplasms of the pancreas are observed in middle-aged and elderly women. This type of tumor rarely requires surgical treatment, whereas mucinous cystic tumors should be resected because of their malignant potential. Nevertheless, some surgeons prefer to resect the serous type as well. In general, the patient's age, overall condition, location of the lesion, and growth over time are factors that help in deciding if surgery is needed [34]. Often any cyst that increases in size, any symptomatic cyst, and cysts in older fit patients are selected for surgery. CT can accomplish preoperative differentiation of the two types in many cases. In serous cystic tumors, traditionally the diagnosis is made if the number of cysts within the tumor is more than six and the diameters of the cysts less than 2 cm [35, 36]. A newer nomenclature calls cysts ≤ 1 cm definitely serous, > 1-2 cm equivocal and > 2 cm definitely mucinous. Grossly, these serous tumors appear either as solid tumors with innumerable tiny cysts, or as honeycombed cystic tumors, depending on the amount of connective tissue. They have a lobulated margin. At times, it is difficult to visualize the cystic areas. Calcifications in serous tumors are central in location and more common than in mucinous tumors. A central enhancing scar may be present and is characteristic of a serous tumor [13].

Mucinous cystic neoplasms of the pancreas (also called cystadenomas and cystadenocarcinomas according to the old nomenclature) have six or fewer cysts, the diameters of the cysts measure more than 2 cm, a central enhancing scar is rarely seen, and calcifications are peripheral [13] (Fig. 3). The margins usually are smooth, and metastatic disease may be present at the time of diagnosis.

Based on the above-mentioned criteria, a correct diagnosis of a serous cystic pancreatic tumor can be made in

62% of cases by CT, in 74% by sonography and in 84% using both modalities [35]. In general, results for mucinous cystic tumors are inferior. Pancreatic pseudocysts and cystic forms of islet cell tumors, ductal carcinomas, solid and papillary tumors and lymphangioma of the pancreas can be indistinguishable from cystic neoplasms on CT. Thus, needle biopsies of the lesions often are necessary.

MRI often can provide better definition of the internal architecture of these cystic neoplasms than CT. Septa and wall thickness of the lesions are well demonstrated by MRI, but calcifications are not always seen. Also, differentiation between serous and mucinous compartments is superior by MRI. MRI is of great help in distinguishing these cystic neoplasms from pseudocysts of the pancreas, particularly if they are multiple. Both MRCP and MDCT with curved planar reconstruction can demonstrate the absence of a connection to the main pancreatic duct.

Intraductal Papillary Mucinous Tumor of the Pancreas

The intraductal papillary mucinous tumor (IPMT, formerly also called ductectatic cystadenoma or ductectatic cystadenocarcinoma) of the pancreas is a rare tumor that is considered a subtype of the mucinous cystic neoplasms of the pancreas. IPMT can be classified as main duct, branch duct (side-branch) or mixed type, depending on the site and extent of involvement [37]. The cystic changes always demonstrate a connection to the pancreatic duct, a diagnostic feature that can be seen on MDCT and MRI. The branch duct tumor consists of cystic dilation of the side branches of the pancreatic duct, usually in the uncinate process. These ducts are lined with atypical, hyperplastic or clearly malignant epithelium. In the late stages, the tumor nodules of the ducts produce copious mucinous secretions, which fill the entire duct. In branch duct IPMT the overall prognosis is good because extension into the parenchyma and beyond occurs relatively late and overall malignant degeneration is rare. Malignancy is present in 25-44% of resected specimens of the other two types. Resection is therefore the treatment of choice in these patients.

CT shows markedly dilated ducts and cystic-appearing structures filled with mucinous material, which has slightly higher attenuation than that of water. MRI can detect the higher signal intensity of mucin on T1-weighted sequences. MRI appears to have a slight advantage over CT because it can visualize the internal architecture of the lesion slightly better than CT, including a solid mass and mural nodules, which are signs of malignancy. EUS also is well suited to detect mural nodules.

Solid and Cystic Papillary Neoplasm of the Pancreas

Papillary solid and cystic tumors, also called solid pseudopapillary tumors of the pancreas, are rare tumors, and are seen almost exclusively in young women and are located mostly in the tail of the pancreas. This tumor is characterized by a solid peripheral area of tumor and a

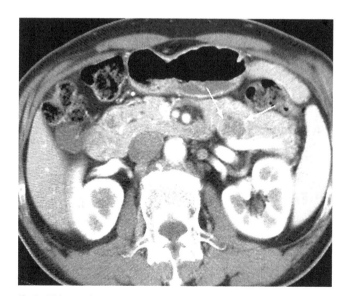

Fig. 3. Thin-section MDCT of serous cystic neoplasm of the pancreas, pancreatic phase. A lobulated and septated cystic mass is present in the body of the pancreas (*arrows*). The individual cysts are small

central zone of degeneration consisting of hemorrhage and cystic spaces filled with necrotic debris that can be visualized by CT and MR. On imaging, these tumors appear as sharply defined, heterogeneous, large cystic pancreatic masses with solid components [38, 39]. Calcifications may be present in the capsule or in the inner portion of the mass. EUS also can be helpful in visualizing the nodules and internal architecture of these masses.

References

1. Bipat S, Phoa SS, van Delden OM et al (2005) Ultrasonography, computed tomography and magnetic resonance imaging for diagnosis and determining resectability of pancreatic adenocarcinoma: a meta-analysis. J Comput Assist Tomogr 29:438-445
2. Schima W, Fugger R, Schober E et al (2002) Diagnosis and staging of pancreatic cancer: comparison of mangafodipir trisodium-enhanced MR imaging and contrast-enhanced helical hydro-CT. AJR Am J Roentgenol 179:717-724
3. Sheridan MB, Ward J, Guthrie JA et al (1999) Dynamic contrast-enhanced MR imaging and dual-phase helical CT in the preoperative assessment of suspected pancreatic cancer: a comparative study with receiver operating characteristic analysis. AJR Am J Roentgenol 173:583-590
4. Tabuchi T, Itoh K, Ohshio G et al (1999) Tumor staging of pancreatic adenocarcinoma using early- and late-phase helical CT. AJR Am J Roentgenol 173:375-380
5. Gangi S, Fletcher JG, Nathan MA et al (2004) Time interval between abnormalities seen on CT and the clinical diagnosis of pancreatic cancer: retrospective review of CT scans obtained before diagnosis. AJR Am J Roentgenol 182:897-903
6. Pamuklar E, Semelka RC (2005) MR imaging of the pancreas. Magn Reson Imaging Clin N Am 13:313-330
7. Gabata T, Matsui O, Kadoya M et al (1994) Small pancreatic adenocarcinomas: efficacy of MR imaging with fat suppression and gadolinium enhancement. Radiology 193:683-688
8. Thoeni RF, Mueller-Lisse UG, Chan R et al (2000) Detection of small, functional islet cell tumors in the pancreas: Selection of MRI Imaging sequences for optimal sensitivity. Radiology 214:483-490
9. Semelka RC, Kroeker MA, Shoenut JP et al (1991) Pancreatic disease: prospective comparison of CT, ERCP, and 1.5 T MR imaging with dynamic Gadolinium enhancement and fat suppression. Radiology 181:785-791
10. Midwinter MJ, Beveridge CJ, Wilsdon JB et al (1999) Correlation between spiral computed tomography, endoscopic ultrasonography and findings at operation in pancreatic and ampullary tumours. Br J Surg 86:189-193
11. McLean AM, Fairclough PD (2005) Endoscopic ultrasound in the localisation of pancreatic islet cell tumours. Best Pract Res Clin Endocrinol Metab 19:177-193
12. Canto MI, Goggins M, Yeo CJ et al (2004) Screening for pancreatic neoplasia in high-risk individuals: an EUS-based approach. Clin Gastroenterol Hepatol 2:606-621
13. Sahani DV, Kadavigere R, Saokar A et al (2005) Cystic Pancreatic Lesions: A Simple Imaging-based Classification System for Guiding Management. Radiographics 25:1471-1484
14. Volmar KE, Vollmer RT, Jowell PS et al (2005) Pancreatic FNA in 1000 cases: a comparison of imaging modalities. Gastrointest Endosc 61:854-861
15. Ardengh JC, de Paulo GA, Ferrari AP (2004) EUS-guided FNA in the diagnosis of pancreatic neuroendocrine tumors before surgery. Gastrointest Endosc 60:378-384
16. Maguchi H (2004) The roles of endoscopic ultrasonography in the diagnosis of pancreatic tumors. J Hepatobiliary Pancreat Surg 11:1-3
17. Lytras D, Connor S, Bosonnet L et al (2005) Positron emission tomography does not add to computed tomography for the diagnosis and staging of pancreatic cancer. Dig Surg 22:55-61
18. Heinrich S, Goerres GW, Schafer M et al (2005) Positron emission tomography/computed tomography influences on the management of resectable pancreatic cancer and its cost-effectiveness. Ann Surg 242:235-243
19. Ruf J, Lopez Hanninen E, Oettle H et al (2005) Detection of recurrent pancreatic cancer: comparison of FDG-PET with CT/MRI. Pancreatology 5:266-272
20. Orlando LA, Kulasingam SL, Matchar DB (2004) Meta-analysis: the detection of pancreatic malignancy with positron emission tomography. Aliment Pharmacol Ther 20:1063-1070
21. Virgolini I, Traub-Weidinger T, Decristoforo C (2005) Nuclear medicine in the detection and management of pancreatic islet-cel tumours. Best Pract Res Clin Endocrinol Metab 19:213-227
22. American Cancer Society 2005: http://www.cancer.org/docroot/STT/stt_0.asp
23. Fletcher JG, Wiersema MJ, Farrell MA et al (2003) Pancreatic malignancy: value of arterial, pancreatic, and hepatic phase imaging with multi-detector row CT. Radiology 229:81-90
24. Imbriaco M, Megibow AJ, Ragozzino A et al (2005) Value of the single-phase technique in MDCT assessment of pancreatic tumors. AJR Am J Roentgenol 184:1111-1117
25. Mitchell DG, Vinitski S, Saponaro S et al (1991) Liver and pancreas: improved spin-echo T1 contrast by shorter echo time and fat suppression at 1.5 T. Radiology 178:67-71
26. Aslanian H, Salem R, Lee J et al (2005) EUS diagnosis of vascular invasion in pancreatic cancer: surgical and histologic correlates. Am J Gastroenterol 100:1381-1385
27. Schumacher B, Lübke HJ, Frieling T et al (1996) Prospective study on the detection of insulinomas by endoscopic ultrasonography. Endoscopy 28:273-276
28. Gouya H et al (2003) CT, EUS combined protocol for preoperative evaluation of pancreatic insulinoma. AJR Am J Roentgenol 181:987-992
29. Semelka RC, Cumming MJ, Shoenut JP et al (1993) Islet cell tumors: comparison of dynamic contrast-enhanced CT and MR imaging with dynamic gadolinium enhancement and fat suppression. Radiology 186:799-802
30. Pisegna JR, Doppman JL, Norton JA et al (1993) Prospective comparative study of the ability of MR imaging and other imaging modalities to localize tumors in patients with Zollinger-Ellison syndrome. Dig Dis Sci 38:1318-1320
31. Tjon A Tham RT, Falke TH et al (1989) CT and MR imaging of advanced Zollinger-Ellison syndrome. J Comput Assist Tomogr 13:821-828
32. Nikou GC, Toubanakis C, Nikolaou P et al (2005) VIPomas: an update in diagnosis and management in a series of 11 patients. Hepatogastroenterology 52:1259-1265
33. Corleto VD, Scopinaro F, Angeletti S et al (1996) Somatostatin receptor localization of pancreatic endocrine tumors. World J Surg 20:241-244
34. Spinelli KS, Fromwiller TE, Daniel RA et al (2004) Cystic Pancreatic neoplasms: Observe or operate. Annals of Surgery 239:651-659
35. Procacci C, Graziani R, Bicego E et al (1997) Serous cystadenoma of the pancreas: report of 30 cases with emphasis on the imaging findings. J Comp Assist Tomogr 21:373-382
36. Gouhiri M, Soyer P, Barbagelatta M et al (1999) Macrocystic serous cystadenoma of the pancreas: CT and endosonographic features. Abdom Imaging 24:72-74
37. Kawamoto S, Horton KM, Lawler LP et al (2005) Intraductal papillary mucinous neoplasm of the pancreas: can benign lesions be differentiated from malignant lesions with multidetector CT? Radiographics 25:1451-1468
38. Buetow PC, Buck JL, Pantongrag-Brown L et al (1996) Solid and papillary epithelial neoplasm of the pancreas: imaging-pathologic correlation on 56 cases. Radiology 199:707-711
39. Merkle EM, Weber CH, Siech M et al (1996) Papillary cystic and solid tumor of the pancreas. Z Gastroenterol 34:743-746

Imaging of Diseases of the Bile Ducts and Gallbladder

C.D. Becker

Diagnostic and Interventional Radiology, University Hospital of Geneva, Geneva, Switzerland

Introduction

Diagnostic imaging plays a key role in the management of diseases of the bile ducts and gallbladder. Although ultrasonography (US) remains the first-line imaging modality for suspected biliary obstruction and even the standard of reference for cholecystolithiasis, it is mainly computed tomography (CT) and, even more, magnetic resonance (MR) imaging that have replaced invasive diagnostic procedures such as endoscopic retrograde cholangiography (ERCP) and percutaneous retrograde cholangiography (PTC) in the majority of diagnostic settings. The different noninvasive and invasive imaging modalities often provide similar or complementary diagnostic information, so the choice of the most appropriate imaging modality for a given indication is often influenced by a variety of factors, including individual patient characteristics, local preferences, local availability, and economic aspects.

This course is intended to provide a practical radiologic approach to biliary diseases and is divided into two parts. In the first part, the diagnostic key elements are reviewed and the advantages and shortcomings of the different modalities are discussed. In the second part, the diagnostic features of selected groups of benign and malignant conditions of the bile ducts and gallbladder are summarized.

Ultrasonography

Real-time US is the method of choice for initial screening of patients with suspected disorders of the gallbladder and the intra- and extrahepatic bile ducts. The main advantages of US are its very high accuracy for the detection of gallbladder disease and dilatation of the intra- and extrahepatic bile ducts, easy availability, and low cost. However, US is an operator-dependent method, and artifacts due to bowel gas and obesity commonly result in insufficient visualization of the distal common bile duct. Therefore, US is not an appropriate test to rule out bile duct calculi. *Endoscopic ultrasonography* (EUS) can be combined with fiberoptic upper GI endoscopy. Although more costly than US and not entirely noninvasive, EUS is

much less influenced by the above limitations. Using high-frequency transducers, EUS can obtain images with very good spatial resolution, although with a very limited depth. In experienced hands, EUS may serve as a valuable complementary tool for the dedicated evaluation of special areas, particularly the intrapancreatic portion of the common bile duct, and the ampullary region.

Computed Tomography (CT)

CT is less limited by artifacts, is less operator-dependent than US and reliably enables visualization of the entire biliary system in virtually all patients. Contrast-material-enhanced mulitslice CT (MSCT) studies with 1-2 mm sections enable multiplanar or curved reformatting, and are thus very suitable for the definition of the exact level of bile duct obstruction and the nature and extent of soft tissue masses causing ductal compression. Image processing with curved reconstructions allows visualization of the common bile duct in its entire length (Fig. 1),

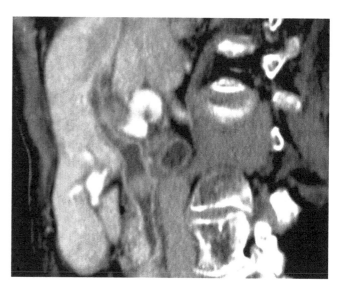

Fig. 1. Choledocholithiasis. MSCT (curved coronal reconstruction) showing a large calculus in the main common bile duct

and minimum intensity algorithms allow the dilated biliary tree visualized with CT to be better delineated (Fig. 2a). It must be recognized, however, that despite its excellent contrast resolution, CT has a limited sensitivity for the detection of cholesterol calculi that are often isodense with the surrounding bile. Therefore, CT cannot be considered as the method of choice to rule out calculous disease. CT-angiography with two-dimensional (2D) and three-dimensional (3D) reconstruction has largely replaced catheter angiography for preoperative delineation of the major arterial and portal venous branches prior to surgery.

Cholangiographic Techniques Using Iodinated Contrast Material

The term *CT cholangiography* refers to MSCT acquisition usually including 2D or 3D reformatted images obtained after the administration of intravenous cholangiographic agents. Since bile duct opacification depends on intact hepatic excretory function, it cannot be used in patients with significant hyperbilirubinemia. For this reason, but also because the cholangiographic agents are unavailable in several countries, CT cholangiography has only a minor role in daily practice.

ERCP and *percutaneous transhepatic cholangiography* (PTC) are used to opacify the biliary system directly by means of contrast material under fluoroscopic vision. Their main diagnostic advantage is the superior spatial resolution of the biliary anatomy, offering maximum anatomic detail (Fig. 2). ERCP is often used as the first-line approach, whereas PTC is mainly used when ERCP fails due to technical reasons or cannot be performed,

e.g., in the presence of surgical anastomoses. The main advantage of ERCP and PTC is that therapeutic interventions may be performed during the same session, which is how these procedures are currently most commonly performed.

MR Imaging

MR cholangiopancreatography (MRCP) is based on the principle that stationary fluids are signal intense on heavily T2-weighted images as opposed to soft tissue structures, solid materials such as calculi, or blood vessels that contain flowing blood. MRCP thus enables the visualization of bile ducts, intraductal calculi, stenoses, and anatomical variants of the biliary system, without the need for contrast material and independent of excretory function. Modern MR techniques enable image acquisition within very short breath-hold intervals (Fig. 3-6). MRCP has rapidly become recognized as an attractive alternative to the established noninvasive imaging techniques for imaging of the biliary system because it has no known side effects and because it has yielded excellent diagnostic results for both bile duct calculi and stenoses. MRCP may now be considered as a very accurate technique for the diagnosis of bile duct calculi and stenoses, provided that the imaging parameters are chosen correctly and that image interpretation is based on both coronal and transverse images. With modern equipment, MR images are acquired in short breath-hold intervals with very consistent quality and excellent resolution. Hepatobiliary contrast materials such as Mangafodipir (Mn-DPDP) are excreted into the bile ducts and allow direct visualization of the biliary tree on

Fig. 2. Primary sclerosing cholangitis (PSC) **a** MSCT image reconstruction with a coronal minimum intensity projection algorithm showing dilated peripheral intrahepatic bile ducts with caliber irregularities. **b** Percutaneous transhepatic cholangiography showing multiple irregularities of the intra- and extrahepatic bile ducts consistent with diffuse inflammatory strictures in the context of advanced PSC

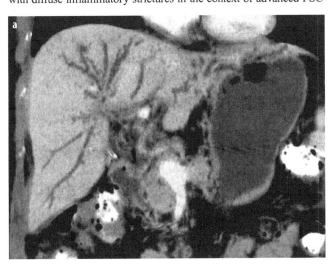

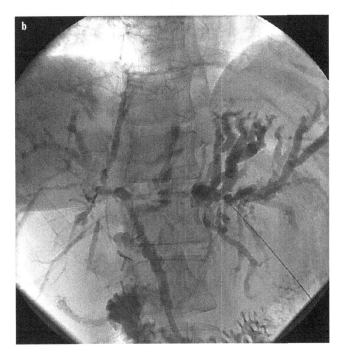

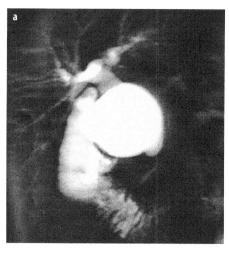

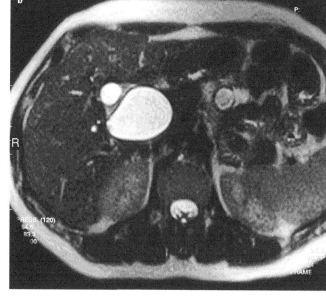

Fig. 3. Choledochal cyst. T2- weighted 'EXPRESS' image in the coronal projection (**a**) and transverse plane (**b**) delineates the morphology and extent of the cystic malformation, making direct cholangiography unnecessary prior to surgery

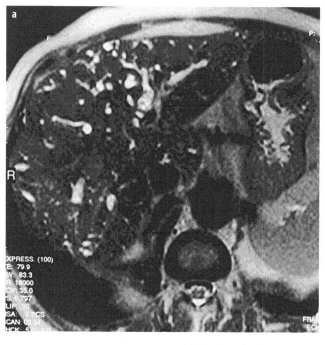

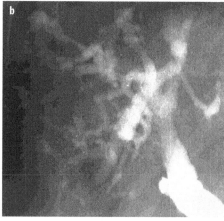

Fig. 4. Caroli's disease. T2-weighted transverse 'EXPRESS' image (**a**) and ERCP image (**b**) show club-like outpouchings of the peripheral intrahepatic bile ducts. Note calculus seen on (**a**)

T1-weighted images. There are some specific clinical indications in the context of bile duct imaging, such as post-operative or post-traumatic bile leaks [1].

Radiologic Diagnosis of Selected Bile Duct Pathologies

Some diagnostic key questions are summarized in Table 1.

Choledocholithiasis is present in approximately 15% of patients undergoing cholecystectomy. The sensitivity of US for bile duct calculi varies widely, from less than 30% to over 70%, but there is a general consensus that US is not sufficiently reliable to rule out bile duct calculi. Although the reported sensitivity of CT is between 80% and 90%, MRCP is superior to CT and may currently be considered the most sensitive noninvasive technique for the detection of bile duct stones; several studies have confirmed that appropriate, modern MRCP technique enables the detection of more than 95% of calculi [2, 3].

Primary sclerosing cholangitis (PSC) is a chronic, noninfectious inflammatory disorder that results in progressive,

Table 1. Diagnostic key elements

- Stone disease (cholecystolithiasis, choledocholithiasis, intrahepatic lithiasis, Mirizzi syndrome)
- Postoperative situations (previous cholecystectomy, sphincterotomy or bilio-digestive anastomosis resulting in enlarged bile ducts, pneumobilia, acute bile leakage, etc.)
- Presence of dilatation of intra- or extrahepatic bile ducts
- Level of bile duct dilatation (intrahepatic/bifurcation/common hepatic, ampulla)
- Cause of bile duct dilatation (stone, solid or cystic mass, stenosis, functional disorder)
- Vascular changes (infiltration/ thrombosis of portal vessels, hepatic arteries)

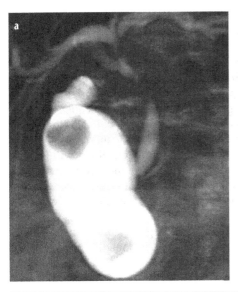

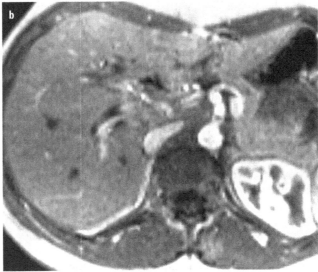

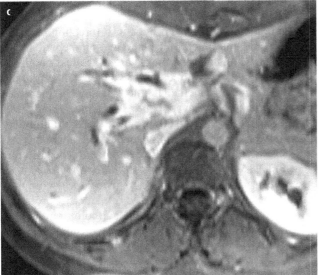

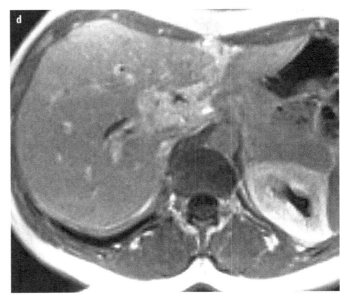

Fig. 5. Cholangiocarcinoma at the level of the common hepatic duct. **a** Breathhold coronary projection (T2-weighted 'EXPRESS') image showing a stenosis of the common hepatic duct, involving the hepatic bifurcation. Dynamic Gadolinium-enhanced T1-weighted GRE images in the arterial phase (**b**), portal venous phase (**c**) and equilibrium phase (**d**) show the tumor as an enhancing, hyperintense mass

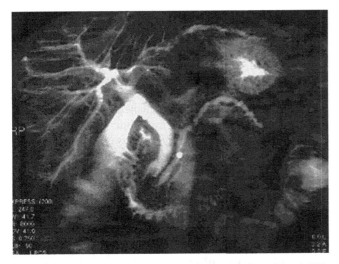

Fig. 6. Adenocarcinoma of the ampullary region. T2-weighted 'EXPRESS' image shows a large mass displacing the duodenum and an intraductal component of the tumor, causing obstruction

multiple stenoses of the intra- and extrahepatic bile ducts, eventually resulting in obliteration of intrahepatic ducts and asymmetrical hepatic atrophy. The etiology is unclear, but there is an association with inflammatory bowel disease and other conditions. Initially, there is edema and proliferation of connective tissue in the periportal spaces and around the bile ducts. Progressive extension of fibrotic proliferation into the hepatic parenchyma eventually results in biliary cirrhosis. Although stenoses of the bile ducts may be solitary, typical cholangiographic features include multifocal stenoses of the bile ducts, often with bilateral intrahepatic involvement. However, dilatation of the peripheral ducts is usually less prominent than with stenosis of other origin because the bile duct walls become thickened and rigid due to the inflammatory process and therefore are less prone to passive dilatation (Fig. 2). PSC significantly predisposes to transformation into cholangiocarcinoma and should therefore be considered a premalignant condition. The distinction between PSC and cholangiocarcinoma may be impossible with imaging tests alone. In the presence of PSC, adenopathy of the hepatoduodenal ligament or in the celiac or pancreaticoduodenal region is often due to reactive inflammation and should not by itself be taken as a strong indicator of malignant degeneration. Cross-sectional imaging techniques are now being primarily used. Although the diagnosis of PSC may be straightforward in the presence of mild, irregular, multisegmental intrahepatic bile duct dilatation without demonstration of a distinct mass, it must be kept in mind that early stages of the disease may be very difficult to detect and that correlation with hepatic biopsy may be required. Besides irregular, multisegmental intrahepatic bile duct dilatation, US may demonstrate focal or generalized thickening and hyperechogenicity of the walls of the intra- and extrahepatic bile ducts. The CT signs of PSC include nodularity and enhancement of the wall of intra- or extrahepatic bile ducts, mild multifocal intra- or extrahepatic biliary dilatation leading to patterns such as skip lesions, pruning, and beading. The typical findings of PSC are also readily recognized with MRCP, and some authors have reported favorable results [4]. Due to its superior resolution, direct cholangiography remains the method of choice, showing, besides typical strictures, an irregular aspect of the biliary mucosa with small outpouchings or microdiverticula.

Bile duct cysts must be distinguished from multiple intrahepatic cysts without connection to the biliary tree. In typical cases, the diagnosis may be readily made with noninvasive imaging studies [5]. Today MRCP is the method of choice for noninvasive delineation of benign cystic biliary disorders (Fig. 3, 4). The absence of ionizing radiation is a major advantage in this benign disorder, which often affects young adults and children. Congenital cystic malformations of the bile ducts may, however, be associated with adult polycystic disease of the liver and kidney. This may sometimes represent a diagnostic challenge, and a complete radiologic workup may then require a cholangiographic study in addition to a standard US or CT examination. Correct diagnosis of cystic biliary malformations is also important because these lesions may predispose to the development of cholangiocarcinoma.

Choledochal cysts may be congenital or acquired, and appear as large cystic masses within the hepatoduodenal ligament, usually along with an abrupt caliber change. They may extend to the intrahepatic level, either unilaterally or bilaterally. Choledochal cysts may be classified according to their location and their concentric or asymmetrical appearance.

Choledochocele is a cyst-like dilatation of the distal portion of the common bile duct with protrusion of the ampullary portion into the duodenal lumen. It may be congenital or acquired, probably due to stone passage. The imaging features of choledochocele include a smooth, club-like cystic mass that protrudes into the duodenal lumen, usually along with moderate dilatation of the extrahepatic common bile duct.

Caroli's disease is a congenital ectasia of the intrahepatic bile ducts. Although it is a benign condition, it is associated with a poor prognosis because it predisposes to intrahepatic sludge and lithiasis with subsequent cholangitis and abscess formation. The typical radiologic features of Caroli's disease include a saccular, cyst-like appearance of the intrahepatic bile ducts along with sludge and/or small calculi. Dilatation of the extrahepatic bile ducts may be primarily associated, but may also develop secondarily due to the passage of calculi.

Malignant neoplasms involving the bile ducts typically present with painless obstructive jaundice [6]. *Primary tumors* originating from the bile ducts are referred to as cholangiocarcinoma. The so-called Klatskin tumor is a scirrhous form of cholangiocarcinoma, which spreads within the ductal tissue without a major mass lesion and is commonly located at the hepatic bifurcation (Fig. 5). The polypoid, intraductal form and the intrahepatic mass-like form of cholangiocarcinoma are much less common. Since advanced cholangiocarcinoma often contains abundant fibrotic components, it may display an increased contrast uptake on delayed, contrast-enhanced CT or MR images. Tumors of the distal bile duct, such as ampullary carcinoma, need to be distinguished from pancreatic carcinoma, since prognosis and treatment may be different (Fig. 6) [7]. A wide variety of *secondary neoplasms* may cause obstructive jaundice due to mechanical compression of the intra- and extrahepatic bile ducts. Carcinoma of the pancreas, gallbladder, stomach, colon and breast, and malignant lymphoma need to be considered in this context.

Gallbladder Disease

US is the method of choice for the diagnosis of gallbladder disease. Its sensitivity for *gallbladder calculi* approaches almost 100%, and it is also very well suited to evaluate changes of the gallbladder wall. *Cholesterol polyps* are small, benign lesions that adhere to the gallbladder wall. They appear as hyperechoic structures of 1-2 mm and may be easily distinguished from calculi, since they cast no shadow and are immobile (Fig. 7).

The diagnosis of *acute cholecystitis* is usually made on the basis of clinical and radiologic criteria. The 'sonographic Murphy's sign' refers to the maximum point of tenderness, which is correlated to the gallbladder at US. Thickening of the gallbladder wall with a hypoechoic layer, enlargement of the gallbladder lumen, and demonstration of an impacted stone in Hartmann's pouch are all useful diagnostic criteria. Acalculous acute cholecystitis is somewhat more difficult to diagnose, particularly if it occurs in patients in the intensive care unit who are fasting and thus display a dilated gallbladder with sludge.

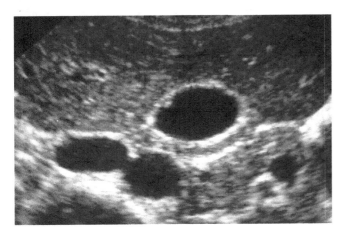

Fig. 7. Cholesterol polyp of the gallbladder. US image showing a small, strongly hyperechoic polyp at the non-dependent portion of the gallbladder wall. Such harmless polyps should not be confused with a neoplastic lesion

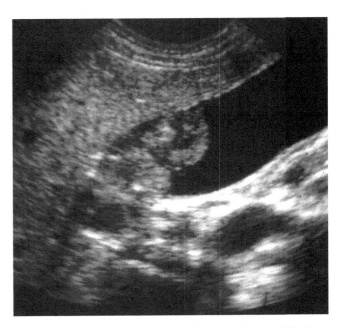

Fig. 8. Gallbladder metastases from malignant melanoma. US shows large, rounded, soft tissue masses bulging into the gallbladder lumen

Chronic cholecystitis is typically associated with cholecystolithiasis, a thickened gallbladder wall and a reduced gallbladder lumen. *Mirizzi's syndrome* is a complication of chronic calculous cholecystitis: a gallstone impacted within the cystic duct or Hartmann's pouch acts as a foreign body and creates an inflammatory reaction. Stenosis or obstruction of the adjacent common hepatic duct may occur either due to this inflammation or due to direct erosion of the stone through the stone into the ductal lumen, with a subsequent bilio-biliary fistula. The imaging features of Mirizzi's syndrome are 1) bile duct obstruction at the level of the common hepatic duct with 2) signs of cholecystolithiasis and chronic gallbladder disease, 3) a stone at the level of obstruction and, occasionally, 4) a hypervascularized (inflammatory) mass at the level of obstruction. The diagnostic features may be demonstrated noninvasively by means of US, CT, and MR cholangiopancreatography. Nonetheless, the preoperative workup should always include direct cholangiography (either ERCP or PTC) because it is the best technique to demonstrate a bilio-biliary fistula. Correct recognition of bilio-biliary fistula is important since it may give rise to postoperative bile leakage if left unrecognized [8].

Gallbladder Carcinoma is strongly associated with long-standing chronic cholecystitis. Since it remains usually asymptomatic until it causes obstructive jaundice due to external compression of the common bile duct, diagnosis is often made only at a late stage, when a large, infiltrating mass is already present. Occasionally, gallbladder carcinoma may be detected on US, CT or

MR imaging as a soft tissue mass within an asymptomatic gallbladder.

Secondary tumors of the gallbladder are uncommon. *Metastases from melanoma* may occur within the gallbladder wall and cause typical, rounded mass lesions (Fig. 8).

References

1. Aduna M, Larena JA, Martin D et al (2005) Bile duct leaks after laparoscopic cholecystectomy: value of contrast-enhanced MRCP. Abdom Imaging 30(4):480-487
2. Becker CD (2003) Multidetector CT and MRI of biliary diseases. J Radiol 84:473-479
3. Becker CD, Grossholz M, Mentha G et al (1997) Choledocholithiasis and bile duct stenosis: diagnostic accuracy of MR cholangiopancreatography. Radiology 205:523-530
4. Revelon G, Rashid A, Kawamoto S et al (1999) Primary sclerosing cholangitis: MR imaging findings with pathologic correlation. AJR Am J Roentgenol 173:1037-1042
5. Krause D, Cercueil JP, Dranssart M et al (2002) MRI for evaluating congenital bile duct abnormalities. J Comput Assist Tomogr 26:541-552
6. Stroszczynski C, Hunerbein M (2005) Malignant biliary obstruction: value of imaging findings. Abdom Imaging 30:314-323
7. Andersson M, Kostic S, Johansson M et al (2005) MRI combined with MR cholangiopancreatography versus helical CT in the evaluation of patients with suspected periampullary tumors: a prospective comparative study. Acta Radiol 46:16-27
8. Becker CD, Hassler H, Terrier F (1984) Preoperative diagnosis of the Mirizzi syndrome: limitations of sonography and computed tomography. AJR Am J Roentgenol 143:591-596

Differential Diagnosis of Diseases of the Gallbladder and Bile Ducts

A.D. Levy

Department of Radiologic Pathology, Armed Forces Institute of Pathology, NW, Washington DC, and Department of Radiology and Nuclear Medicine, Uniformed Services University of the Health Sciences, Bethesda, Washington DC, USA

The opinions and assertions contained herein are the private views of the authors and are not to be construed as official or as representing the views of the Department of the Army or the Department of Defense.

Introduction

Patients with gallbladder and biliary disease may present with complaints of the right upper quadrant or mid-epigastric pain, fever, jaundice, pruritis, nausea, vomiting, or may be asymptomatic with only laboratory abnormalities. Technological advances in ultrasound (US), multidetector computed tomography (MDCT), and magnetic resonance imaging (MRI) have greatly improved the noninvasive evaluation of patients with signs and symptoms of gallbladder and biliary disease. In many instances, noninvasive imaging establishes the diagnosis prior to endoscopic or surgical intervention. The differential diagnosis for these patients is broad and includes infectious, noninfectious inflammatory, neoplastic, and congenital disorders of the liver, gallbladder, and bile ducts. This course uses a patterned approach to differential diagnosis to discuss and review pathologic processes that affect the gallbladder and bile ducts.

Gallbladder Wall Thickening

Focal or diffuse gallbladder wall thickening is most commonly caused by cholecystitis. Noninflammatory conditions that may produce gallbladder wall thickening include heart failure, cirrhosis, hepatitis, hypoalbuminemia, and renal failure. Gallbladder carcinoma should be suggested when there are features of focal mass, lymphadenopathy, extension of the process to adjacent organs, hepatic metastases, or biliary obstruction at the level of the porta hepatis [1]. Xanthogranulomatous cholecystitis (XGC) is a pseudotumoral inflammatory condition of the gallbladder that radiologically simulates gallbladder carcinoma. There is a significant overlap in the CT features of XGC and gallbladder carcinoma. Both entities may demonstrate wall thickening, infiltration of the surrounding fat, hepatic involvement, and lymphadenopathy [2, 3]. Adenomyomatous

hyperplasia is a common tumor-like lesion of the gallbladder, with no malignant potential [4]. It may produce focal, segmental, or diffuse mural thickening. Sonographically, adenomyomatous hyperplasia is characterized by focal or diffuse gallbladder wall thickening with echogenic foci and ring down artifact emanating from the gallbladder wall [5]. The echogenic foci represent bile salts, cholesterol crystals, or small stones in Rokitansky-Aschoff sinuses. On MR, Rokitansky-Aschoff sinuses are best visualized on breathhold T2-weighted sequences. Accordingly, MR can be useful to distinguish adenomyomatous hyperplasia from gallbladder carcinoma (Fig. 1) [6, 7].

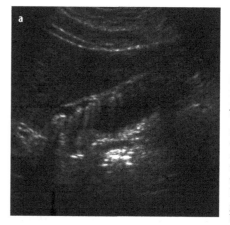

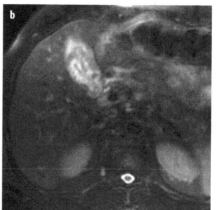

Fig. 1. A 48-year-old man evaluated for jaundice was found to have a benign stricture in the distal common bile duct and adenomyomatous hyperplasia of the gallbladder. **a** Longitudinal sonogram of the gallbladder shows mural thickening along the anterior gallbladder wall and echogenic foci in the gallbladder wall that produce ring-down reverberation artifact. **b** Single shot fast spin echo T2-weighted MR image with fat saturation shows multiple hyperintense foci within the thickened gallbladder wall consistent with adenomyomatous hyperplasia

Gallbladder Polypoid Mass

Polypoid gallbladder masses are commonly demonstrated by US as incidental findings when the gallbladder is imaged on sonography. Polyps are estimated to be present in approximately 3% of gallbladders. The differential diagnosis for a gallbladder polyp includes cholesterol polyp, adenoma, adenomyomatous hyperplasia, inflammatory polyp, heterotopia, neurofibroma, carcinoma, carcinoid tumor, lymphoma, and metastasis. The majority of gallbladder polyps are benign. The management of gallbladder polyps is based on the risk of malignancy, which increases for polyps greater than 10 mm in size and in patients over the age of 60. The incidence of malignancy in polyps greater than 10 mm ranges from 37% to 88% [8]. Therefore, it has been recommended that patients undergo cholecystectomy for symptomatic polyps greater than 10 mm. Polyps less than 10 mm should be followed periodically by US. At sonography, careful attention should be paid to other features that suggest malignancy, such as thickening or nodularity of the gallbladder wall, evidence of hepatic invasion, such as an indistinct margin between the liver and gallbladder, biliary duct dilatation, and peripancreatic hepatoduodenal ligament adenopathy [1].

Cystic Dilatation of the Extrahepatic Bile Duct

Mechanical biliary obstruction is the most common cause of extrahepatic bile duct dilatation. Upon initial imaging, an obstructive lesion should be sought. Once an obstructive lesion is excluded, congenital etiologies of bile duct dilatation should be considered. Choledochal cysts, unlike obstructive dilatation, generally have more focal extrahepatic bile duct dilatation or are typically more expansive than is usually encountered in mechanical dilatation (Fig. 2). It may be more difficult to differentiate a choledochal cyst that has mild or fusiform dilatation of the extrahepatic duct from a duct that is dilated secondary to an obstructing lesion. In these cases, magnetic resonance cholangiopancreatography (MRCP) and/or endoscopic retrograde cholangiopancreatography (ERCP) are useful to exclude an obstructing lesion and to evaluate the pancreaticobiliary junction [9]. An anomalous pancreaticobiliary junction is commonly observed in patients with choledochal cyst. Occasionally, pancreatic pseudocysts, echinococcal cysts, and cystic biliary neoplasms such as biliary cystadenoma or biliary cystadenocarcinoma may occur in or around the porta hepatis, simulating a biliary dilatation and choledochal cyst. The appearance of rim-like calcification and enhancing septations or mural nodules should help to establish the diagnosis of a biliary cystadenoma or cystadenocarcinoma. Likewise, echinococcal cysts generally have evidence of inner membranes, daughter cysts, or rim-like peripheral calcification. MR of echinococcal cysts may show a low-

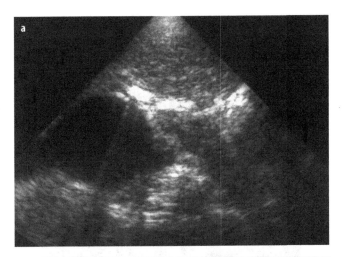

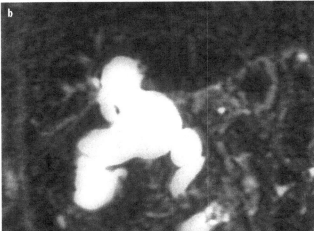

Fig. 2. Choledochal cyst in a three-year-old boy evaluated for a palpable right upper quadrant mass. **a** Transverse sonogram at the level of the pancreatic head shows dilatation of the common bile duct. **b** MRCP shows a Todani Type IV choledochal cyst with marked extrahepatic bile duct dilatation extending into the right and left hepatic ducts, cystic duct, and gallbladder

signal intensity fibrous capsule and membranes on T2-weighted images.

Cystic Dilatation of Intrahepatic Bile Ducts

Similar to extrahepatic duct dilatation, a mechanical biliary obstruction is the most common cause of intrahepatic bile duct dilatation. Intrahepatic biliary dilatation in mechanical obstruction is generally tubular and lacks focal stricture formation. Caroli disease, recurrent pyogenic cholangitis, polycystic liver disease, primary sclerosing cholangitis, choledochal cyst, and peribiliary cysts should be included in the differential diagnosis of cystic intrahepatic biliary dilatation. Caroli disease is suggested by focal or diffuse biliary dilatation that is cystic or fusiform in character (Fig. 3) [10, 11]. When diffuse involvement is present, the bile ducts converge

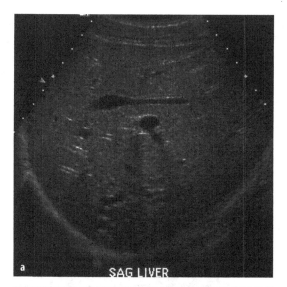

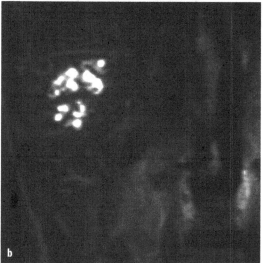

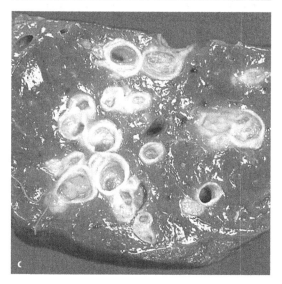

Fig. 3. Caroli disease in a 23-year-old man who complained of abdominal pain. **a** Sagittal sonogram of the liver shows multiple cystic spaces in the posterior right lobe. **b** MRCP shows high signal intensity within these cysts. **c** Photograph of the resected liver shows focal cystic dilatation of the intrahepatic bile ducts

toward the porta hepatis. Echogenic intraductal sludge or inflammatory debris may be present, as well as echogenic stones with posterior acoustic shadowing. The most important differential diagnosis for patients with suspected Caroli disease is recurrent pyogenic cholangitis, which is characterized by biliary dilatation with intrahepatic stone formation. The left hepatic lobe is more commonly involved than the right in recurrent pyogenic cholangitis. Polycystic liver disease may mimic Caroli disease. However, in most cases, the bile ducts in polycystic liver disease are intrinsically normal; only rarely do cysts communicate with the bile ducts.

Although intrahepatic bile duct dilatation is a feature of primary sclerosing cholangitis, the duct dilatation is typically fusiform and isolated. The degree and extent of duct dilatation in primary sclerosing cholangitis is not as severe as that in obstructive biliary dilatation, Caroli disease, or recurrent pyogenic cholangitis because fibrosis, stricture formation, and secondary cirrhosis are the major features of primary sclerosing cholangitis.

Choledochal cyst should be considered in the differential diagnosis when both intrahepatic and extrahepatic duct dilatations are present. In general, patients with choledochal cyst will have more severe extrahepatic dilatation when compared to the degree of intrahepatic dilatation.

Multiple peribiliary cysts in sequence may simulate bile duct dilatation that has a beaded or saccular appearance [12]. The bile ducts adjacent to peribiliary cysts are normal. Therefore, correct diagnosis depends upon visualization of a normal bile duct. Peribiliary cysts are usually associated with various hepatic diseases such as cirrhosis, polycystic liver disease, portal hypertension, portal vein obstruction, and metastatic disease.

Biliary Stricture

Focal narrowing or structuring in the biliary ducts may be secondary to neoplasia, inflammation, trauma (iatrogenic or noniatrogenic), or mass effect from adjacent processes [13, 14]. The location of biliary strictures narrows the differential diagnosis. Strictures at the level of the porta hepatis (in or near the confluence of the right and left hepatic ducts) may be secondary to hilar cholangiocarcinoma (Klatskin tumor) (Fig. 4), inflammation, or vascular impressions. Strictures in the mid portion of the extrahepatic bile duct are commonly related to diseases of the gallbladder, such as carcinoma that has invaded the cystic duct and hepatoduodenal ligament, or inflammatory conditions, such as impaction of a stone in the cystic duct (Mirrizi syndrome). Distal extrahepatic strictures may be due to inflammatory or neoplastic diseases of the pancreas, primary carcinomas of the bile duct or ampulla, sphincter of Oddi dysfunction, or less commonly, infectious papillitis that may be seen in AIDS cholangiopathy.

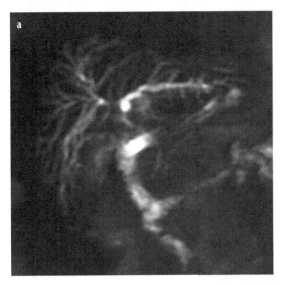

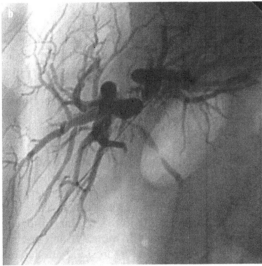

Fig. 4. Hilar cholangiocarcinoma in a 40-year-old man who complained of abdominal pain. Coronal MRCP (**a**) and percutaneous transhepatic cholangiogram (**b**) show a hilar stricture and mild intrahepatic biliary dilatation

Conclusions

A patterned approach to differential diagnosis of gallbladder and biliary duct disease is useful and may be applied to findings identified with all the noninvasive imaging techniques.

References

1. Levy AD, Murakata LA, Rohrmann CA, Jr. (2001) Gallbladder carcinoma: radiologic-pathologic correlation. Radiographics 21:295-314
2. Chun KA, Ha HK, Yu ES et al (1997) Xanthogranulomatous cholecystitis: CT features with emphasis on differentiation from gallbladder carcinoma. Radiology 203:93-97
3. Goodman ZD, Ishak KG (1981) Xanthogranulomatous cholecystitis. Am J Surg Pathol 5:653-659
4. Albores-Saavedra J, Hensen DE, Klimsta DS (2000) Tumors of the gallbladder, extrahepatic bile ducts, and ampulla of vater. In: Atlas of tumor pathology. Fasc 27, ser 3. Armed Forces Institute of Pathology, Washington, DC
5. Raghavendra BN, Subramanyam BR, Balthazar EJ et al (1983) Sonography of adenomyomatosis of the gallbladder: radiologic-pathologic correlation. Radiology 146:747-752
6. Haradome H, Ichikawa T, Sou H et al (2003) The pearl necklace sign: an imaging sign of adenomyomatosis of the gallbladder at MR cholangiopancreatography. Radiology 227:80-88
7. Yoshimitsu K, Honda H, Jimi M et al (1999) MR diagnosis of adenomyomatosis of the gallbladder and differentiation from gallbladder carcinoma: importance of showing Rokitansky-Aschoff sinuses. AJR Am J Roentgenol 172:1535-1540
8. Ishikawa O, Ohhigashi H, Imaoka S et al (1989) The difference in malignancy between pedunculated and sessile polypoid lesions of the gallbladder. Am J Gastroenterol 84:1386-1390
9. Levy AD, Rohrmann CA Jr (2003) Biliary cystic disease. Curr Probl Diagn Radiol 32:233-263
10. Guy F, Cognet F, Dranssart M et al (2002) Caroli's disease: magnetic resonance imaging features. European Radiology 12:2730-2736
11. Levy AD, Rohrmann CA Jr, Murakata LA, Lonergan GJ (2002) Caroli's disease: radiologic spectrum with pathologic correlation. AJR Am J Roentgenol 179:1053-1057
12. Baron RL, Campbell WL, Dodd GD 3rd (1994) Peribiliary cysts associated with severe liver disease: imaging-pathologic correlation. AJR Am J Roentgenol 162:631-636
13. Baron RL, Tublin ME, Peterson MS (2002) Imaging the spectrum of biliary tract disease. Radiol Clin North Am 40:1325-1354
14. Schulte SJ, Baron RL, Teefey SA et al (1990) CT of the extrahepatic bile ducts: wall thickness and contrast enhancement in normal and abnormal ducts. AJR Am J Roentgenol 154:79-85

Imaging the Adrenal Glands

R.H. Reznek[1], G.P. Krestin[2]

[1] Cancer Imaging, St Bartholomew's Hospital, West Smithfield, London, United Kingdom
[2] Department of Radiology, Erasmus MC, University Medical Center Rotterdam, Rotterdam, The Nederlands

Introduction

Clinically, one can distinguish two major settings of adrenal disorders: a small group of patients with clinical and laboratory findings of adrenal endocrinopathy, and a second, much larger group of patients, with an incidentally found enlargement of the adrenal glands. The diagnostic approach to these two groups is totally different; in the first category imaging methods are used for localization of an adrenal pathology, while in the second group the lesion is found in the course of a routine imaging examination or while staging a malignant primary tumor [1-5].

Adrenal masses are seen at autopsy in 2-10% of all patients and metastases are found postmortem in the adrenal glands in up to 26% of patients with primary extra-adrenal malignancies. It is thus not surprising that adrenal mass lesions are quite common incidental findings during imaging of the abdomen. However, even in an oncologic setting, many adrenal lesions are benign, mostly non-hyperfunctioning adenomas, resulting in the need for a reliable method to discriminate between these lesions and malignant masses [6-7].

Normal Radiological Anatomy of the Adrenal Glands

The adrenal glands are enclosed within the perinephric fascia and are usually surrounded by a sufficient amount of fat for identification on computed tomography (CT) or magnetic resonance imaging (MRI). The right adrenal gland lies immediately posterior to the inferior vena cava (IVC). The left adrenal gland lies anteromedial to the upper pole of the left kidney and posterior to the pancreas and splenic vessels. The shape of the adrenals can vary, depending on the orientation of the gland and the level of the image, but the normal adrenal gland has an arrowhead configuration, with a body and medial and lateral limbs. The normal adrenals extend over 2-4 cm in the craniocaudal direction, and on CT the thickness of the normal adrenal body and limbs does not exceed 10-12 and 5-6 mm, respectively [8].

Computed Tomography

Unenhanced CT

At CT, certain imaging findings indicate a higher likelihood of lesion malignancy. Lesions greater than 5 cm in diameter tend to be either metastases or primary adrenal carcinomas. However, size alone is poor at discriminating between adenomas and non-adenomas. Using 3.0 cm as the size cut-off, the specificity of such a discrimination is only 79% and the sensitivity is 84% [9].

Rapid change in size suggests malignancy because adenomas are slow-growing lesions. Although it has been suggested that adenomas have a smooth contour, whereas malignant lesions have an irregular shape, there is a very large overlap between the two groups, and shape is therefore not a helpful differentiating feature.

Adenomas have a high intra-cellular lipid content, which lowers their attenuation value. If an adrenal mass measures 0 HU or less (with a threshold attenuation value of 0 HU), the specificity of the mass being an adenoma is 100%, but the sensitivity is an unacceptable 47%. Boland et al. [9] performed a meta-analysis of ten studies, and demonstrated that if a threshold attenuation value of 10 HU was adopted, the specificity was 98% and the sensitivity increased to 71%. Therefore, in clinical practice, 10 HU is the most widely used threshold attenuation value for the diagnosis of an adrenal adenoma [9].

Contrast-enhanced CT

Contrast-enhanced CT is a CT scan acquired after the administration of intravenous contrast medium. CT contrast media contain iodine with a very high density and hence a high attenuation value. The contrast medium is usually administered into an antecubital vein and injected at variable rates. The CT images are acquired at variable time intervals after the administration of contrast medium, and uptake of the contrast medium is termed 'contrast enhancement'. Contrast enhancement is directly proportional to the vascularity of the enhancing structure. The increase in attenuation values of adrenal masses after contrast administration is a direct measurement of their contrast enhancement properties.

On non-contrast-enhanced CT, up to 30% of benign adenomas have an attenuation value greater than 10 HU and are considered to be lipid poor. Malignant lesions are also lipid poor. Characterization of adrenal masses using contrast-enhanced CT utilizes the different physiological perfusion patterns of adenomas and metastases. Adenomas enhance rapidly after contrast administration and also demonstrate a rapid loss of contrast medium – a phenomenon termed contrast washout. Metastases also enhance rapidly but show a slower washout of contrast medium (Fig. 1). In a standard abdominal CT obtained for staging patients with cancer, the CT images are acquired 60 seconds after contrast administration. Attenuation values of adrenal masses obtained 60 seconds after contrast medium injection show too much overlap between adenomas and malignant lesions to be of clinical value. Adrenal masses with CT attenuation value measuring less than 30 HU, on delayed images obtained 10-15 minutes after contrast enhancement are almost always adenomas. However, the percentage of contrast washout between initial enhancement (at 60 seconds) and delayed enhancement (at 15 minutes) can be used to differentiate adenomas from malignant lesions. Measurement of the attenuation value of the mass before injection of contrast medium, at 60 seconds after injection of contrast medium and then again at 10-15 minutes, are made using an electronic cursor. These absolute contrast medium enhancement washout values are only applicable to relatively homogeneous masses without large areas of necrosis or hemorrhage. It has been shown that washout of contrast from adenomas occurs much faster than from metastases. Both lipid-rich and lipid-poor adenomas behave similarly, because this property of adenomas is independent of their lipid content [10-15].

The percentage of absolute enhancement washout can be thus calculated:

$$\% \text{ washout} = \frac{\text{enhanced attenuation value} - \text{delayed attenuation value}}{\text{enhanced attenuation value} - \text{non-enhanced attenuation value}} \times 100$$

The enhanced attenuation value is the attenuation value of the mass, measured in HU, 60 seconds after contrast administration. The delayed attenuation value is the attenuation value of the mass, measured in HU, 10-15 minutes after contrast administration [10-11].

If the percentage absolute enhancement washout is 60% or higher, this has a sensitivity of 88% and a specificity of 96% for the diagnosis of an adenoma. However, the measurement of this absolute contrast medium enhancement washout requires an unenhanced image. Frequently in clinical practice, only post-contrast images are available. In these patients, the percentage 'relative' enhancement washout can be thus calculated:

$$\% \text{ relative washout} = \frac{\text{enhanced attenuation value} - \text{delayed attenuation value}}{\text{enhanced attenuation value}} \times 100$$

The enhanced and delayed attenuation values are measured as described previously.

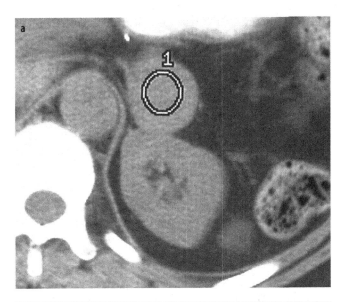

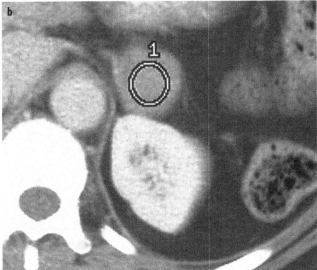

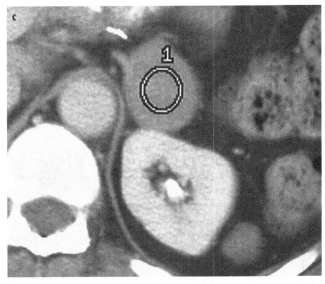

Fig. 1. Adrenal metastasis. (**a**) A 3 cm left adrenal mass measures 34 HU on the unenhanced scan. (**b**) After contrast administration it enhances to 64 HU. (**c**) The mass measures 59 HU on delayed images

At 15 minutes, if a relative enhancement washout of 40% or higher is achieved, this has a sensitivity of 96-100% and a specificity of 100% for the diagnosis of an adenoma. Therefore a combination of unenhanced CT and enhancement washout characteristics correctly separates nearly all adrenal masses as adenomas or metastases [15].

Magnetic Resonance Imaging

Conventional Spin-echo Imaging

Early reports were enthusiastic about the ability of MRI to differentiate benign from malignant adrenal masses on the basis of signal intensity (SI) differences on T2-weighted spin-echo images. In general, metastases and carcinomas have a higher fluid content than adenomas and therefore are of higher SI on T2-weighted images than the surrounding normal adrenal gland. Adenomas are homogeneously iso- or hypo-intense compared with the normal adrenal gland. However, considerable overlap exists between the signal intensities of adenomas and other lesions, and up to 31% of lesions remain indeterminate [16-18].

Gadolinium-enhanced Magnetic Resonance Imaging

The accuracy of MRI in differentiating benign from malignant masses can be improved after intravenous gadolinium injection on gradient echo sequences. As with CT, adenomas show enhancement after administration of gadolinium with quick washout, whereas malignant tumours and pheochromocytomas show strong enhancement and slower washout. Uniform enhancement (capillary blush) on post-gadolinium capillary phase has been reported in up to 70% of adenomas, but is rare in other masses. In addition, adenomas often show a thin rim of enhancement in the late phase of gadolinium-enhanced images. Metastases frequently have heterogeneous enhancement. However, as with signal characteristics, there is considerable overlap in the characteristics of benign and malignant masses, limiting the clinical applicability of this technique to distinguish adenomatous from malignant masses [19-20].

Chemical-shift Imaging

Chemical-shift imaging (CSI) relies on the fact that, within a magnetic field, protons in water molecules oscillate or precess at a slightly different frequency than the protons in lipid molecules. As a result, water and fat protons cycle in- and out-of-phase with respect to one another. By selecting appropriate sequencing parameters, images can be acquired with the protons oscillating in and out of phase. The SI of a pixel on an in-phase image is derived from the signal of water plus fat protons, if water and fat are present in the same pixel. On out-of-phase sequences, the SI is derived from the difference of the signal intensities of water and fat protons. Therefore, adenomas that contain intracellular lipid lose SI on out-of-phase images compared with in-phase images (Fig. 2), whereas metastases that lack intracellular lipid remain unchanged [21-23].

There are several ways of assessing the degree of loss of SI. Quantitative analysis can be made using a variety of ratios, essentially comparing the loss of signal in the adrenal mass with that of liver, paraspinal muscle or spleen on in-phase and out-of-phase images. However, fatty infiltration of the liver (particularly in oncology patients receiving chemotherapy) and iron overload make the liver an unreliable internal standard. Fatty infiltration might also affect skeletal muscle, although to a lesser ex-

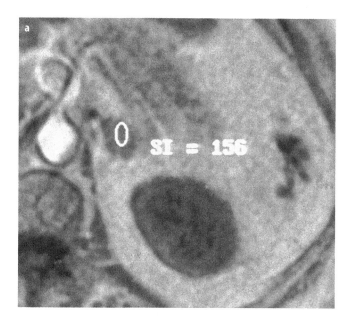

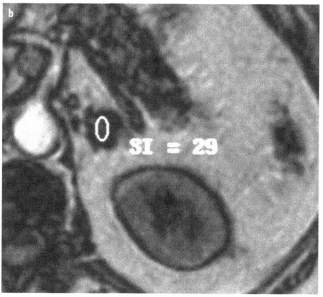

Fig. 2. Left adrenal adenoma in a patient with lung cancer. Chemical-shift MRI shows significant signal decrease on opposed phase (**b**), compared to the in-phase image (**a**)

tent. The spleen has been shown to be the most reliable internal standard, although this might also be affected by iron overload [21].

To calculate the adrenal lesion to spleen ratio (ASR), regions of interest are used to acquire the SI within the adrenal mass and the spleen from in-phase and out-of-phase images. The ASR reflects the percentage signal drop-off within the adrenal lesion compared with the spleen and it can be calculated as follows:

$$\text{ASR} = \frac{\text{SI lesion (out-of-phase)} / \text{SI spleen (out-of-phase)}}{\text{SI lesion (in-phase)} / \text{SI spleen (in-phase)}} \times 100$$

An ASR ratio of 70 or less has been shown to be 100% specific for adenomas but only 78% sensitive [21-23].

Simple visual assessment of relative signal intensity loss is just as accurate, but quantitative methods might be useful in equivocal cases. A signal intensity loss within an adrenal mass on out-of-phase images of greater than 20% is diagnostic of an adenoma [24].

The combination of spin-echo signal characteristics, gadolinium enhancement and CSI is currently 85-90% accurate in distinguishing adenomas from non-adenomas.

There are few direct comparisons between CT and MRI. Evidence from one histological study showed that because both non-contrast CT alone and CSI rely upon the same property of adenomas, namely their lipid content, the techniques correlate.

Positron Emission Tomography

Whole body positron emission tomography (PET) with 18-F-fluorodeoxyglucose (18-FDG) allows malignant adrenal lesions to be recognized. The contribution of 18-FDG PET has been well evaluated in large studies in relation to lung cancer, and is highly accurate in differentiating benign non-inflammatory lesions from malignant disease. Using 18-FDG PET, these studies have shown a 100% sensitivity and specificity for the diagnosis of malignant adrenal mass when CT or MRI identify enlarged adrenal glands or a focal mass. Recent studies have reported false positive results as a result of 18-FDG uptake by pheochromocytomas and benign adenomas. For the diagnosis of a malignant adrenal tumour, the positive predictive value of 18-FDG PET was 100% and the negative predictive value (NPV) to rule out malignancy was also 100%. Within these study populations, 18-FDG PET also has the ability to detect metastatic lesions in non-enlarged adrenal glands, but its accuracy in this situation has not been fully evaluated. In addition, 18-FDG PET has the advantage of simultaneously detecting metastases at other sites. However, in some countries, PET is not readily available. Nevertheless, it is a useful tool for evaluating masses that are indeterminate by both CT and MRI. PET can substitute for percutaneous biopsy and has the advantage of being non-invasive and therefore a safer investigation for the patient [25].

Percutaneous Adrenal Biopsy

With improved imaging and recent techniques, such as contrast medium washout measurement on CT and chemical-shift MRI, only a small proportion of adrenal masses cannot be characterized accurately and require percutaneous biopsy for diagnosis. However, before percutaneous biopsy, the possibility of a pheochromocytoma must be excluded because of the risk of an adrenal crisis induced by the biopsy. In a recent study by Harisinghani et al. [26], the NPV of adrenal biopsies was shown to be between 98% and 100%. In this study, 225 CT-guided biopsies were evaluated, where no malignant lesion was missed on the first biopsy. It was concluded that a single negative biopsy for malignancy can be regarded as a true negative, and there is no necessity to repeat the biopsy. Percutaneous CT-guided adrenal biopsy is a relatively safe procedure in patients with a known extra-adrenal malignancy. Minor complications of adrenal biopsy include abdominal pain, hematuria, nausea and small pneumothoraces. Major complications, generally regarded as those requiring treatment, occur in 2.8-3.6% of cases and include pneumothoraces requiring intervention, and hemorrhage. There are also isolated reports of adrenal abscesses, pancreatitis and seeding of metastases along the needle track [26].

References

1. Korobkin M, Francis IR (1995) Adrenal Imaging. Semin Ultrasound CT MR 16:317-330
2. Krestin GP (1999) Genitourinary MR: kidneys and adrenal glands. Eur Radiol 9:1705-1714
3. Reznek RH, Armstrong P (1994) The adrenal gland. Clinical Endocrinology 40:561-576
4. Pender SM, Boland GW, Lee MJ (1998) The incidental non-hyperfunctioning adrenal mass: an imaging algorithm for characterization. Clin Radiol 53:796-804
5. Dunnick NR, Korobkin M (2002) Imaging of adrenal incidentalomas: current status. AJR Am J Roentgenol 179:559-568
6. Glazer HS, Weyman PJ, Sagel SS et al (1982) Nonfunctioning adrenal masses: Incidental discovery on computed tomography. AJR Am J Roentgenol 139:81-85
7. Mitnick JS, Bosniak MA, Megibow AJ, Naidich DP (1983) Non-functioning adrenal adenomas discovered incidentally on computed tomography. Radiology 148:495-499
8. Vincent JM, Morrison ID, Armstrong P, Reznek RH (1994) The size of normal adrenal glands on computed tomography. Clinical Radiology 49:453-455
9. Boland GW, Lee MJ, Gazelle GS et al (1998) Characterization of adrenal masses using unenhanced CT: an analysis of the CT literature. AJR Am J Roentgenol 171:201-204
10. Korobkin M, Brodeur FJ, Francis IR et al (1998) CT time-attenuation washout curves of adrenal adenomas and nonadenomas. AJR Am J Roentgenol 170:747-752
11. Szolar DH, Kammerhuber F (1997) Quantitative CT evaluation of adrenal gland masses: a step forward in the differentiation between adenomas and nonadenomas? Radiology 202:517-521
12. Boland GW, Hahn PF, Peña C, Mueller PR (1997) Adrenal masses: characterization with delayed contrast-enhanced CT. Radiology 202:693-696

13. Caoili EM, Korobkin M, Francis IR et al (2000) Delayed enhanced CT of lipid-poor adrenal adenomas. AJR Am J Roentgenol 175:1411-1415
14. Peña CS, Boland GW, Hahn PF et al (2000) Characterization of indeterminate (lipid-poor) adrenal masses: use of washout characteristics at contrast-enhanced CT. Radiology 217:798-802
15. Korobkin M (2000) CT characterization of adrenal masses: the time has come. Radiology 217:629-632
16. Baker ME, Blinder R, Spitzer C et al (1989) MR evaluation of adrenal masses at 1.5 T. AJR Am J Roentgenol 153:307-312
17. Heinz-Peer G, Hönigschnabl S, Schneider B et al (1999) Characterization of adrenal masses using MR imaging with histopathologic correlation. AJR Am J Roentgenol 173:15-22
18. Peppercorn PD, Reznek RH (1997) State-of-the-art CT and MRI of the adrenal gland. Eur Radiol 7:822-836
19. Krestin GP, Friedman G, Fischbach R et al (1991) Evaluation of adrenal masses in oncologic patients: dynamic contrast-enhanced MR vs CT. J Comput Assist Tomogr 15:104-110
20. Krestin GP, Steinbrich W, Friedmann G (1989) Adrenal Masses: Evaluation with fast gradient-echo MR imaging and Gd-DTPA-enhanced dynamic studies. Radiology 171:675-680
21. Mitchell DG, Crovello M, Matteucci T et al (1992) Benign adrenocortical masses: diagnosis with chemical shift MR imaging. Radiology 185:345-351
22. Outwater EK, Siegelman ES, Radecki PD et al (1995) Distinction between benign and malignant adrenal masses: Value of T1- weighted chemical-shift MR imaging. AJR Am J Roentgenol 165:579-583
23. Tsushima Y, Ishizaka H, Matsumoto M (1993) Adrenal masses: differentiation with chemical shift, fast low-angle shot MR imaging. Radiology 186:705-709
24. Korobkin M, Lombardi TJ, Aisen AM et al (1995) Characterization of adrenal masses with chemical shift and gadolinium enhanced MR imaging. Radiology 197:411-418
25. Maurea S, Mainolfi C, Bazzicalupo L et al (1999) Imaging of adrenal tumors using FDG PET: comparison of benign and malignant lesions. AJR Am J Roentgenol 173:25-29
26. Harisinghani MT, Maher MM, Hahn PF et al (2002) Predictive value of benign percutaneous adrenal biopsies in oncology patients. Clin Radiol 57:598-901

Radiologic Approach to Solid and Cystic Renal Masses

S.G. Silverman[1], D.S. Hartman[2]

[1] Division of Abdominal Imaging and Intervention, Department of Radiology, Brigham and Women's Hospital, Boston, MA, USA
[2] Department of Radiology, Penn State University, Hershey, PA, USA

Introduction

Renal mass-like lesions are ubiquitous. Fortunately, most are benign. The most common renal mass is a benign cyst. In fact, pathologic investigations have shown that approximately one-half of the population over the age of 50 has one or more renal cysts [1]. Computed tomography (CT) investigations show that one-quarter to one-third of patients over 50 years of age has at least one cyst [2]. Renal cell carcinoma (RCC) is most commonly identified because of the widespread use of cross-sectional imaging in the abdomen, either by CT or ultrasound (US), usually performed for a non-renal complaint [3]. With advances in CT and US technology, radiologists are detecting more masses and characterizing cysts as small as 5 mm [4]. Similarly, small solid masses may be also characterized with confidence.

To determine whether a solid or cystic renal mass is benign or malignant, the mass is initially examined by US, CT, magnetic resonance imaging (MRI), or a combination of these techniques [5]. Occasionally, percutaneous biopsy is needed [6]. For lesions considered indeterminate after an imaging evaluation, there are many factors that contribute to the management of an individual case, including patient needs, co-morbidity, equipment availability, and the experience of the radiologist and urologist [4].

The differential diagnosis of mass-like lesions of the kidney includes pseudotumors, cysts, inflammatory lesions, and neoplasia. Pseudotumors refers to normal variants that mimic renal masses, and include persistent fetal lobation, column of Bertin, and hypertrophied parenchyma. These entities might cause a renal contour abnormality that mimics a renal mass. However, these entities are generally identified at CT by noting that they are iso-dense compared to normal renal parenchyma at all phases of the examination. Inflammatory lesions are caused by infection, vascular infarction, and trauma. These lesions are often diagnosed in the appropriate clinical setting but may also be identified on the basis of their radiologic appearance. Thickening of Gerota's fascia and perinephric stranding may be indicative of an inflammatory etiology. Pseudotumors and inflammatory lesions should always be considered first when a mass-like lesion is en-countered in the kidney. After their exclusion, solid and cystic renal masses may be considered. This article focuses on solid and cystic renal masses and summarizes an approach that is useful in clinical practice.

Solid Renal Masses

Solid renal masses contain little or no liquid components, and when examined with CT or MRI, usually (but not always) consist of predominantly enhancing tissue. Enhancement is an important feature; the presence of unequivocal enhancement by CT or MRI signifies that the lesion has a blood supply and is solid. Solid tumors may be benign or malignant. Benign entities encountered in clinical practice include angiomyolipoma and oncocytoma. RCC is the most common malignant tumor of the kidney, but other entities such as transitional cell carcinoma, lymphoma, and metastases may present as solitary, solid renal masses.

Although most solid renal masses in adults are due to RCC, a substantial fraction of solid renal masses are benign. A recent study of 2,770 resections of solid renal masses found that 12.8% were benign [7]. When stratified by size, benign masses represented 25% of those smaller than 3 cm, 30% of masses less than 2 cm, and 44% of masses smaller than 1 cm. Most benign solid renal masses were angiomyolipomas and oncocytomas.

When a solid renal mass is encountered on US, CT, or MRI, a diagnosis of angiomyolipoma should be considered first – well before other entities are contemplated. These lesions are benign and should remain untreated. Large (> 3 cm) lesions may bleed, and therefore should be noted in the patient's medical record, but the risk of bleeding is not high enough to warrant either surgery of frequent follow-up. Most angiomyolipomas can be diagnosed with confidence by identifying the presence of fat, indicated by a CT attenuation of less than -10 HU, within a non-calcified renal mass [8]. There have been case reports of fat within calcified [9-12] and non-calcified [13] RCC and atypical Wilms' tumors [14], and investigators have cautioned that large malignant renal tumors may appear to contain fat because they have engulfed sinus or perirenal fat [15, 16]. Approximately 5% of angiomyolipomas contain little or no fat cells, and therefore do not show evidence of fat in imaging studies. Most angiomyolipomas with minimal or no fat present as small (≤ 3 cm) hyperdense, homogeneously enhancing renal masses [17] (Fig. 1). However, masses with these features also may represent RCC (particularly the papillary subtype) (Fig. 2). Therefore, discriminating angiomyolipomas with minimal or no fat, from renal cancers (short of resection) requires a percutaneous biopsy. Biopsy can be used to diagnose renal cancers and angiomyolipomas [6]. Small, hyperdense, enhancing masses are referred to radiologists for ablation and it is in this clinical setting that biopsy has been found to be useful [18].

Oncocytomas are generally considered as benign tumors [19, 20]. Homogeneous enhancement and a central scar have been described [21, 22], but are not pathognomonic. These features have also been described in oncocytic RCC. These features may suggest an oncytoma or an oncocytic RCC, which means that less aggressive approaches (e.g., partial nephrectomy, percutaneous tumor ablation) may be considered.

Excluding angiomyolipomas and oncocytomas, the majority of solid renal masses are RCC. Therefore, a solid renal tumor (after a benign tumor is excluded) is typically treated with surgical resection. Percutaneous ablation may be considered for small (≤ 3 cm) tumors, or larger tumors in patients who need nephron-sparing surgery such as those with co-morbid disease [23].

Percutaneous biopsy plays an important role in the evaluation of the solid renal mass [6]. There are six clinical scenarios which may merit biopsy when a solid mass is identified with imaging. First, biopsy is indicated in patients with an extra-renal primary malignancy and a solid renal mass which may be considered both a renal metastasis and a RCC (second primary). Second, biopsy provides a tissue diagnosis and allows therapy to be instituted in patients who have unresectable RCC. Third, renal mass biopsy should be considered in patients with renal mass-like lesions of potentially infectious origin, but which cannot be diagnosed clinically. The fourth indication is in a patient with a solitary kidney, renal insufficiency, or other medical co-morbidities, and pathology confirmation is needed before a partial nephrectomy (with its attendant surgical morbidity and potential for compromising renal function) is performed. The fifth indication is somewhat controversial. As described above, when encountering a small, homogeneously enhancing renal mass,

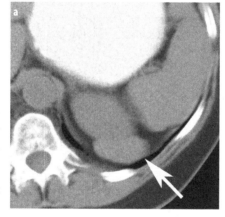
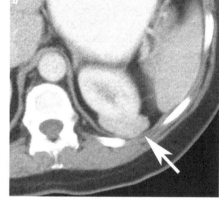

Fig. 1. Incidental, hyperdense mass in a 59-year-old female. (**a**) Transverse unenhanced CT shows a 4 cm hyperdense (56 HU) mass (*arrow*) in the upper pole of the left kidney with no evidence of fat. (**b**) Transverse CT shows enhancement of the mass (128 HU) (*arrow*). Angiomyolipoma with minimal fat was found at partial nephrectomy

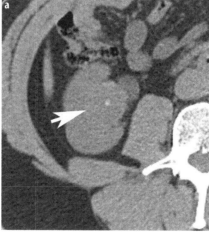
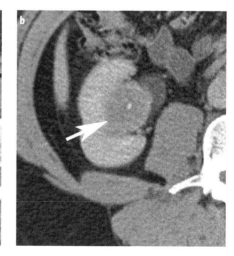

Fig. 2. Small, hyperdense, enhancing mass in a 55-year-old male with bladder carcinoma. (**a**) Transverse unenhanced CT of the mass shows a 3 cm mass (*arrow*) in the upper pole of the right kidney with an attenuation of 43 HU and a central calcification. (**b**) Transverse CT shows enhancement of the mass (*arrow*) to 62 HU. Papillary renal cell carcinoma was found at nephrectomy

biopsy may be used to diagnose angiomyolipomas so that these patients do not unnecessarily undergo surgical resection or ablation. Similarly, biopsy should be used to diagnose renal masses prior to ablation. Patients referred for ablation might have benign masses [18].

Cystic Renal Masses

Approximately 10% of cases of RCC present as a fluid-filled, cystic mass [24-26]. Simple, uncomplicated cysts can be accurately diagnosed by US, CT or MRI. Although uncommon, these simple cysts may be complicated by hemorrhage, infection, or ischemia. As part of the reparative process, complicated cysts demonstrate acute and chronic inflammatory changes with granulation tissue that may include neovascularity and calcification (Fig. 3). On gross examination, a complicated cyst is often indistinguishable from cystic RCC. The precise differentiation of cystic renal carcinoma from complicated cyst is performed by microscope. RCC is best treated by surgical excision or by ablation. A cyst is not simple if it has any of the following: calcification, hyperdensity/high signal, septations, multiple locules, en-

hancement, nodularity or wall thickening (Fig. 4). Although microscopic evaluation is required for precise diagnosis, there are certain radiological findings that are reliable for differentiation of a complicated cyst from a cystic RCC. The goal of the radiologist is to categorize each cystic renal mass as nonsurgical (i.e. benign) or as surgical. Although most cystic renal masses can thus be appropriately classified and correctly managed, there is a subset of cystic masses that are probably benign but do not fulfill either the benign or the surgical criteria and thus should be followed.

When following cystic lesions that are probably benign, surgery can be avoided in many patients [25]. When a lesion is to be followed, it is important to communicate to the referring physician and to the patient the importance of complying with the follow-up recommendations. Follow-up time for these lesions has not been definitively determined, but an initial re-examination after three to six months, followed by an annual examination is reasonable. The total time for follow-up is also subjective. Five year follow-up is probably adequate in older patients, whereas a longer follow-up is prudent in younger patients. When evaluating for changes, it is important to compare the current study to the *earliest* images, not on-

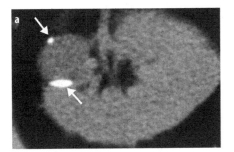
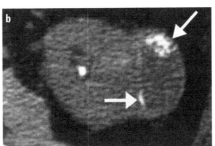
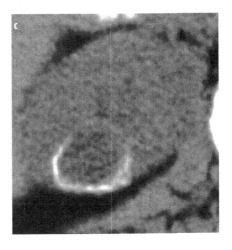

Fig. 3. Patterns of calcification. (**a**) Punctate (*upper arrow*), milk of calcium (*lower arrow*). (**b**) nodular (*upper arrow*), septal (*lower arrow*). (**c**) Peripheral. Reprinted with permission from [26]

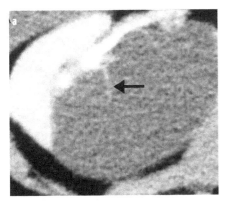
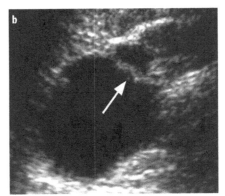
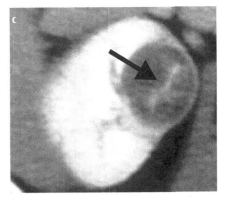

Fig. 4. Patterns of septation within a cystic mass. (**a**) Thin (*arrow*). (**b**) Thick (*arrow*). (**c**) Irregular and enhancing (arrow). Fig. 4a. Reprinted with permission from [26]

ly the most recent. Change is often slow and only recognized by comparing the oldest and current images.

Table 1 presents the guidelines for cystic renal masses: ignore, excise or follow. When evaluating cystic renal masses, it is always important to consider the patient's pretest probability for disease (e.g. Von Hippel Lindau disease) and the patient's ability to tolerate uncertainty, especially if a lesion is to be followed.

Percutaneous biopsy of indeterminate cystic renal masses remains controversial at best. Indeterminate cystic renal masses that are benign usually represent complicated cysts that contain inflammatory changes [27]. As a result, biopsy specimens obtained from the cyst's wall or fluid typically contains only renal epithelial cells, inflammatory cells, and fibrous tissue, material which cannot be used for a specific benign diagnosis [28]. Retrieving no malignant cells still leaves the radiologist, referring physician, and patient with the possibility that the lesion was improperly sampled or missed. Therefore, complete surgical resection is the only procedure that allows a definitive tissue diagnosis to be obtaineid. However, follow-up is not definitive because there is no known period of follow-up that can result in a confirmation of the benign diagnosis based on the lack of growth or change in appearance of the mass. As many indeterminate cystic renal masses are benign, proceeding directly to surgery would result in unnecessary surgery in many patients. Furthermore, some patients have co-morbidities that place the patient at risk for surgery. Recently it was shown that biopsy was avoided in 39% of patients with co-morbid disease and an indeterminate cystic renal mass [29]. Therefore, biopsy may be helpful in selected circumstances, such as patients who have co-morbidities that increase the risk of surgical exploration. In these patients, biopsy results serve as additional data that can be combined with imaging data to render a probable clinical diagnosis. However, it should be emphasized to the patient and referring physician that cystic renal mass biopsy results, particularly in the absence of malignant cells, are typically not definitive alone.

References

1. Kissane JM (1997) Congenital malformations. In: Hepinstall RH (ed) Pathology of the kidney. Little, Brown and Company, Boston, pp 69-119
2. Tada S, Yamagishi J, Kobayashi H et al (1983) The incidence of simple renal cyst by computed tomography. Clin Radiol 34:437-439
3. Smith SJ, Bosniak MA, Megibow AJ et al (1989) Renal cell carcinoma: earlier discovery and increased detection. Radiology 170:699-703
4. Jinzaki M, McTavish JD, Zou KH, Silverman SG (2004) Small (< 3 cm) renal masses improved detection and characterization with multidetector CT (MDCT). Radiology 183:223-228
5. Bosniak MA (1991) The small (less than or equal to 3.0 cm) renal parenchymal tumor detection diagnosis and controversies. Radiology 179:307-317
6. Silverman SG, Gan YU, Mortele KJ et al (2006) Renal masses in the adult patient: the role of percutaneous biopsy. Radiology (in press)
7. Frank I, Blute ML, Cheville JC et al (2003) Solid renal tumors: an analysis of pathological features related to tumor size. J Urol 170:2217-2220
8. Bosniak MA, Megibow AJ, Hulnick DH et al (1998) CT diagnosis of renal angiomyolipoma: the importance of detecting small amounts of fat. AJR Am J Roentgenol 151:497-501
9. Strotzer M, Lehner KB, Becker K (1993) Detection of fat in a renal cell carcinoma mimicking angiomyolipoma. Radiology 188:427-428
10. Helenon O, Chretien Y, Paraf F et al (1993) Renal cell carcinoma containing fat: demonstration with CT. Radiology 188:429-430
11. Castoldi MC, Dellafiore L, Renne G et al (1995) CT demonstration of liquid intratumoral fat layering in a necrotic renal cell carcinoma. Abdom Imaging 20:483-485

Table 1. Cystic renal masses: ignore, excise or follow

Finding	Ignore	Excise	Follow
Calcification	Small amount Smooth Wall or septum Milk of calcium	Associated enhancement	Thick Nodular No enhancement
Hyperdense	Sharp margin Homogeneous No enhancement < 3cm 25% extrarenal	Irregular margin Heterogeneous Enhancement Solid on US	> 3 cm Totally intrarenal
Septations	Thin Smooth No nodularity Small number	Thick Irregular Nodular Large number	'Greater than hairline'
Multiloculated		ALL	
Enhancement		ALL	
Nodularity		ALL enhancing	Small non-enhancing
Wall Thickening		ALL non-infected	

12. Lesavre A, Correas J, Merran S et al (2003) CT of papillary renal cell carcinomas with cholesterol necrosis mimicking angiomyolipomas. AJR Am J Roentgenol 181:143-145

13. Schuster TG, Ferguson MR, Baker DE et al (2004) Papillary renal cell carcinoma containing fat without calcification mimicking angiomyolipoma on CT. AJR Am J Roentgenol 183:1402-1404

14. Parvey LS, Warner RM, Callihan TR, Magill HL (1981) CT demonstration of fat tissue in malignant renal neoplasms: atypical Wilms' tumors. J Comput Assist Tomogr 5:851-854

15. Curry NS, Schabel SI, Garvin AJ, Fish G (1990) Intratumoral fat in a renal oncocytoma mimicking angiomyolipoma AJR Am J Roentgenol 154:307-308

16. Prando A (1991) Intratumoral fat in a renal cell carcinoma. AJR Am J Roentgenol 156:871

17. Jinzaki M, Tanimoto A, Narimatsu Y et al (1997) Angiomyolipoma: imaging findings in lesions with minimal fat. Radiology 205:497-502

18. Tuncali K, vanSonnenberg E, Shankar S et al (2004) Evaluation of patients referred for percutaneous ablation of renal tumors: importance of a preprocedural diagnosis. AJR Am J Roentgenol 183:575-582

19. Dechet CB, Bostwick DG, Blute ML et al (1999) Renal oncocytoma: multifocality, bilateralism, metachronous tumor development and coexistent renal cell carcinoma. J Urol 62:40-42

20. Chao DH, Zisman A, Pantuck AJ et al (2002) Changing concepts in the management of renal oncocytoma. Urology 59:635-642

21. Harmon WJ, King BF, Lieber MM (1996) Renal oncocytoma: magnetic resonance imaging characteristics. J Urol 155:863-867

22. Quinn MJ, Hartman DS, Friedman AC et al (1984) Renal oncocytoma: new observations. Radiology 153:49-53

23. Silverman SG, Tuncali K, vanSonnenberg E et al (2005) Renal tumors: MRI-guided percutaneous cryotherapy: initial experience in 23 patients. Radiology 236:716-724

24. Bosniak MA (1986) The current radiological approach to renal cysts. Radiology 158:1-10

25. Israel GM, Bosniak MA (2003) Follow up CT of moderately complex cystic lesions of the kidney (Bosniak category IIF). AJR Am J Roentgenol 181:627-633

26. Hartman DS, Choyke PL, Hartman MS (2004) A practical approach to cystic renal masses. Radiographics 24:S101-S115

27. Kissane JM (1976) The morphology of renal cystic disease. Perspect Nephrol Hypertens 4:31-63

28. Renshaw AA, Granter SR, Cibas ES (1997) Fine-needle aspiration of the adult kidney. Cancer 81:71-88

29. Harisinghani MG, Maher MM, Gervais DA et al (2003) Incidence of malignancy in complex cystic renal masses (Bosniak category III): should imaging-guided biopsy precede surgery? AJR Am J Roentgenol 180:755-758

Urinary Tract Obstruction and Infection

R.J. Zagoria[1], J.R. Fielding[2]

[1] Abdominal Radiology Section, Department of Radiology, Wake Forest University Baptist Medical Center, Winston-Salem, NC, USA
[2] Division of Abdominal Imaging, University of North Carolina at Chapel Hill, Chapel Hill, NC, USA

Urinary Tract Obstruction

In most patients, ureteral obstruction results from an acute process with associated symptoms. Some controversy exists as to which imaging studies are best for investigating suspected ureteral obstruction. In most hospitals in the United States, non-contrast helical computed tomography (CT) is preferred because it is safe and extremely rapid, and the accuracy rate for detecting ureteral stones, the most common cause of ureteral obstruction, exceeds that of other imaging studies. Other causes of acute abdominal pain, such as appendicitis, leaking aortic aneurysm, and diverticulitis, can also be readily diagnosed and occur in 13-19% of cases. Non-contrast helical CT has an overall accuracy of 97% for diagnosing ureteral stone disease [1-8]. This far exceeds the accuracy of intravenous urography (IVU) or ultrasonography (US) (See Table 1). Regardless of composition, virtually all ureteral stones have high attenuation values, making them readily detectable with CT. Nonmineralized matrix stones and some drug-related stones (due, for example, to protease inhibitors) may not be visible on CT images, but are rarely encountered.

The proper technique for performing noncontrast helical CT to detect ureteral stone disease using a helical scanner includes 5 mm collimation scanning from the top of the kidneys to the base of the bladder without intravenous or oral contrast material. Scans should be obtained during a single breath hold or in clusters. A pitch of 1-1.5 is preferable. Using a 16 slice MDCT, collimation of 1.5 mm is appropriate. In order to reduce radiation dose, a variable mA is used for each slice, based on beam attenuation. For the obese patient, a fixed mA equal to his/her weight in pounds will usually suffice. The expected dose is 30-40 mSv. Review of the images in cine mode on a workstation facilitates continuous identification of the ureter and workflow. Three-dimensional (3D) reconstructions are usually not necessary.

In addition to direct visualization of the ureteral stone, secondary signs of ureteral obstruction include unilateral nephromegaly, perinephric stranding, hydronephrosis, and periureteral stranding. The combination of perinephric stranding and unilateral hydronephrosis has a positive predictive value of 96% for the presence of stone disease. The absence of both of these signs has a negative predictive value of 93% for excluding stone disease. CT also gives information that determines therapy. Stones that are 5 mm or less in size, of smooth shape, and located within the distal third of the ureter are likely to pass spontaneously [9].

The major pitfall of noncontrast helical CT evaluation of the urinary tract for stone disease is the difficulty in distinguishing pelvic phleboliths from ureteral calculi. The presence of a tissue 'rim' sign usually indicates that the calcification is a stone rather than a phlebolith. Alternatively, the absence of the tissue rim sign, or pres-

Table 1. Diagnostic performance for CT, US, and IVU for detection of ureteral stones

Lead author	Year of publication	N	Stone +	Test	Sensitivity	Specificity
Catalano	2002	181	82	CT	.92	.96
				US/plain radiography	.77	.96
Boulay	1999	51	49	CT	1.0	.96
Sheley	1999	180	87	CT	.86	.91
Sourtzis	1999	36	36	CT	1.0	1.0
				IVU	.66	1.0
Yilmaz	1998	97	64	CT	.94	.97
				US	.19	.97
				IVU	.52	.94
Smith	1996	210	100	CT	.97	.96

N, Number of subjects; *Stone +*, Number of subjects with ureteral stone

ence of a 'comet tail' sign strongly suggests that the calcification is a phlebolith rather than a stone. In practice, the presence of two or more secondary signs of obstruction, even without clear visualization of a calcification within the ureter, indicates obstruction. If there is no history of recent stone passage, a cistoscopy and contrast-enhanced study of the upper tracts may be needed to exclude neoplasm.

Intravenous urography is an alternative technique for the detection of urinary tract obstruction [10]. It is safe, relatively inexpensive, and allows evaluation of the entire urinary tract with some functional information. Abnormalities may be subtle during the earliest phases of obstruction. Dilatation of the urinary tract may be minimal or even absent. Delayed opacification of the collecting system, asymmetric persistent nephrograms, and columnization of the ureteral contrast material down to the level of obstruction, indicate ongoing obstruction. Delayed films may be necessary to delineate the level of obstruction using IVU. The accuracy of IVU in diagnosing ureteral obstruction is unknown, but small studies suggest that it is significantly lower than the accuracy derived by noncontrast helical CT studies. Extraurinary causes of acute abdominal pain are not usually detectable with intravenous urography.

US, usually combined with a plain film, is an alternative method for evaluating the obstructed or dilated urinary tract. Although US allows for excellent evaluation of the renal parenchyma and the collecting system to the ureteropelvic junction, it is limited in the evaluation of the ureter and of soft-tissue lesions within the collecting system. The use of renal US in the evaluation of suspected acute ureteral obstruction is limited because dilatation often does not develop for hours, or even days. In these cases, US findings are normal in up to 50% of patients. The use of US Doppler-derived resistive indices may be helpful in detecting acute obstruction before dilatation develops. The usefulness of this finding is controversial [11-14]. Identification of jets at the ureterovesical junctions indicates that obstruction is incomplete and may be used to guide therapy [15].

In diuresis renography, radionuclides are injected to evaluate the urinary tract for obstruction. Considerably less anatomic detail is available with this test than with other radiographic examinations, so it is less useful in the acute setting than for follow-up or evaluation of chronic urinary tract obstruction. Diuresis renography does have the advantage of yielding objective data regarding the significance of hydronephrosis and also allows for evaluation of the function of each kidney. Administration of a diuretic, usually furosemide, augments the standard renogram and is useful in evaluating dilated urinary systems.

Magnetic resonance urography (MRU), using rapid scanning techniques such as HASTE or single-shot fast spin echo sequences, is beginning to be used for evaluation of the urinary tract [16, 17]. The kidneys and dilated ureters are very bright on T2-weighted images and their stable position allows for clear imaging of the level of ob-

struction. Unfortunately, stones appear as signal voids and can be difficult to identify and measure.

Most stones are radiodense, meaning that confirmation of stone location during conservative therapy is best performed using plain films [18]. US is useful in identifying persistent hydronephrosis or cortical atrophy.

In dealing with the pregnant patient with flank pain, fetal age and estimated radiation dose is of paramount importance. Right hydronephrosis is commonly encountered as the enlarging uterus turns slightly to the right, compressing the ureter. When an obstructing stone is suspected in either the right or left system, ultrasound should first be performed. Some urologists will place a stent based on clinical findings and severe hydronephrosis. If more imaging information is needed, a limited IVU using a plain scout film followed by a 10 minute post infusion delayed film yields the least radiation in the first trimester patient. After 20-24 weeks, IVU becomes difficult to interpret because of the enlarging uterus, and CT should be considered [19]. The expected fetal dose is approximately 16 mSv, well below that expected to cause anomalies.

Urinary Tract Infection

Acute Pyelonephritis

Acute pyelonephritis is usually an ascending infection spread from the bladder, and is seen predominately in females. Rarely, the source of infection is hematogenous bacteremia. Diagnosis is usually made on clinical grounds and with urine analysis. Imaging may be needed to detect complications or sequela of pyelonephritis. When clinical pyelonephritis persists for greater than three days after antibiotic therapy has been initiated, then imaging is recommended. CT is the imaging technique of choice to evaluate the kidneys for possible complications of pyelonephritis, such as abscess or obstruction. CT is the most sensitive and specific test for detecting the changes of acute pyelonephritis and its complications. Typical CT findings of pyelonephritis include unilateral nephromegaly, renal striations, wedge-shaped defects, and perinephric inflammatory changes [20]. Areas of liquefaction within the renal parenchyma indicate the development of a renal abscess. CT is more sensitive for the detection of renal abscess than other techniques, such as IVU or US.

In males with a urinary tract infection (UTI) and/or suspected pyelonephritis, US is valuable to identify common causes of UTI such as epididymitis, orchitis and prostatitis. Patients with a neurogenic bladder secondary to a spinal cord injury pose a difficult problem as the urine is usually colonized. Development of systemic symptoms should prompt rapid imaging as these patients may not be sensate to pain and a devastating abscess can develop quickly [21]. Finally, in order to diminish radiation dose to pregnant patients, US with power Doppler may be attempted prior to CT to detect areas of aberrant blood flow. This has been shown to be useful in children [22, 23].

Sequela of pyelonephritis includes changes of reflux nephropathy. These changes include renal scarring and calyceal blunting due to reflux of urine through the ducts of Bellini, resulting in parenchymal scarring. Changes of reflux nephropathy include broad-based scars centered over clubbed calyces, predominately occurring in the poles of the kidneys. Overall renal function of the affected kidney is best evaluated with radionuclide renography.

Emphysematous Pyelonephritis

This life-threatening infection with a gas-producing organism has a mortality rate of up to 90% without nephrectomy. The infection is usually caused by a strain of *E. coli* in diabetic patients. The diagnosis of emphysematous pyelonephritis is made when gas is seen in the renal parenchyma. CT is the most accurate technique for diagnosing emphysematous pyelonephritis and for differentiating this entity from emphysematous pyelitis or perinephric emphysematous infections. CT is also most accurate for differentiating localized from diffuse emphysematous pyelonephritis. Localized emphysematous pyelonephritis has been successfully treated with percutaneous drainage in combination with systemic antibiotic management.

Granulomatous Renal Infections

Tuberculosis, xanthogranulomatous pyelonephritis (XGP), malacoplakia, and fungal infections can all affect the urinary tract. Renal tuberculosis is usually spread hematogenously from the lungs seeding the kidneys. Symptomatic renal tuberculosis results from secondary, reactivation tuberculosis. Symptoms typically include hematuria and sterile pyuria. The earliest signs of renal tuberculosis include focal papillary necrosis and inflammation of the calyces. With progression, areas of fibrosis and calcification may develop. Long-standing tuberculosis may result in numerous fibrotic strictures, ureteral wall thickening, hydronephrosis, and autonephrectomy.

XGP, an inflammatory condition with a marked female predominance, is associated with recurrent UTIs caused by proteases, or *E. coli* bacteria. An infection-based stone is seen in the majority of cases. The classic radiographic triad includes reniform enlargement of the kidney, a renal stone, and markedly decreased or absent renal function in the affected kidney. Localized XGP occurs in 20% of cases and can mimic renal neoplasms on imaging studies [24].

Both malacoplakia and fungal infections have nonspecific appearances. They are often multifocal, but a tissue diagnosis is required to exclude neoplasm. A feature of malacoplakia is congregated histiocytes. It is more commonly seen in the bladder and ureter than the kidney. The microscopic hallmark of malacoplakia is the Michaelis-Gutman inclusion body seen within the abnormal histiocytes. When malacoplakia involves the ureter or bladder, multiple submucosal masses are usually identified.

Imaging findings are nonspecific and tissue is required for definitive diagnosis. Fungal infections are usually seen in immunocompromised patients, including diabetics. Debris, often present within the renal collecting system forms a 'hand-in-glove' filling defect of the contrast-opacified calyces.

AIDS Nephropathy

Autoimmune deficiency syndrome (HIV/AIDS) nephropathy constitutes a variety of renal pathologies. Findings are generally nonspecific, but patients with an HIV infection, renal failure, and hyperechoic nephromegaly likely have AIDS nephropathy. These sonographic findings in an AIDS patient usually indicate that the patient will develop irreversible renal failure.

Pyonephrosis

Pyonephrosis constitutes a bacterial infection of the urine associated with ureteral obstruction. If untreated, this can lead to rapid demise and irreversible damage to the kidney, and septicemia. Pyonephrosis is best diagnosed with US. Any febrile patient with hydronephrosis should be suspected of harboring pyonephrosis. Other findings that suggest pyonephrosis include echogenic urine, and debris within the hydronephrotic calyces. Prompt urinary tract drainage, preferably using percutaneous nephrostomy techniques, is required for treatment of pyonephrosis. This is accompanied by systemic antibiotic administration.

Schistosomiasis

Schistosomiasis of the urinary tract is caused by infection with *Schistosoma hematobium*. This parasite is endemic in Egypt. The infection usually arises in the bladder, but may spread to the ureters and kidneys via reflux to the upper tracts. Dystrophic calcifications in the wall of the bladder and ureter are typical findings and are caused by calcification of the dead ova. Typical radiographic findings include mural calcifications, ureteral strictures, and vesicoureteral reflux. These patients have a markedly increased risk for development of squamous cell carcinoma of the urinary tract.

Ureteral Pseudodiverticulosis

This uncommon abnormality is caused by overgrowth of the urothelial lamina propria. Although cellular atypia is commonly seen in association with ureteral pseudodiverticulosis, it is thought to be a benign lesion. However, the presence of ureteral pseudodiverticulosis should be considered a warning sign for the development of transitional cell carcinoma. There appears to be high risk of synchronous transitional cell carcinomas, or later development of transitional cell carcinoma in the urothelial field affected by the pseudodiverticulosis. Close radiographic follow-up is warranted in these patients.

References

1. Sourtzis S, Thibeau JF, Damry N et al (1999) Radiologic investigation of renal colic: unenhanced helical CT compared with excretory urography. AJR Am J Roentgenol 172:1491-1494
2. Yilmaz S, Sindel T, Arslan G et al (1998) Renal colic: comparison of spiral CT, US and IVU in the detection ureteral calculi. Eur Radiol, pp 8212-8217
3. Catalano O, Nunziata A, Altei F et al (2002) Suspected ureteral colic: primary helical CT versus selective helical CT after unenhanced radiography and sonography. AJR Am J Roentgenol 178:379-387
4. Levine JA, Neitlich J, Verga M et al (1997) Ureteral calculi in patients with flank pain: correlation of plain radiography with unenhanced helical CT. Radiology 204:27-31
5. Olcott EW, Sommer FG, Napel S (1997) Accuracy of detection and measurement of renal calculi: in vitro comparison of three-dimensional spiral CT, radiography, and nephrotomography. Radiology 204:19-25
6. Remer EM, Herts BR, Streem SB et al (1997) Spiral noncontrast CT versus combined plain radiography and renal UR after extracorporeal shock wave lithotripsy; cost-identification analysis. Radiology 204:33-37
7. Zagoria RJ, Khatod E, Chen MYM (2001) Abdominal radiography after positive CT stone study: a method to predict utility based on stone size and CT attenuation. AJR Am J Roentgenol 176:1117-1122
8. Smith RC, Verga M, McCarthy S et al (1996) Diagnosis of acute flank pain:value of unenhanced helical CT. AJR Am J Roentgenol 166:97-101
9. Fielding JR, Silverman SG, Samuel S et al (1998) Unenhanced helical CT of ureteral stones: a replacement for excretory urography in planning treatment. AJR Am J Roentgenol 171:1051-1053
10. Dyer RB, Chen MYM, Zagoria RJ (2001) Intravenous urography: technique and interpretation. Radiographics 21:799-824
11. Platt JF, Ellis JH, Rubin JM (1995) Role of renal Doppler imaging in the evaluation of acute renal obstruction. AJR Am J Roentgenol 164:379-380
12. Platt JF, Rubin JM, Ellis JH (1989) Distinction between obstructive and nonobstructive pyelocaliectasis with duplex Doppler sonography. AJR Am J Roentgenol 153:997-1000
13. Cronan JJ (1992) Contemporary concepts for imaging urinary tract obstruction. Urol Radiol 14:8-12
14. Older RA, Stoll HL III, Omary RA et al (1997) Clinical value of renovascular resistive index measurement in the diagnosis of acute obstructive uropathy. J Urol 157:2053-2055
15. Burge HJ, Middleton WD, McClennan BL et al (1991) Ureteral jets in healthy subjects and in patients with unilateral ureteral calculi: comparison with color Doppler US. Radiology 180:437-442
16. Aerts P, Van Hoe L, Bosmans H et al (1996) Breath-hold MR urography using the HASTE technique. AJR Am J Roentgenol 166:543-545
17. Rothpearl A, Frager D, Subramanian A et al (1995) MR urography: technique and application. Radiology 194:125-130
18. Assi Z, Platt JF, Francis IR et al (2000) Sensitivity of CT scout radiography and abdominal radiography for revealing ureteral calculi on helical CT: implications for radiologic follow-up. AJR Am J Roentgenol 175:333-337
19. Fielding JR, Washburn D (2005) Imaging the pregnant patient: a uniform approach. J Women's Imaging 7:16-21
20. Zagoria RJ, Dyer RB (1991) Radiology of renal infectious disease. Contemp Diagn Radiol 8:1-6
21. Rubenstein JN, Schaeffer AJ (2003) Managing complicated urinary tract infections. The urologic view. Infect Dis Clin N Am 17:333-351
22. Dacher J, Pfister C, Monroc M et al (1996) Power Doppler sonographic pattern of acute pyelonephritis in children: comparison with CT. AJR Am J Roentgenol 166:1451-1455
23. Majd M, Nussbaum Blask AR, Markle BM et al (2001) Acute pyelonephritis: comparison with Tc99m-DMSA SPECT, spiral CT, MR imaging, and power Doppler US in an experimental pig model. Radiology 218:101-108
24. Parker MD, Clark RL (1989) Evolving concepts in the diagnosis of xanthogranulomatous pyelonephritis. Urol Radiol 11:7-15

Diseases of the Female Genital Tract I

S.M. Ascher

Department of Radiology, Georgetown University Hospital, NW, Washington, DC, USA

Introduction

Transvaginal Sonography (TVS) is often the initial imaging exam used when evaluating the female genital tract. However, if the TVS is suboptimal or non-diagnostic, or if additional information is needed, magnetic resonance imaging (MRI) should be considered. MRI is advantageous because of its multiplanar capability, high spatial and contrast resolution and lack of ionizing radiation. For the evaluation of a possible pelvic abnormalities, MRI is able to address the following clinical questions: (1) where is it? (e.g., uterine or ovarian); (2) what is it? (neoplastic or non-neoplastic, malignant or benign, congenital or acquired); and (3) how does the information impact patient management (e.g., selection of appropriate candidates for different therapies and patient monitoring following treatment).

MRI Technique

Pelvic MRI is best performed on high field strength systems ($\geq$ 1.5 T) using a torso phased-array body coil. This set-up affords the greatest signal-to-noise ratios and spatial resolution. Patient preparation is negligible. In our practice, patients are asked to fast for 4-6 hours prior to the exam in order to limit bowel peristalsis. Patients are also asked to void immediately before imaging to increase their comfort during the course of the exam.

A bare bones examination includes orthogonal T2-weighted (W) fast spin echo sequences (FSE), axial T1-W sequences, with and without fat suppression, and when indicated, sagittal dynamic contrast-enhanced 3D fat-suppressed T1-W sequences. Most of our sequences are performed in a breath hold (e.g., T2-W single shot FSE [SS FSE]). Breath hold sequences are advantageous because they eliminate respiratory artifacts, limit peristatic artifacts and shorten exam times, leading to greater patient satisfaction. We reserve high resolution (512 matrix), non-breath hold T2-W FSE sequences to determine tumor extent in patients with gynecologic malignancies.

The Uterus: Benign Conditions

Leiomyoma

Leiomyomas are benign tumors of smooth muscle origin. They are the most common uterine tumors, with a prevalence of 20% in women over the age of 35. The prevalence is even higher in women of African descent. The tumors are estrogen-dependent and often regress with menopause.

Leiomyomas may be located intramurally (most common), submucosally or subserosally. They tend to be well-demarcated and may undergo some degree of degeneration (e.g., hyaline, cystic, fatty or carneous). Calcification is common in leiomyomas of older women. Rare complications include infection, torsion and sarcomatous degeneration (< 1%). Symptoms associated with leiomyomas include menorrhagia, dysmenorrhea, infertility (especially submucosal leiomyomas that may impede the implantation of fertilized ova) and bulk-related symptoms (mass effect on the bladder or bowel).

MRI can accurately diagnose leiomyomas [1-3]. It is also accurate for determining their size, number and location. This information is important to help match the appropriate patients with symptomatic leiomyomas with the different therapies available. For example, a patient with multiple intramural and/or submucosal hypervascular leiomyomas is a good candidate for uterine artery embolization (UAE), whereas a patient with a pedunculated subserosal leiomyoma may be better served by myomectomy. Similarly, hysteroscopic resection may be the best therapeutic option in a patient with a single submucosal leiomyoma that does not significantly extend into the underlying myometrium. Detection of significant ovarian artery supply to the pre-UAE uterus may be a predictor of treatment failure or fibroid recurrence following UAE [4]. MRI can also be used to follow patients post-UAE and may help with imaging any complications [5].

T2-W images provide optimal contrast between leiomyomas and adjacent uterine tissue (Fig. 1). Most leiomyomas are well-circumscribed, low signal intensity (SI) masses. If there is associated degeneration, they may exhibit high SI components [6]. T1-W images provide information about the type of degeneration (e.g., high SI to

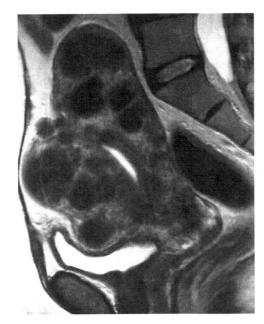

Fig. 1. Leiomyomas. Sagittal T2 SS FSE with multiple well-circumscribed low signal intensity intramural and subserosal leiomyomas

The symptoms of adenomyosis are non-specific and may mimic leiomyomas. However, it is important to establish the correct diagnosis pre-operatively, because uterine-conserving therapy is possible with leiomyomas, whereas hysterectomy is the definitive treatment for debilitating adenomyosis.

MRI is an accurate, non-invasive modality for the diagnosis of adenomyosis, differentiation of adenomyosis from other gynecologic disorders, and planning for appropriate therapy [10]. Several studies have found MRI to be very accurate in diagnosing adenomyosis, with a sensitivity and specificity ranging from 86-100% [11-13].

Adenomyosis is diagnosed when the junctional zone is greater than, or equal to, 12 mm (Fig. 2). Ancillary findings

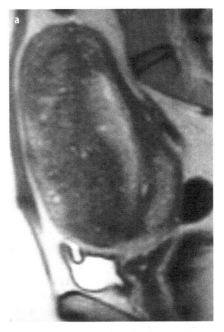

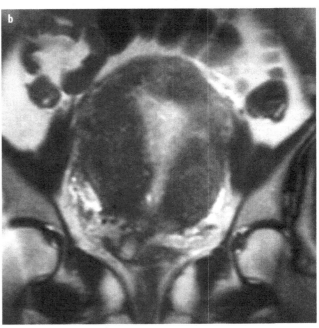

Fig. 2. Adenomyosis. Sagittal (**a**) and coronal (**b**) T2 SS-FSE images with junctional zone widening, striations and the punctuate foci of adenomyosis

diagnose hemorrhage). Additionally, T1-W sequences can aid in differentiating a pedunculated subserous leiomyoma from an ovarian mass. Contrast-enhanced T1-W sequences are optional, but do provide information about blood supply to, and viability of, a leiomyoma, which may be important for planning treatment and follow-up [7].

Prospectively differentiating a leiomyosarcoma from a degenerated benign leiomyoma is difficult. Reported MRI findings are variable and include lobulated mass of high SI on T2-W images, a sharply marginated mass of low SI on T2-W images, or a mass with focally infiltrative margins [8]. In a study of 12 patients (nine with leiomyosarcoma and three with smooth muscle tumors of uncertain malignant potential), the majority of malignant tumors had more than 50% high signal on T2-W images, the presence of many small high signal areas of T1-W images and well-demarcated, non-enhancing regions [9]. While these imaging characteristics are non-specific, any fibroid that demonstrates marked interval growth or change in appearance may suggest the possibility of leiomyosarcoma.

Adenomyosis

Adenomyosis is common uterine condition affecting up to one third of hysterectomy specimens. It is defined as the presence of ectopic endometrial glands and stroma within the myometrium. Adenomyosis is also associated with myometrial hyperplasia. Cyclic hemorrhage is unusual in adenomyosis because of the predomination of the zona basalis endometrial layer. This zone is relatively unresponsive to hormonal stimuli. Two types of adenomyosis exist: diffuse adenomyosis and focal adenomyosis (adenomyoma). Diffuse adenomyosis is more common and typically affects the posterior uterine wall.

include high SI foci on T1- and/or T2-W images. These may represent islands of ectopic glands, cystically dilated glands and/or hemorrhagic fluid. In some patients, linear high SI striations can be seen radiating from the endometrium into the myometrium. Following contrast, adenomyosis may have a 'swiss cheese' appearance, with foci of signal void that represent ectopic endometrial glands. Adenomyomas may be separate from the junctional zone and image as ill-defined, low SI masses on T2-W sequences.

Occasionally, the imaging appearance of submucous leiomyomas and adenomyosis overlap. Features favoring the diagnosis of adenomyosis include lesions that: (1) are poorly marginated; (2) elliptical lesions with minimal mass effect relative to their size; (3) have linear striations that originate in the endometrium and extend into the myometrium; and (4) do not have dilated vessels at their margins [10, 14, 15].

Congenital Anomalies

The incidence of congenital uterine anomalies among women of reproductive age ranges from 0.1-0.5%. The clinical significance of such anomalies is an increased likelihood of infertility, pregnancy wastage (e.g., recurrent miscarriage, premature labor, intrauterine growth retardation) and menstrual disorders.

The uterus, fallopian tubes and upper two thirds of the vagina originate from paired mullerian ducts. The ducts migrate caudally and then fuse. Subsequently, the intervening tissue (septum) resorbs to form the endometrial, endocervical and endovaginal canals. This process, which begins at approximately 10 weeks of gestation, may be interrupted at any stage in development. Failure of the paired ducts to develop results in various degrees of agenesis (or hypoplasia). Absent or incomplete fusion leads to didelphys or bicornuate uteri, respectively. Complete or partial failure of resorption following fusion results in a septate uterus. Congenital anomalies are classified according to the American Fertility Society classification, which divides anomalies into classes with similar features, prognoses and treatment options [16, 17]. It is important to note however, that congenital uterine anomalies are a spectrum of disorders and occasionally it may be impossible to assign a malformation to one particular class. This fact underscores the importance of imaging to highlight the affected anatomy. MRI is the most accurate modality for identifying uterine anomalies: it is more specific than ultrasound (US) or hysterosalpingography (HSG), and it is less invasive and less costly than laparoscopic evaluation [18]. In addition to depicting genital anomalies, MRI's large field of view allows the abdomen and pelvis to be surveyed for associated urinary tract anomalies (e.g., renal agenesis, ectopia).

Class I: Segmental Agenesis/Hypoplasia
This class of anomalies may affect just a portion of genital tract, or combined abnormalities may be present. Agenesis/hypoplasia may occur as part of a syndrome, as a result of chromosomal defects, or in isolation. Patients with vaginal agenesis but with patent endometrial and endocervical canals are treated with vaginoplasty to allow egress of menses. Hysterectomy is reserved for patients without a cervix, as a neocervix or uterovaginal fistula is unable to successfully sustain a pregnancy, nor can it prevent retrograde menses and endometriosis.

Class II: Unicornuate Uterus
These anomalies result from the failure of one of both of the paired mullerian ducts. If no rudimentary horn is present, usually no further treatment is required. Similarly, no intervention is needed if there is a rudimentary horn that does not contain endometrium. However, if a rudimentary horn contains endometrium, regardless of whether it communicates with the main uterine cavity, surgical excision is recommended to prevent retrograde menses or ectopic pregnancy.

Class III: Uterus Didelphys
This anomaly results from failure of mullerian duct fusion, leading to two uteri and two cervices. In the majority of cases there is a transverse vaginal septum. If the septum is obstructive, hematocolpometra results. Resection of the septum establishes normal egress of menses via the vagina.

Class IV: Bicornuate Uterus
This class of anomalies results from incomplete fusion of the mullerian ducts. A fundal cleft of more than 1 cm distinguishes a bicornuate uterus from a septate uterus (see Class V). Bicornuate uteri rarely require surgery. However, if a patient is symptomatic, a transabdominal metroplasty can be performed.

Class V: Septate Uterus
This class of anomaly results from a failure of resorption of the central intervening tissue, septum, between the two endometrial canals. Complete and incomplete forms exist. In the former, the septum extends into the cervix (Fig. 3),

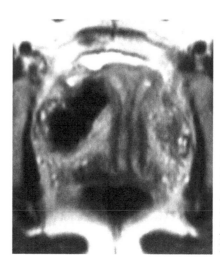

Fig. 3. Complete Septate Uterus. Coronal T2 SS FSE of the uterus with fundal notch < 1 cm, and two endometrial and endocervical canals separated by a low signal intensity septum. Both ovaries are normal

whereas in the latter it is confined to the uterine body. Septate uteri have a flat, convex or minimally concave fundal contour. Septate uteri have the highest incidence of fetal wastage and can be successfully treated with hysteroscopic removal of the septum.

Class VI: Arcuate Uterus

This anomaly is more appropriately termed a normal variant, as there is a slight fundal indentation. Patients are asymptomatic and do not require treatment.

Class VII: Diethystilbesterol (DES) Exposure in Utero

Approximately half of the women exposed to DES *in utero* have a congenital uterine anomaly. The most common abnormality is a T-shaped uterus, which often results in cervical incompetence. In these instances, pregnant women are treated with cervical cerclage.

The Uterus: Malignant Conditions

Cervical Cancer

Patients with cervical cancer are staged according to the classification of the International Federation of Gynecology and Obstetrics (FIGO) (Table 1). Unfortu-nately, FIGO staging is based primarily on clinical exam (neither cross-sectional imaging, nor lymph node status is routine), and staging errors of 15-24% for patients with Stage IB disease and 45-58% for patients with Stages IIA and IIB disease have been reported [19, 20]. MRI is the best single modality for the pre-operative staging of cervical cancer: it is cost minimizing and it can alter therapy [21-23]. In a retrospective study, Hricak et al. found that women with cervical cancer > 2 cm whose initial staging examination was MR required fewer tests and fewer procedures compared to the standard work-up [22]. MR imaging correlates for FIGO staging have been developed and are summarized in Table 1.

T2-W images consistently demonstrate the relatively high SI tumors, and are 93% accurate in determining tumor size compared with surgical specimens [24]. The overall staging accuracy of MR imaging ranges from 87-92% [24, 25].

Moreover, the negative predictive value for parametrium invasion, 95%, makes MR imaging an attractive modality for selecting appropriate therapy [21, 24, 25].

The morbidity associated with radiation therapy (RT) is increased after surgery, resulting in a preference for pre-operative RT followed by surgery. Moreover, conventional RT in combination with brachytherapy is as effec-

Table 1. Cervical cancer: FIGO staging with corresponding MR imaging findings[1]

Stage	Findings
FIGO Stage	
Stage 0	Carcinoma *in situ*
Stage I	Tumor confined to cervix
Stage IA	Microscopic tumor (preclinical tumor)
Stage IB	Clinically visible invasive tumor > 5 mm
Stage II	Tumor invades beyond uterus but not to pelvic wall or lowest third of vagina
Stage IIA	Vaginal invasion
Stage IIB	Parametrial invasion
Stage III	Tumor extends to pelvic wall and/or involves lowest third of vagina and/or hydronephrosis, non-functioning kidney
Stage IIIA	Invasion of lowest third of vagina
Stage IIIB	Pelvic sidewall invasion, hydronephrosis, non-functioning kidney
Stage IV	Tumor invades outside true pelvis and/or invades bladder or rectal mucosa
Stage IVA	Invasion of bladder or rectal mucosa
Stage IVB	Distant metastasis
MR imaging findings[2]	
Stage 0	No tumor present
Stage IA	No tumor present or localized widening of the endocervical canal with a small tumor mass
Stage IB	Partial or complete disruption of low-signal-intensity stromal ring, intact tissue surrounding tumor
Stage IIA	Segmental disruption of low-signal-intensity stromal ring with tumor extending into parametrium
Stage IIB	Complete disruption of low-signal-intensity stromal ring with tumor extending into parametrium
Stage IIIA	Segmental disruption of low-signal-intensity vaginal wall (lowest third)
Stage IIIB	Tumor extends to obturator internus, piriformis, levator ani muscles; dilated ureter
Stage IVA	Signal loss of low-signal-intensity bladder or rectal wall
Stage IVB	Tumor in distant organs

[1] T2-weighted or contrast-enhanced T1-weighted images.
[2] Modified from [26]

tive as surgery for FIGO stage IB (2) disease [27]. That is, patients with less than 5 mm stromal invasion (Stage IA1/2), or patients without evidence of a bulky tumor (> 4 cm) confined to the cervix (Stage IB1) may be amenable to surgical cure. Patients with bulky tumors (> 4 cm) confined to the cervix (Stage IB2) or patients with parametrial invasion (Stage IIB, tumor extends beyond the low SI cervical stroma and smooth muscle into the parametrium), or patients with more advanced disease are better treated with RT (Fig. 4). As a practical issue, when trying to distinguish Stage IB tumors from IIB tumors, it is better to overcall, sparing patients the added morbidity of RT after surgery [28]. The National Cancer Institute recommends that many patients with cervical cancer benefit from concurrent chemotherapy [29-31]. Chemotherapy decreases the relative risk of death, decreases tumor bulk and controls micrometastases.

There is some debate concerning the need for gadolinium in the evaluation of cervical cancers. Some reports found that delayed gadolinium-enhanced T1-W sequences were less accurate in depicting stromal invasion compared to T2-W sequences, while others have found that dynamic gadolinium-enhanced images are superior to both T2-W and delayed contrast-enhanced studies for assessing stromal invasion [32-34]. For the most part, cervical cancers enhance more than adjacent fibrocervical stroma immediately following contrast administration. This relationship reverses with delayed imaging. Dynamic contrast-enhanced MRI has also been advocated to predict tumor response to therapy, both prior to the institution of therapy and during the course of treatment [35].

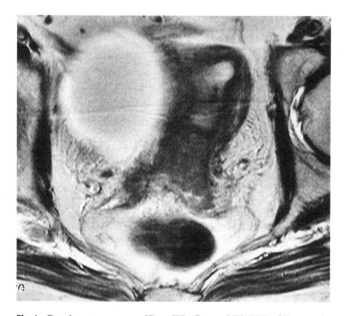

Fig. 4. Cervix cancer: stage IB vs IIB. Coronal T2 FSE of the cervix with effacement of normal zonal anatomy. While it is difficult to identify direct extension into the parametrium, upstaging is preferred in cases where the distinction between IB (1) and IIB tumor is controversial. An incidental simple right adnexal cyst is seen

For lymph node assessment, MR relies on size criteria. For para-aortic, iliac and obturator lymph nodes, a short axis of more than 1 cm is used to detect disease. For parametrial lymph nodes, most experts agree that those lymph nodes greater than 5 mm are suspicious for metastatic disease. While SI has no predictive value, central necrosis may imply involvement. Unfortunately, relying on lymph node size is imperfect. Using a 1 cm short axis as indicative of involvement has a modest sensitivity (45-60%). Ultra-small paramagnetic iron-oxide particles (USPIO) MR or positron emission tomography computed tomography (PET CT) will likely change lymph node assessment in patients with cervical cancer.

Conditions where MR imaging should be recommended in women with cervical cancer include:
– Transverse diameter > 2 cm, based on physical exam
– Tumor that is endocervical or predominantly infiltrative that cannot be accurately assessed clinically
– Tumor that is clinically suspected to be stage II disease
– Patients who are pregnant or have concomitant uterine lesions (e.g., leiomyomas), making assessment by other means difficult.

Endometrial Cancer

MRI has been gaining widespread acceptance for the evaluation of women with diagnosed endometrial cancer. MR correlates of surgical FIGO staging have been described (Table 2). The overall staging accuracy of MRI ranges from 83-92% [36-38]. Studies have found MRI to be 74-91% accurate for differentiating early superficial endometrial cancer (stages IA and IB) from cancers with deep myometrial invasion (stage IC). MRI examination of women with endometrial cancer should include dynamic intravenous gadolinium administration. Intravenous contrast improves the following: (1) detection of endometrial abnormalities; (2) distinguishing viable tumor from debris; and (3) assessment of depth of myometrial and cervical invasion [39-41]. A recently published meta-analysis comparing the utility of CT, US and MR for staging endometrial cancer found that contrast-enhanced MRI tended to perform better than CT or US in assessing depth of myometrial invasion [40]. This has important economic implications for the identification of a subset of patients that might benefit from referral to a tertiary care center for more aggressive management by a gynecologic oncologist.

Endometrial cancer images on T2-W sequence as either diffuse or focal widening of the endometrial canal [1, 37, 38 ,42] (Fig. 5). The hormonal milieu determines the normal endometrial width (approximately 13 mm for reproductive age women or post-menopausal women on hormone replacement therapy (HRT) vs 3 mm for post-menopausal women not on HRT). Disruption or irregularity of the junctional zone signifies myometrial invasion. Invasion is further classified as superficial, ≤ 50%,

Table 2. Endometrial cancer: FIGO staging with corresponding MR imaging findings[1]

Stage	Findings
FIGO Stage	
Stage 0	Carcinoma *in situ*
Stage I	Tumor confined to corpus
Stage IA	Tumor limited to endometrium
Stage IB	Invasion < 50% of myometrium
Stage IC	Invasion > 50% of myometrium
Stage II	Tumor invades cervix but does not extend beyond uterus
Stage IIA	Invasion of endocervix
Stage IIB	Cervical stromal invasion
Stage III	Tumor extends beyond uterus but not outside true pelvis
Stage IIIA	Invasion of serosa, adnexa, or positive peritoneal cytologic findings
Stage IIIB	Invasion of vagina
Stage IIIC	Pelvic or para-aortic lymphadenopathy
Stage IV	Tumor extends outside true pelvis or invades bladder or rectal mucosa
Stage IVA	Invasion of bladder or rectal mucosa
Stage IVB	Distant metastases (includes intra-abdominal or inguinal lymphadenopathy)
MR imaging findings[2]	
Stage 0	Normal or thickened endometrial stripe
Stage IA	Thickened endometrial stripe with diffuse or focal abnormal signal intensity; endometrial stripe may be normal; intact junctional zone with smooth endometrial-myometrial interface
Stage IB	Signal intensity of tumor extends into myometrium < 50%; partial- or full-thickness disruption of junctional zone with irregular endometrial-myometrial interface
Stage IC	Signal intensity of tumor extends into myometrium > 50%; full-thickness disruption of junctional zone; intact stripe of normal outer myometrium
Stage IIA	Internal os and endocervical canal are widened; low signal of fibrous stroma remains intact
Stage IIB	Disruption of fibrous stroma
Stage IIIA	Disruption of continuity of outer myometrium; irregular uterine configuration
Stage IIIB	Segmental loss of hypointense vaginal wall
Stage IIIC	Regional lymph nodes greater than 1.0 cm in diameter
Stage IVA	Tumor signal disrupts normal tissue planes with loss of low signal intensity of bladder or rectal wall
Stage IVB	Tumor masses in distant organs or anatomic sites

[1] T2-weighted or contrast-enhanced T1-weighted images.
[2] Modified from [26]

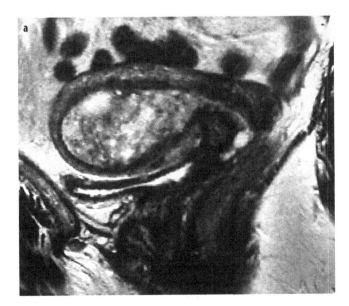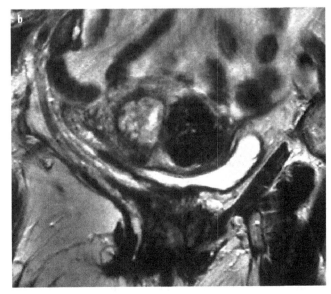

Fig. 5. Endometrial cancer: stage IB. Sagittal (**a**) and coronal (**b**) T2 FSE of the uterus with distended heterogeneous endometrial canal. The tumor myometrial interface is irregular, a sign of superficial invasion

or deep, > 50%, depending on penetration into the underlying myometrium.

Current recommendations for MR imaging in women with endometrial cancer include instances where:

– There is a high pretest probability for lymph node metastases (e.g., high grade tumor, papillary or clear cell tumor) (CT is equivalent)
– There is a high pretest probability for cervical invasion
– There is a need for multi-factorial assessment of myometrial, cervical and lymph node involvement.

The Ovary

The main role of MRI in evaluating ovarian abnormalities is that of tissue characterization [43, 44]. MRI is a problem-solving tool for determining the origin of a mass and providing information on its make-up.

Benign Conditions

The most commonly encountered benign ovarian condition is physiologic cysts. These are round, smooth-walled and lack solid elements or debris. These simple cysts are low in SI on T1-W sequences and get progressively higher in SI on T2-W images. Hemorrhagic cysts, which contain methemoglobin, tend to have high SI intensity on both T1- and T2-W sequences, whereas endometriomas are multilocular masses that are high in SI on T1-W sequences and show shading on T2-W sequences [45, 46] (Fig. 6). This shading reflects rebleeding into the cysts and consequently the presence of blood products of varying chronicity. T1-W fat-suppressed sequences improve the conspicuity of endometriomas [47, 48]. In one study, the sensitivity and specificity for detecting endometriomas ≥ 1 cm was 91% and 94%, respectively [49]. T1-W fat suppressed sequences also help differentiate fat-containing lesions (e.g., cystic teratomas) from blood-containing lesions [50] (Fig. 7).

Malignant Conditions: Ovarian Carcinoma

The sensitivity of MR for detecting adnexal pathology parallels that of US and CT, ranging from 87-100%. However, it is the tissue characterization potential of MRI that makes it robust for evaluating the adnexa [51]. In fact, for characterizing an ovarian mass as benign or malignant the accuracy of MR ranges from 83-95% compared to US and CT, which range from 53-88% and 66-94%, respectively [52-54]. In the largest prospective trial evaluating ovarian masses imaged with transvaginal sonography, MRI was more accurate than CT or Doppler sonography for diagnosing malignancy [55]. Once the diagnosis of malignancy is made, CT of the abdomen and pelvis is typically performed. The accuracy of CT and MR staging is comparable, approaching 90% [56]. Neither modality can supplant staging laparotomy because of their limited ability to detect small intraperitoneal implants, although MRI

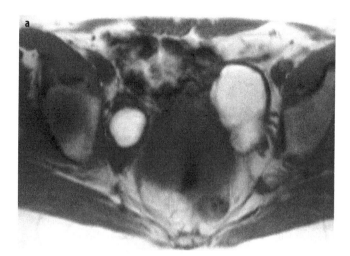

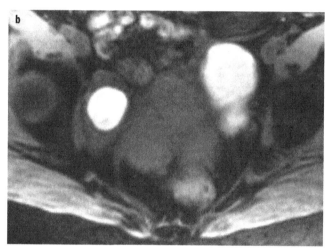

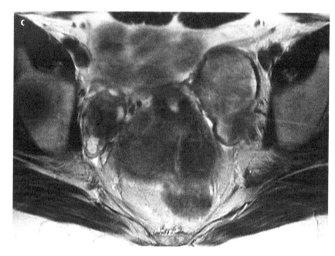

Fig. 6. Endometriomas. Axial T1 without fat supression (**a**), T1 with fat suppression (**b**) and T2 FSE (**c**) of bilateral ovarian masses that retrain high signal intensity on the T1 fat-suppressed technique and demonstrate loss of signal shading, on T2 FSE

may aid surgical treatment planning. MRI is also adept at identifying patients with bulky non-resectable disease and can spare patients the morbidity of surgical staging. The positive and negative predictive values for

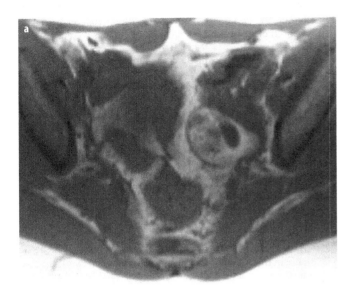

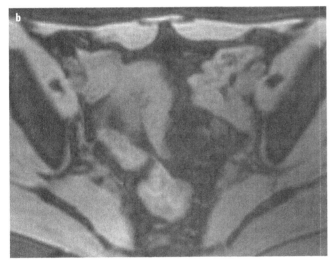

Fig. 7. Dermoid. Axial T1 without fat suppression, and T1 with fat suppression, of left ovarian mass. High signal intensity elements on T1 image without fat suppression fall in signal with the addition of chemically selective fat suppression

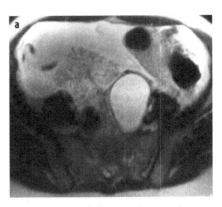

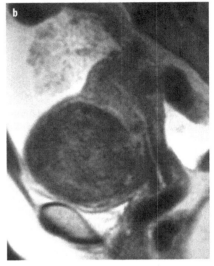

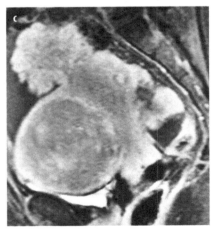

Fig. 8. Ovarian cancer. Axial (**a**) and sagittal (**b**) T2 SSFSE and sagittal gadolium-enhanced T1 with fat suppression (**c**) of complex ovarian mass. Incidental note is made of large anterior uterine corpus leiomyoma

diagnosing non-resectability are 91% and 97%, respectively [57].

Ovarian cancers are typically large heterogeneous masses with both cystic and solid components (Fig. 8). Owing to their complexity, their SI on T1 and T2-W sequences is variable. Rather than predicting the exact histology of an ovarian cancer, the real strength of MRI is in suggesting whether or not a lesion is malignant. Both primary and ancillary criteria have been formulated for this determination. These criteria are up to 95% accurate in correctly characterizing an adnexal mass as benign or malignant [52]. Primary criteria include size greater than 4 cm, solid or predominantly solid lesion, wall thickness greater than 3 mm, septae greater than 3 mm, nodularity, and presence of necrosis. Ancillary criteria include involvement of pelvic organs or sidewall, peritoneal, mesenteric or omental disease, ascites and lymphadenopathy.

Results of a multivariate analysis found that necrosis within a solid lesion, vegetations within a cystic lesion, ascites and peritoneal metastases are the features most predictive of malignancy [52].

Current imaging recommendations for MRI of the adnexa include:

- Evaluation of an equivocal or non-diagnostic transvaginal sonogram
- Characterization of a known ovarian mass
- Determination of resectability in women with the diagnosis of ovarian cancer.

Conclusions

The role of MRI in many gynecologic disease states is established, while in others it is expanding. As with most advanced technologies, MRI is a moving target. MR hardware and software upgrades, coupled with an increasing emphasis on evidence-based medicine, will help refine both the protocols and interpretation models for imaging women with gynecologic conditions.

References

1. Reinhold C, Gallix BP, Ascher SM (1997) Uterus and Cervix. In: Semelka RC, Ascher SM, Reinhold C (eds) MRI of the abdomen and pelvis: a text atlas. 1st ed, Wiley-Liss, New York, NY, pp 585-660
2. Weinreb JC, Barkoff MD, Megibow A, Demopoulos R (1990) The value of MR imaging in distinguishing leiomyomas from other solid pelvic masses when sonography is indeterminate. AJM Am J Roentgenol 154:295-299
3. Hricak H, Tscholakoff D, Heinrichs L et al (1986) Uterine leiomyomas: Correlation of MR histopathologic findings, and symptoms. Radiology 158:385-391
4. Pelage JP, Cazejust J, Pluote E et al (2005) Uterine fibroid vascularization and clinical relevance to uterine fibroid embolization. Radiographics 25:S99-S117
5. Kitamura Y, Ascher SM, Cooper C et al (2005) Imaging manifestations of complications associated with uterine artery embolization. Radiographics Suppl 1:S119-S132
6. Ueda H, Togashi K, Konishi I et al (1999) Unusual appearances of uterine leiomyomas: MR imaging findings and their histopathologic backgrounds. Radiographics 19:S131-S145
7. Jha RC, Ascher SM, Imaoka I, Spies JB (2000) Magnetic resonance imaging of the uterus pre- and post uterine artery embolization. Radiology 217:228-235
8. Kido A, Togashi K, Takashi K et al (2003) Diffusely enlarged uterus: evaluation with MR imaging. Radiographics 23:1423-1439
9. Tanaka YO, Nishida M, Tsunoda H et al (2004) Smooth muscle tumors of uncertain malignant potential and leiomyosarcomas of the uterus: MR findings. JMR I6:998-1007
10. Tamai K, Togashi K, Tsuyoshi I et al (2005) MR Imaging findings of adenomyosis: Correlation with histopathologic features and diagnostic pitfalls. Radiographics 25:21-40
11. Togashi K, Nishimura K, Itoh K et al (1988) Adenomyosis: diagnosis with MR imaging. Radiology 166:111-114
12. Ascher SM, Arnold LL, Patt RH et al (1994) Adenomyosis: prospective comparison of MR imaging and transvaginal sonography. Radiology 190:803-806
13. Reinhold C, McCarthy S, Bret P et al (1996) Diffuse adenomyosis: comparison of endovaginal US and MR imaging with histopathologic correlation. Radiology 199:151-158
14. Mark AS, Hricak H, Heinrichs LW et al (1987) Adenomyosis and leiomyoma: differential diagnosis with MR imaging. Radiology 163:527-529
15. Togashi K, Ozasa H, Konishi I et al (1989) Enlarged uterus: differentiation between adenomyosis and leiomyoma with MR imaging. Radiology 171:531-534
16. Buttram VC Jr, Gibbons WE (1979) Muellerian anomalies: a proposed classification (an analysis of 144 cases). Fertil Steril 32:40-46
17. Buttram VC (1983) Muellerian anomalies and their management. Fertil Steril 40:159-163
18. Pellerito JS, McCarthy SM, Doyle MB et al (1992) Diagnosis of uterine anomalies: relative accuracy of MR imaging, endovaginal sonography, and hysterosalpingography. Radiology 183:795-800
19. Matsuyama T, Inoue I, Tsukamoto N et al (1984) Stage IB, IIA and IIB cervix cancer, postsurgical staging and prognosis. Cancer 54:3072-3077
20. VanNagell JR, Roddick JW, Lowin DM (1971) The staging of cervical cancer: inevitable discrepancies between clinical staging and pathologic findings. Am J Obstet Gynecol 110:973-978
21. Subak LL, Hricak H, Powell CB et al (1995) Cervical carcinoma: computed tomography and magnetic resonance imaging for pre-operative staging. Obstet Gynecol 86:46-50
22. Hricak H, Powell CB, Yu KK et al (1996) Invasive cervical carcinoma: role of MR imaging in pretreatment work-up-cost minimization and diagnostic efficacy analysis. Radiology 198:403-409
23. Durfee SM, Zou KH, Muto MG et al (2000) The role of magnetic resonance imaging in treatment planning of cervical carcinoma. Journal of Women's Imaging 2:63-68
24. Hricak H, Lacey CG, Sandles LG et al (1988) Invasive cervical carcinoma: comparison of MR imaging and surgical findings. Radiology 166:623-631
25. Lien HH, Blomlie V, Kjorstad K et al (1991) Clinical stage I carcinoma of the cervix: value of MR imaging in determining degree of invasiveness. AJR Am J Roentgenol 156:1191-1194
26. Ascher SM (1999) Female pelvis: malignant disease. RSNA Categorical Course in Diagnostic Radiology. Body MRI, pp 85-94
27. Herzog TJ (2003) New approaches for the managemet of cervical cancer. Gynecol Oncol 90:S22-S27
28. Sironi S, Belloni C, Taccagni GL, Del Maschio A (1991) Carcinoma of the cervix: value of MR imaging in detecting parametrial invasion. AJR Am J Roentgenol 156:753-756
29. Rose PG, Bundy BN, Watkins EB et al (1999) Concurrent cisplatin-based radiotherapy and chemotherapy for locally advanced cervical cancer. New Engl J Med 340:1144-1153
30. Morris M, Eifel PJ, Lu J et al (1999) Pelvic radiation with concurrent chemotherapy compared with pelvic and para-aortic radiation for high-risk cervical cancer. New Engl J Med 340:1137-1143
31. Keys HM, Bundy BN, Stehman FB et al (1999) Cisplatin, radiation, and adjuvant hysterectomy compared with radiation and adjuvant hysterectomy for bulky stage IB cervical carcinoma. New Engl J Med 340:1137-1143
32. Hricak H, Hamm B, Semelka RC et al (1991) Carcinoma of the uterus: use of gadopentetate dimeglumine in MR imaging. Radiology 181:95-106
33. Sironi S, De Cobelli F, Scarfone G et al (1993) Carcinoma of the cervix: value of plain and gadolinium enhanced MR imaging in assessing degree of invasiveness. Radiology 188:797-801
34. Yamashita Y, Takahashi M, Sawada T et al (1992) Carcinoma of the cervix: dynamic MR imaging. Radiology 182:643-648
35. Yamashita Y, Baba T, Baba Y et al (2000) Dynamic contrast-enhanced MR imaging of uterine cervical cancer: pharmacokinetic analysis with histopathologic correlation and its importance in predicting the outcome of radiation therapy. Radiology 216:803-809
36. Hirano Y, Kubo K, Hirai Y et al (1992) Preliminary experience with gadolinium-enhanced dynamic MR imaging for uterine neoplasms. Radiographics 12:243-256
37. Hricak H, Rubinstein LV, Gherman GM, Karstaedt N (1991) MR imaging evaluation of endometrial carcinoma: results of an NCI cooperative study. Radiology 179:829-832

38. Lien HH, Blomlie V, Trope C et al (1991) Cancer of the endometrium: value of MR imaging in determining depth of invasion into the myometrium. AJR Am J Roentgen 157:1221-1223

39. Frei KA, Kinkel K, Bonel HM et al (2000) Prediction of deep myometrial invasion in patients with endometrial cancer: clinical utility of contrast-enhanced MR imaging – a meta analysis and bayesian analysis. Radiology 216:444-449

40. Seki H, Takan T, Sakai K (2000) Value of dynamic MR imaging in assessing endometrial carcinoma involvement of the cervix. AJR Am J Roentgenol 175:171-176

41. Kinkel K, Kaji Y, Yu KK et al (1999) Radiological staging in patients with endometrial cancer: a meta-analysis. Radiology 212:711-718

42. Takahashi S, Murakami T, Narumi Y et al (1998) Preoperative staging of endometrial carcinoma: diagnostic effect of T2-weighted fast spin echo MR imaging. Radiology 206:539-547

43. Ascher SM, Outwater EK, Reinhold C (1997) Adnexa. In: Semelka RC, Ascher SM, Reinhold C (eds) MRI of the abdomen and pelvis: a text-atlas. 1st ed. Wiley-Liss, New York, NY pp 661-715

44. Outwater EK, Dunton CJ (1995) Imaging of the ovary and adnexa: clinical issues and applications of MR imaging. Radiology 194:1-18

45. Arrive L, Hricak H, Martin MC (1989) Pelvic endometriosis: MR imaging. Radiology 171:687-692

46. Zawain M, McCarthy SM, Scoutt L, Comite F (1989) Endometriosis: appearance and detection on MR imaging. Radiology 171:693-696

47. Sugimura K, Okizuka H, Imaoka I et al (1993) Pelvic endometriosis: detection and diagnosis with chemical shift MR imaging. Radiology 188:435-438

48. Ha HK, Lim YT, Kim HS et al (1994) Diagnosis of pelvic endometriosis. Fat-suppressed T1-weighted vs conventional MR images. AJR Am J Roentgenol 163:127-131

49. Ascher SM, Agrawal R, Bis KG et al (1995) Endometriosis: appearance and detection with conventional and contrast-enhanced fat suppressed spin echo techniques. J Magn Reson Imaging 5:251-257

50. Stevens SK, Hricak H, Campos Z (1993) Teratomas versus cystic hemorrhagic adnexal lesions: differentiation proton-selective fat saturation MR imaging. Radiology 186:481-488

51. Siegelman ES, Outwater EK (1999) Tissue characterization in the female pelvis by means of MR imaging. Radiology 212:5-18

52. Stevens SK, Hricak H, Stern JL (1991) Ovarian lesions: detection and characterization with gadolinium-enhanced MR imaging at 1.5 T. Radiology 181:481-488

53. Komatsu T, Konishi I, Mandai M et al (1996) Adnexal masses: transvaginal US and Gadolinium-enhanced MR imaging assessment of intratumoral structure. Radiology 198:109-115

54. Yamashita Y, Torashima M, Hatanaka Y et al (1995) Adnexal masses: accuracy of characterization with transvaginal US and precontrast and postcontrast MR imaging. Radiology 194:557-565

55. Kurtz AB, Tsimikas JV, Tempany CMC et al (1999) Diagnosis and staging of ovarian cancer: comparative values of Doppler and Conventional US, CT and MR imaging correlated with surgery and histopathologic analysis. Report of the radiology diagnostic oncology group. Radiology 212:19-27

56. Amendola MA (1985) The role of CT in evaluation of ovarian malignancy. Crit Rev Diag Imaging 24:329-368

57. Forstner R, Hricak, Occhipinti KA et al (1995) Ovarian cancer: staging with CT and MR imaging. Radiology 197:619-626

Diseases of the Female Genital Tract II

R.A. Kubik

Department of Radiology, Kantonsspital Baden, Baden, Switzerland

Introduction

While transabdominal or transvaginal ultrasound remain the imaging modalities of first choice for the initial evaluation of any suspected pathologic condition of the female genital tract, technical advances in cross-sectional imaging have opened up many diagnostic applications in female pelvic pathology. Computed tomography (CT) is usually employed in an emergency situation, such as in an acute abdomen caused by ovarian torsion, as well as for the diagnosis of metastatic spread in oncologic patients. Compared to CT, magnetic resonance imaging (MRI) provides improved soft tissue contrast and is thus better suited to evaluate female genital organs. Further advantages of MRI over CT include that it does not employ ionizing radiation and has no teratogenic effects. MRI is thus well suited for imaging women of reproductive age and especially during pregnancy, e.g., for MR pelvimetry and, more recently, as an adjunct to sonography for fetal imaging. MRI nowadays plays an increasing role in preoperative characterization and staging of gynecologic tumors and is also used as a problem-solving tool in benign conditions, e.g., in patients with uterine malformations or leiomyoma, or to select appropriate candidates for therapies such as myomectomy and uterine embolization.

Normal MR Anatomy of the Female Genital Organs

The uterus is best depicted using T2-weighted sagittal sequences. In women of reproductive age, the uterus is approximately 6-9 cm in length. In the premenopausal woman, three distinct zones are recognized: (1) the high-signal intensity endometrium of varying thickness, depending on the menstrual cycle; (2) the hypointense junctional zone, anatomically corresponding to the innermost layer of the myometrium; and (3) the outer layer of the myometrium of intermediate signal intensity. Four zones are distinguished in the cervix by high-resolution MRI: (1) the hyperintense mucous within the endocervical canal, (2) the cervical mucosa of intermediate to high signal intensity, (3) the hypointense cervical stroma surrounding the mucosa, and, (4) an additional layer of in-

termediate signal intensity in continuity with the uterine myometrium representing smooth muscle (Fig. 1). In postmenopausal patients, the uterine corpus, but not the cervix, regresses and decreases in size.

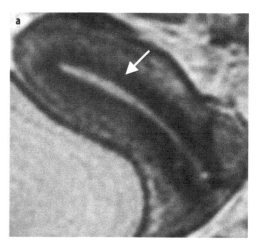

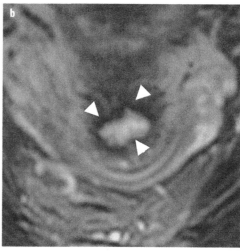

Fig. 1. Normal MR anatomy (T2-weighted images) of the uterus and cervix. **a** Three zones are recognized in the uterus: the hyperintense endometrium, the hypointense junctional zone (*arrow*) and the outer layer of the myometrium of intermediate signal intensity. **b** Four zones are distinguished in the cervix: the hyperintense mucous within the endocervical canal, the cervical mucosa, the hypointense cervical stroma (*arrowheads*), and an additional layer of smooth muscle

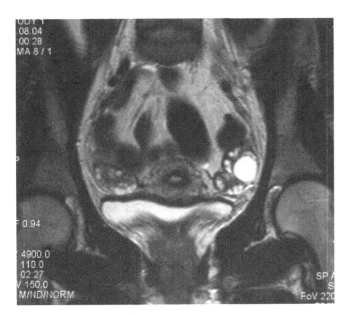

Fig. 2. Normal MR anatomy (coronal T2-weighted image) of ovaries. Multiple follicular cysts are seen in both ovaries

Normal ovaries measure between 1.5 and 3 cm during reproductive age while their size decreasing after menopause. They can be easily diagnosed by the presence of T2-weighted hyperintense follicles (Fig. 2).

Congenital Anomalies of the Uterus

Congenital malformations of the uterus, also termed Müllerian duct anomalies (MDA), are a relatively uncommon, but often treatable, cause of infertility. The incidence of congenital MDA among women of reproductive age is estimated to be up to 0.5%. However, since normal pregnancies can occur in women with MDA and the anomalies are discovered in most cases in patients presenting with infertility, the reported prevalence of MDA in the general population is probably underestimated. Uterine malformations can be associated with subfertility, pregnancy wastage, and menstrual disorders. Congenital malformations of other organ systems may be present - most frequently renal malformations like renal agenesis or ectopia - whereas bony malformations, such as fusion of the vertebral column, are less commonly seen. Whereas transvaginal ultrasound and hysterosalpingography are the primary imaging modalities, MRI is currently used as a problem-solving modality in inconclusive cases, e.g., in the differentiation between septate and bicornuate uterus, and is widely accepted as the leading imaging modality for further surgical planning. MRI provides high resolution images of the entire uterine anatomy (internal and external contour) and allows diagnosis of secondary findings like renal malformation. If possible, patients undergoing MRI for suspected MDA should be scheduled in the second half of the menstrual cycle, since the thickness of the endometrial stripe increases during the follicular and

secretory phase and thus the normal zonal anatomy of the uterus can be better appreciated.

According to the classification of the American Fertility Society, MDAs can be classified into seven different classes (Fig. 3, 4, 6). The classification describes

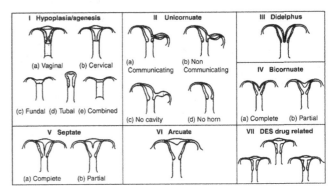

Fig. 3. Classification system of Müllerian duct anomalies according to the American Fertility Society

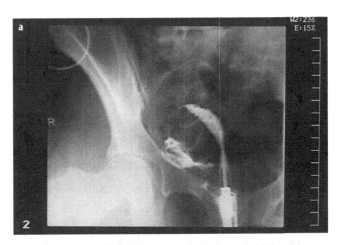

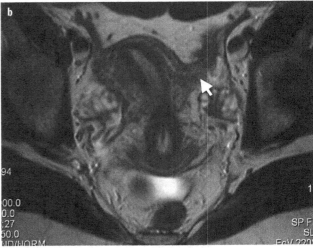

Fig. 4. A 28-year-old woman with a history of infertility. **a** Hysterosalpingography. **b** Axial T2-weighted MR image. An unicornuate uterus with a rudimentary left horn without endometrial cavity (*arrow*) is seen

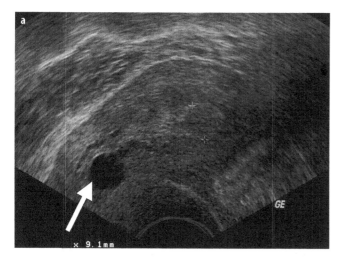

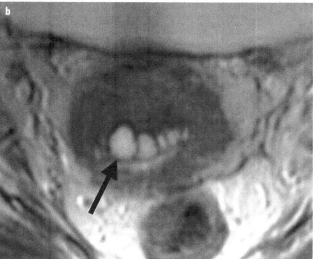

Fig. 5. Nabothian cysts (*arrows*) of the cervix. **a** Ultrasound **b** T2-weighted MR image

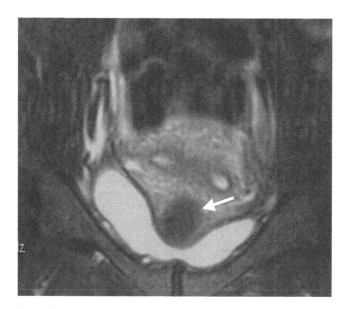

Fig. 6. Coronal T2-weighted FSE MR image. Small hypointense leiomyoma (*arrow*) in a bicornuate uterus

primarily the uterine defects, because of the wide variability and overlap of associated cervical and vaginal anomalies, whereas the cervico-vaginal defects are added separately in the form of a subset.

Benign Conditions of the Vagina, Cervix and Uterus

Bartholin's cysts are caused by retained secretions within the vulvo-vaginal glands, mostly as a result of chronic inflammation or trauma. They are located in the posterolateral parts of the lower vagina and vulva, whereas *Nabothian Cysts* are retention cysts of the cervical glands and clefts.

Leiomyomas (also known as fibroids and fibromyomas) are benign neoplasms of smooth-muscle cell origin and are the most common uterine tumors (Fig. 5-7).

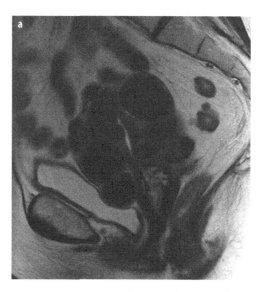

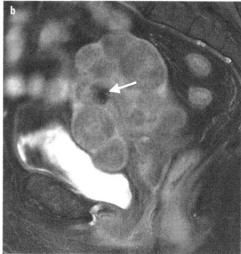

Fig. 7. Multiple uterine leiomyomas. Sagittal T2-weighted and contrast-enhanced T1-weighted image. The multiple lesions are sharply demarcated. They present as hypointense lesions on the T2-weighted sequence. Contrast-enhancement is less pronounced compared to the adjacent normal myometrium. A signal void is indicative of calcification (*arrow*)

The lesions must be differentiated from focal adeno-myosis (Fig. 8). Ultrasound remains the primary imaging modality for clinically suspected leiomyomas, and in the vast majority of routine clinical presentations no additional investigation is needed. MRI is recommended in selected cases as a problem-solving modality, e. g., to distinguish between a pedunculated leiomyoma and a solid ovarian mass, to demonstrate the exact size and location of the lesion (subserosal, intramural, submucosal) before uterine-sparing surgery or for selecting candidates for uterine artery embolization, as well as to distinguish leiomyoma from adenomyoma.

Most leiomyomas have a typical appearance on MRI. They are depicted as sharply marginated, hypointense lesions not only on T1-, but also on T2-weighted sequences. Low-signal intensity on T2-weighted images permits differentiation from malignant tumors. Leiomyomas, especially when large and during pregnancy, may undergo degenerative changes such as necrosis, resulting in various, non-specific MR appearances.

Malignant Tumors of the Cervix and Uterus

Invasive *cervical carcinoma* is the third most common malignancy of the female genital tract. Early detection of cervical carcinoma due to gynecologic examination and the Pap smear has led to a significant reduction in mortality. At histology, squamous cell carcinoma is found in over 90% of cases. Imaging is not used for tumor detection, but for staging of cytologically proven disease. Transvaginal ultrasound is usually the first imaging modality employed. Additional cross-sectional imaging is especially useful if the tumor volume is large. MRI was shown to be superior to CT in the local staging of cervical carcinoma.

T2-weighted MR sequences are most helpful for local staging of cervical disease. The tumor presents with high signal intensity compared with the low intensity cervical stroma. Stage-IB International Federation of Gynecology and Obstetrics (FIGO) carcinoma is restricted to the cervix and presents on T2-weighted images with a fully preserved hypointense rim of normal cervical stroma surrounding the tumor (Fig. 9), whereas in patients with parametrial invasion (stage FIGO IIB), i.e., one of the most important criteria influencing therapeutic decision making, the normal stroma is disrupted. Contrast-enhanced sequences are not routinely used for the staging of cervical carcinoma. They may be useful in selected cases with suspected invasion of the bladder or rectum.

In patients with *endometrial carcinoma* proven by fractional abrasion, MRI is the imaging modality of choice for preoperative staging. It is used to assess the depth of myometrial invasion and to identify invasion of the cervix or extrauterine spread. It was shown to be especially helpful in the subpopulation of patients in whom the extent of tumor growth may alter the surgical approach or in patients in whom concomitant lesions, such as leiomyomas, make clinical assessment difficult.

Signal intensities of small endometrial tumors are similar to that of normal endometrium on T2-weighted sequences, limiting the ability of tumor delineation, whereas larger tumors result in the widening of the endometrial cavity. It should be kept in mind that endometrial hyperplasia and endometrial polyps are benign entities also resulting in a thickened endometrium that have therefore to be distinguished from endometrial carcinoma (Fig. 10).

A disruption of the junctional zone by a hyperintense

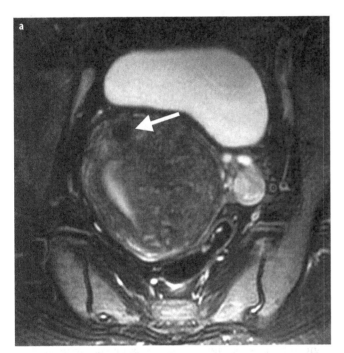

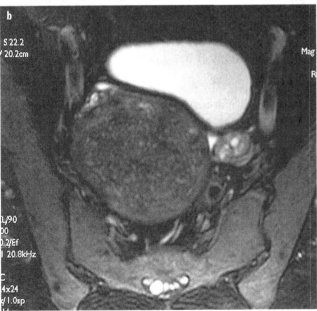

Fig. 8. Focal adenomyosis (T2-weighted images). Enlarged uterus with diffusely thickened junctional zone with multiple hyperintense foci indicative of adenomyoma. A small leiomyoma can also be seen (*arrow*)

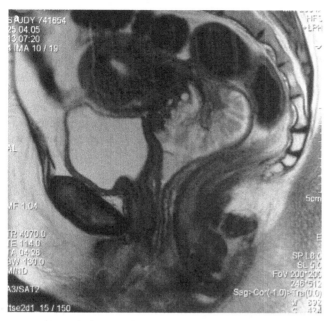

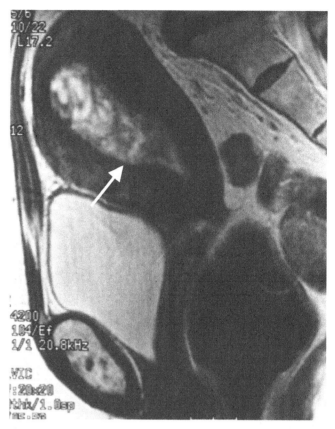

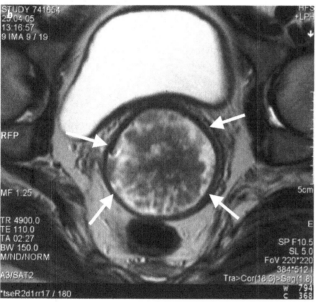

Fig. 10. Endometrial Carcinoma stage FIGO IA (sagittal T2-weighted MR Image). The endometrial stripe is thickened due to the presence of tumor, while the junctional zone (*arrow*) remains intact

Fig. 9. Cervical carcinoma stage FIGO IB. **a** Sagittal T2-weighted MR image. **b** Axial oblique T2-weighted MR image. Although the tumor volume is rather large, the cervical stroma (*arrows*) is not disrupted

Most uterine tumors are adenocarcinomas; other histologic subtypes like leiomyosarcoma or endometrial stromal tumors are rare.

Benign Conditions of the Ovaries

Follicular cysts are the most common benign ovarian masses. Other non-neoplastic adnexal lesions include endometrioma, adnexal torsion and tubo-ovarian abscess. Paraovarian cysts, also termed Gartner's duct cysts, are remants of the Wolffian body and are found in the mesosalpinx in the hilum of the ovary.

Those non-neoplastic masses should be distinguished from benign and malignant ovarian neoplasm.

Ultrasound is again the primary imaging modality for assessment of suspected ovarian lesions. However, due to its multiplanar imaging capabilities and high soft tissue contrast, MRI is superior to ultrasound for demonstrating the origin of a lesion (e.g., distinguishing a subserosal leiomyoma from a solid ovarian mass), as well as in lesion characterization, and is thus employed in unclear cases for tissue characterization or surgical planning. MRI is able to diagnose certain benign ovarian lesions that can have misleading sonographic features, such as endometrioma or mature cystic teratoma (also known as dermoid cyst). The

endometrial tumor is indicative of myometrial invasion. The junctional zone, however, cannot always be delineated in postmenopausal women, which makes correct imaging interpretation difficult in these cases. Deep myometrial invasion is suggested by the presence of hyperintense tumor in the outer half of the myometrium. Intravenous administration of gadolinium compounds is helpful for MR staging of endometrial carcinoma, with the cancer demonstrating less pronounced contrast-enhancement compared with the surrounding tissues. Contrast-enhanced images further improve the differentiation of vital tumor from necrosis or hematometra.

latter are very common ovarian neoplasms and belong to the group of germ cell tumors. Evidence of intralesional fat, independent of the size of the lesion, is indicative of this being a benign entity (Fig. 11).

Primary criteria of malignancy on MRI include a diameter of greater than 4-6 cm, intralesional solid elements or septations, wall thickening, and necrosis (Fig. 12). Ancillary criteria are enlarged lymph nodes, ascites, and infiltration of neighboring structures.

In patients with ovarian carcinoma, preoperative cross-sectional imaging may help in preoperative planning by providing information on tumor spread. Currently, CT re-

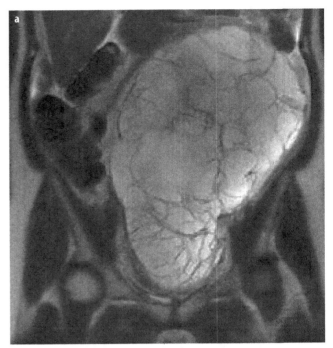

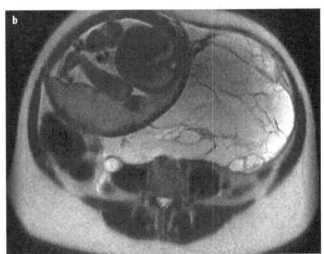

Fig. 12. Mucinous ovarian cystadenocarcinoma with ascites in a pregnant patient (coronal and axial TruFisp sequence). A large multiloculated lesion is seen

mains, in our opinion, the imaging modality of choice for this indication, having similar staging accuracy, but being more widely available and cost efficient.

Up to 10% of ovarian tumors are metastatic. Rarely, the ovarian lesion may be the first manifestation of disease. Primaries most commonly originate from the gastrointestinal tract, breast, uterus, or thyroid.

MRI in Obstetrics

There is no clinical or experimental evidence of teratogenic or other adverse fetal effects from MRI in pregnancy, and the technique is thus well suited for imaging of

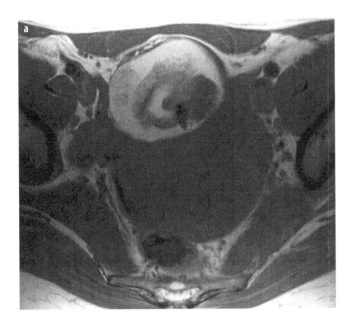

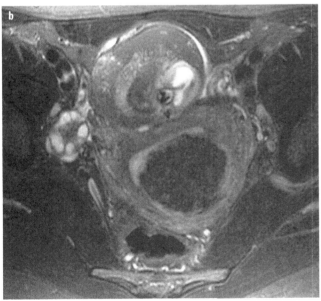

Fig. 11. Benign mature teratoma. **a** Precontrast T1-weighted image. **b** T2-weighted fat-saturated image. Parts of the lesion were hyperintense on T1- (**a**) and T2-weighted images (not shown) and showed a signal decrease after fat saturation (**b**). The presence of fat is indicative of a benign ovarian lesion.

pregnant women for maternal or fetal reasons (Fig. 12).

MR pelvimetry is indicated in pregnant women with a history of pelvic trauma, previous cesarean section, or in women who desire a trial of labor when the fetus is in breech presentation. The use of X-ray pelvimetry has decreased steadily in recent years. MRI offers the benefit of accurate measurement of the maternal pelvic dimensions without exposure to ionizing radiation.

More recently, technical advances in ultrafast MRI have revolutionized our ability to image the fetus. MRI is most likely to become an important tool for intrauterine *fetal imaging* as an operator-independent supplement to prenatal ultrasound in the near future.

Suggested Reading

Anonymous (1988) The American Fertility Society classifications of adnexal adhesions, distal tubal occlusion, tubal occlusion secondary to tubal ligation, tubal pregnancies, mullerian anomalies and intrauterine adhesions. Fertil Steril 49:944-955

Hamm B, Kubik-Huch RA, Fleige B (1999) MR imaging and CTof the female pelvis: radiologic-pathologic correlation (pictorial review). Eur Radiol 9:3-15

Hricak H, Powell CB, Yu KK et al (1996) Invasive cervical carcinoma: role of MRI in pretreatment work-up: cost minimization and diagnostic efficacy analysis. Radiology 198:403-409

Hricak H, Rubinstein LV, Gherman et al (1991) MR imaging evaluation of endometrial carcinoma: results on NCI cooperative study. Radiology 179:829-832

Keller TM, Michel SCA, Fröhlich J et al (2004) USPIO-enhanced MRI for preoperative staging of gynecological pelvic tumors – preliminary results. Eur Radiol 14:937-944

Keller TM, Rake A, Michel SCA et al (2003) Obstetric MR pelvimetry: reference values and evaluation of inter- and intraobserver error and intraindividual variability. Radiology 227:37-43

Kubik-Huch RA, Wisser J, Stallmach T, Marincek B (1998) Prenatal diagnosis of fetal malformation by ultrafast magnetic resonance imaging. Prenatal Diagn 18:1205-1208

Levine D, Barnes PD, Edelman RR (1999) State of the art. Obstetric MR imaging. Radiology 211:609-617

Mark AS, Hricak HH, Heinrichs LW et al (1987) Adenomyosis and leiomyoma. Differential diagnosis with MR imaging. Radiology 163:527-529

Outwater EK, Dunton CJ (1995) Imaging of the ovary and adnexa. Clinical issues and applications of MR imaging. Radiology 194:1-18

Saleem SN (2003) MR imaging diagnosis of uterovaginal anomalies: current state of the art. Radiographics 23:e13

Scoutt LM, McCauley TR, Flynn SD et al (1993) Zonal anatomy of the cervix: correlation of MR imaging and histologic examination of hysterectomy specimen. Radiology 186:159-162

Stevens SK, Hricak H, Campos Z (1993) Teratomas versus cystic hemorrhagic adnexal lesions: differentiation with proton-selective fast saturation MR imaging. Radiology 186:481-488

Tamai K, Togashi T, Morisawa N (2005) MR imaging findings of adenomyosis: Correlation with histopathologic features and diagnostic pitfalls. Radiographics 25:21-40

Troiano RN, McCarthy SM (2004) Mullerian duct anomalies: imaging and clinical issues. Radiology 233:19-34

Yamashita Y, Mizutani H, Torashima M et al (1993) Assessment of myometrial invasion by endometrial carcinoma: transvaginal sonography vs contrast-enhanced MR imaging. AJR Am J Roentgenol 161:595-599

Yamashita Y, Torashima M, Hatanaka Y et al (1995) Adnexal masses: accuracy of characterization with transvaginal US and precontrast and postcontrast MR imaging. Radiology 194:557-565

Imaging of the Male Pelvis

J.O. Barentsz[1], B.J. Wagner[2], E. Abouh-Bieh[3]

[1] Department of Radiology, University Medical Center St Radboud, Nijmegen, The Netherlands
[2] Department of Radiology, The Reading Hospital and Medical Center, West Reading, PA, and Armed Forces Institute of Pathology, Washington, DC, USA
[3] Department of Radiology, Urology and Nephrology Center, Mansoura, Egypt

Part I: MRI of Prostate Cancer*

Introduction

Prostate cancer continues to be the leading cancer among American men, with 184,500 new cases annually [1]. It has been estimated that 39,200 men died of prostate cancer in the U.S.A. in 1998. This makes prostate cancer the second cause of cancer-related death in men [2, 3]. Furthermore, the probability of developing prostate cancer from birth to death is 20% [3]. Treatment selection is dependent on patient age and health, cancer stage and grade, morbidity and mortality of treatment, as well as patient and physician preference. The mainstay for organ-confined disease is either radical surgery or curative radiotherapy [4, 5]. This is only considered an option in the absence of seminal vesicle infiltration (SVI), extension through the prostatic capsule (extracapsular extension, ECE) or metastatic disease. Therefore, the purpose of staging is the possible detection of extraprostatic disease. Clinical staging by digital rectal examination (DRE) and prostate specific antigen (PSA) remains as yet inaccurate. Imaging modalities such as transrectal ultrasound (TRUS) and magnetic resonance (MR) imaging can be used to increase staging accuracy. This review deals with the current possibilities and limitations of MR imaging in the staging of prostate cancer.

Clinical Staging Methods

Accurate staging of prostate cancer is important because treatment decisions are mainly based on the local extent of prostate cancer (ECE, SVI) and the presence of metastatic disease (lymphatic or hematogenous). DRE is not an accurate staging method, as there are no gross characteristics that are reliable to distinguish benign from malignant nodules [6]. Furthermore, the interobserver agreement among urologists for detection of prostate cancer by DRE is only fair [7]. Data accumulated from carefully examined prostatectomy specimens revealed that DRE underestimates the local extent of cancer in 40-60% of the cases [8, 9]. PSA is the most accurate marker to screen for

prostate cancer, but has limited accuracy in staging because there is a substantial overlap in PSA concentrations and pathologic stages. Nevertheless, the combination of serum PSA concentration and other variables such as tumour grade, volume and clinical stage, significantly enhance the predictive value of serum PSA for the pathological stage [10, 11]. The probability of ECE, SVI and nodal involvement can be predicted by using the normograms of Partin [10] that are based on clinical stage, Gleason score and serum prostate specific antigen (PSA).

MR Imaging

MR imaging of the prostate is still in an exploratory phase and is not yet advocated as a routine staging procedure. Prostate MR imaging should be performed in centers where at least 25-50 patients per year are examined and the results can be compared with histology, preferably whole mount specimen [12]. Currently, the major clinical indication for MR imaging is detection of ECE, SVI, nodal and bone marrow metastases, which are contraindications for radical prostatectomy [13]. Prostate cancer is usually visible as a low signal intensity lesion in a bright peripheral zone on a T2-weighted image (Fig. 1). The differential diagnosis of low signal intensity areas includes cancer, hemorrhage, prostatitis, effects of hormonal or radiation treatment, benign prostate hyperplasia (BPH), scar, calcifications, smooth muscle hyperplasia, and fibromuscular hyperplasia [14]. Hemorrhage, mostly a result from biopsy, can be differentiated from cancer by evaluation of T1-weighted images (Fig. 2). Hemorrhage is hyperintense on these images, whereas cancer has the same intensity compared to adjacent normal tissue. BPH, smooth muscle hyperplasia and fibromuscular hyperplasia are located mostly in the central zone (CZ) and transitional zone (TZ), whereas cancer is primarily located in the peripheral zone (PZ). Calcifications are common in all locations of the prostate; however, these may be differentiated from cancer based on their distinct oval form. Scars are rare. Detection of cancer in the CZ and TZ is generally not possible, as this area is commonly replaced by BPH, which has an identical signal.

---

* J.O. Barentsz

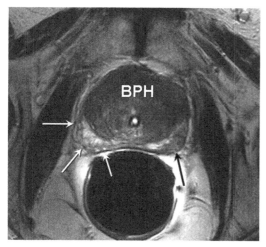

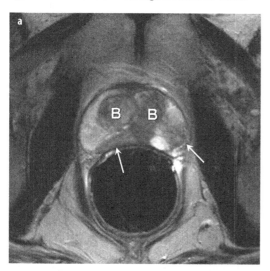

Fig. 1. Stage T2a prostate cancer. On axial T2 weighted MR image normal peripheral zone has high SI (*white arrows*), prostate cancer (*black arrow*) and benign prostatic hyperplasia (*BPH*) have low SI. Centrally, a bladder catheter with high SI urine is visible

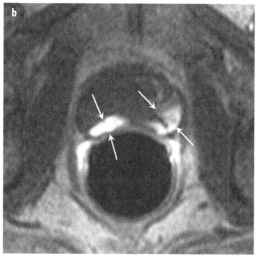

Fig. 2. Biopsy hematoma and BPH (**a**) T2-weighted and (**b**) T1-weighted axial images two weeks post biopsy. **a** Both hematoma (*arrows*), and benign prostatic hypertrophy (*B*) cannot be differentiated from tumor as all have low SI. **b** However, hematomas (*arrows*) have high SI, and can be separated from BPH and cancer

A review of existing literature revealed that an optimal imaging protocol includes turbo/fast spin echo, at least two imaging planes, high-resolution images, and the use of an endorectal phased array coil. Reading should (preferably) be performed in consensus, using experienced readers.

Staging

Several MR imaging criteria for ECE have been used. Table 1 presents commonly used criteria for ECE with its specificity and sensitivity. Most frequent used criteria are asymmetry of the neurovascular bundle, obliteration of the rectoprostatic angle, and bulging of the prostate capsule (Fig. 3). SVI is detected by an abnormal, asymmetric, low signal intensity within the lumen on T2-weighted images (Fig. 4) [15]. It should be noted that amyloid deposits, stones or blood could also cause low signal intensity of the seminal vesicles on T2-weighted images [14-17].

In staging, MR imaging should have a high specificity for periprostatic extension, to ensure that only few patients will be deprived of a potentially curative therapy [18]. Sensitivity for periprostatic extension is of minor importance, because even a low sensitivity is an improvement on clinical staging [18]. MR imaging is considered cost-effective if performed in a subgroup of patients with a prior-probability of ECE of at least 30%; that is, a PSA greater than 10 or a Gleason grade greater than 7 [19].

The initial accuracy in 1990 for the staging of prostate cancer with MR imaging was 69% [20]. Since then the most prominent change was the development of an endorectal coil (ERC), which resulted in faster imaging and improved spatial resolution. Accuracy for ECE with the ERC has a wide range, between 58-90% [21-24]. Several reasons for this wide range can be given. Firstly, due to the rapidly developing MR imaging technique, different studies used different imaging protocols. Secondly, due to inexperience with this new method, considerable interobserver variation may be present. A third important reason is that different studies use different criteria for ECE (Table 3) resulting in different accuracies. Although this variation remains, the use of an ERC is considered to be an improvement of the conventional MR examination [23-25]. Although major developments have changed the MR imaging technique, it is still not possible to detect microscopic ECE [20, 22, 26, 27]. The detection of SVI is generally not

Table 1. Criteria to predict extracapsular extension of prostate cancer

Criteria for capsular penetration	Acc	Spec	Sens	PPV
Asymmetry of neurovascular bundle	70%	95%	38%	–
Obliteration of rectoprostatic angle	71%	88%	50%	–
Bulge	72%	79%	46%	28%
Overall impression	71%	72%	68%	32%
Extracapsular tumor	73%	90%	15%	34%

Acc, accuracy; *Spec*, specificity; *Sens*, sensitivity; *PPV*, positive predictive value; –, no data available

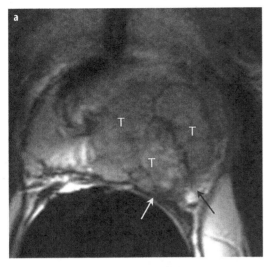

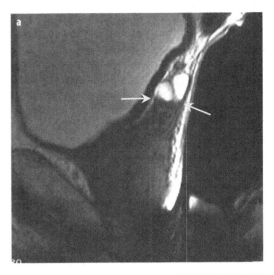

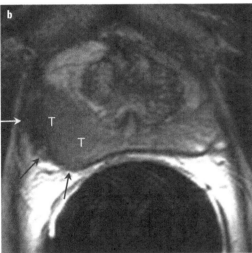

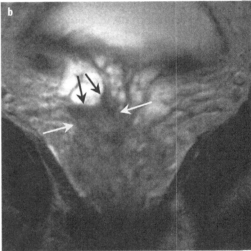

Fig. 3. Two stage T3a prostate cancers (extracapsular invasion), T2-weighted axial MR image. **a** Large cancer is replacing about two thirds of the left prostate (T). There is extracapsular extension at the site of the neurovascular bundle (*arrows*). Clear asymmetry of neurovascular bundles. Normal neurovascular bundle on right. **b** Large tumor (*T*) in right peripheral zone. There is bulging and extracapsular tumor spread (*arrows*)

Fig. 4. Stage T3b prostate cancer (seminal vesicle infiltration). On sagittal (**a**) and coronal (**b**) T2-weighted images, low SI area is present representing tumor with seminal vesicle invasion (*arrows*)

a problem using the ERC, which has an accuracy range between 81-96% [21, 23, 24, 26]. T1- and T2-weighted images should be acquired at least two weeks after the prostate biopsy, as hemorrhage decreases staging accuracy [28].

Beside its role in staging, MR imaging is useful in reducing the number of false negative prostate biopsies in patients with elevated PSA and repeated negative (TRUS-guided) biopsies. With MR imaging, prostate cancer can be detected and then a MR-directed biopsy can be performed. Using MR imaging as a method to detect cancer lesions in a group of 36 patients with negative biopsies and elevated PSA values, an accuracy of 78%, a positive predictive value of 74%, and a negative predictive value of 84% was achieved [29].

In summary, the role of MR imaging in local staging is not yet clearly defined, however, it is considered to be

cost-effective in a selected group of patients. SVI can be detected with high accuracy, which is an advantage in comparison with TRUS alone.

Metastatic Disease

CT and MR imaging are reported to be the most accurate non-invasive methods of detecting pelvic lymph node metastases. Scheidler et al. [30] concluded that CT and two-dimensional MR imaging perform similarly for the detection of lymph node metastasis, with a trend towards an improved accuracy for MR imaging. Therefore, both MR imaging and CT are recommended, because unlike lymphangiography (LAG), they are non-invasive. A recent study using MR imaging with a three-dimensional technique has revealed a specificity of 98% and a positive predictive value of 94% in the detection of nodal metastasis in bladder and prostate cancer [31]. This is clinically relevant because this can facilitate the indication for (MR-guided) biopsy [32], which can avoid an invasive pelvic lymph node dissection in the case of a positive biopsy. The multi-planar reconstructions obtained with this technique allow the evaluation of not only nodal size, but also nodal shape. This is important because the cut-off point between normal and metastatic nodes differ for round and oval nodes. The smallest lymph node diameter that can be detected by this method is 2 mm. Different sensitivities and specificities are acquired depending on the selection of cut-off size [31, 33, 34].

An important limitation of CT and MR imaging in the evaluation of nodal metastasis is that both imaging methods depend on enlargement of lymph nodes as a criterion for metastasis. The problem is that metastasis may also be present in normal sized nodes, thus causing low sensitivities (36-60%) [35]. Due to their high cost, CT and MR imaging in detection of nodal metastasis should only be performed in a selected group of patients with high risk for nodal metastases, which can be predicted by DRE, PSA and biopsy Gleason score [10, 31, 35].

Hematogenous metastases are most common in the axial skeleton. Currently, the mainstay for the detection of bone metastases is a radionuclide bone scan. However, it is well known that bone scans can yield false-negative findings, especially in cases of very aggressive metastases. Furthermore, the technique has a high false-positive rate, mainly due to degenerative disease, healing fractures and various metabolic disorders and their complications (e.g., osteoporosis and osteomalacia). It has been demonstrated that bone scintigraphy is unnecessary in the evaluation of newly diagnosed, untreated prostate cancer with no clinical signs of bone pathology and serum PSA levels of less than 10 ng/ml [36]. In patients with an elevated PSA (> 10 ng/ml) or with locally advanced tumours, bone scans are considered worthwhile for detecting both asymptomatic and symptomatic metastasis. MR imaging is more sensitive in detecting bone marrow metastases compared to radionuclide bone scanning [37]. Therefore, MR imaging can be useful in the evaluation of patients suspected of having vertebral metastases with equivocal or negative bone scans. Thanks to its high spatial resolution, MR imaging may also guide needle biopsy procedures. Plain radiographs are the least sensitive in evaluating the axial skeleton for metastases. 50% of bone mineral content must be altered before evidence of metastasis is visible.

In summary, MR imaging has a major role in detecting nodal and bone marrow metastases in patients with bladder or prostate cancer with high risk for metastatic disease.

Future Developments

Recent developments in MR imaging include contrast-enhanced fast dynamic MR imaging, magnetic resonance spectroscopy (MRS), the use of nano-particles and 3T.

Fast Dynamic Imaging

Cancer can be differentiated from normal tissue by fast dynamic contrast-enhanced MR imaging because of typical tumour enhancement characteristics. On contrast-enhanced MR imaging, prostate cancer shows a typical early and rapid enhancement with a higher peak enhancement and wash-out of contrast compared to normal tissues [38-39]. This can be used to improve tumour localisation detection (Fig. 5). Also, when one knows where the tumour is locat-

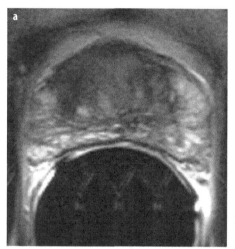

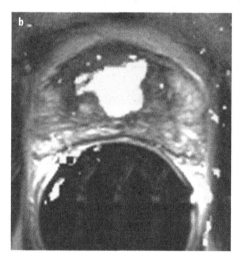

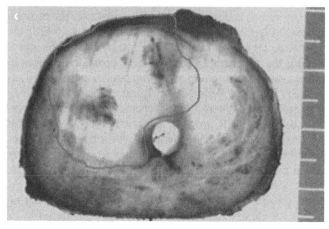

Fig. 5. Patient with previous negative biopsies. **a** Axial T2-weighted image shows low SI region in central gland, but not specific for tumor. **b** Wash-out image, same slice level as **a** shows wash-out of contrast in the central gland. Biopsy directed to this area was positive and stage T2B prostate cancer was confirmed at prostatectomy (**c**) within lined area

ed, staging results will improve. This has been shown to be especially valuable for inexperienced readers [40]. Other fields where dynamic MR imaging may have a potential role are therapy monitoring and the prediction of therapy success of systemic therapy of prostate cancer [41]. Current problems of detection with dynamic MR imaging of prostate carcinoma involve the large variation in enhancement patterns among patients with prostate carcinoma and the overlapping enhancement pattern of BPH, prostatic intraepithelial hyperplasia (PIN) and inflammation. However, using fast sequences and quantitative or semiquantitative parameters, like wash-out of the contrast agent in cancer, makes differentiation from BPH possible [42].

MRS

Image-guided proton MRS (^{1}H MRS) is a technique that provides metabolic information about the prostate gland, which may be used for in situ characterisation, diagnosis and therapy evaluation of prostate cancer (Fig. 6). Although the examination is comparable with MR imaging, the spatial resolution is lower (down to 0.24 cm^3 has been reported for the prostate) [43] and the information obtained is related to metabolites rather than anatomy. It has been shown that prostate cancer is characterised by a decreased level of citrate and an increased level of (phospho)choline [44]. Especially in the PZ, tumour tissue can be identified by an increased choline/citrate (or choline+creatine/citrate) signal-ratio [44, 45]. Correlations have been reported between metabolite ratios and the histologic grade in human prostate cancers [46]. The addition of ^{1}H MRS to (dynamic) MR imaging can improve tumour visualisation and spatial extent [43, 47]. Potential areas of

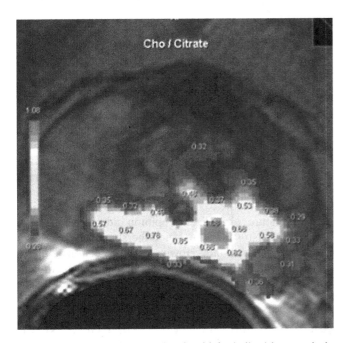

Fig. 6. MRSI. Metabolic map showing high choline/citrate ratio in left peripheral zone. Prostatectomy confirmed cancer

prostate cancer management that may benefit from the ^{1}H MRS information include targeted TRUS-guided biopsies for patients with PSA levels indicative of cancer but negative previous biopsies, therapy monitoring (watchful waiting) and guiding focal prostate cancer therapies [48].

Nodal Staging Using Nano-Particles [48, 49]

New MR contrast agents with ultra small super paramagnetic iron oxide (USPIO) particles are currently under investigation. In normal lymph nodes with functioning macrophages, the iron oxide particles are phagocytosed and thereby decrease the signal intensity on MR imaging. Metastatic nodes, lacking macrophages, do not take up the contrast agent and hence show no change in signal on post contrast images. These agents may increase sensitivity for nodal metastasis, by detection of metastasis in normal sized nodes. When using high resolution MR-technique, small metastases (3-7 mm) can be prospectively recognised in small (5-10 mm) size lymph nodes. These small lymph nodes would be considered to be benign in plain MRI or CT examinations. In addition, hyperplastic enlarged nodes can be correctly recognised as non-metastatic, based on their low signal intensity. Using USPIO, MRI patients may be reliably selected for prostatectomy or radiotherapy without the need for invasive and costly procedures such as open and laparoscopic pelvic lymphadenectomy (PLND). Furthermore, USPIO can identify large malignant nodes and extracapsular extension. If the node is not too small the presence of a malignancy can be confirmed by image-guided biopsy in 70% of the cases, and thus also avoid PLND in these patients. Finally, Fowler and Whitmore showed that 12% of all positive-node patients or 5% of all patients subjected to PLND will have the positive nodes missed, because they are located in the internal iliac or common iliac region only and thus are not included in the modern modified PLND for prostate cancer. With USPIO MRI all pelvic nodes are visualised. Harisinghani et al. [49] showed that in 9 of their 80 patients with prostate cancer in which post USPIO MRI suggested metastases outside the classical field of lymph node resection (Fig. 7), and who underwent more extensive exploration, true metastases were confirmed at these sites.

3T

It is feasible to perform endorectal MR imaging at 3T in patients with prostate cancer, with the potential advantages of increased spatial resolution of T$_2$-weighted and contrast enhanced MR images, increased temporal resolution of dynamic contrast-enhanced MR imaging and increased spectral resolution and signal-to-noise (SNR) of MRSI [50]. It is likely that imaging with an endorectal coil at a magnetic field strength of 3T will expand potential clinical applications in evaluating the prostate. The reported sensitivity and specificity for detecting extracapsular disease was 88% and 96% respectively, which is an improvement compared to 1.5T (Fig. 8) [51].

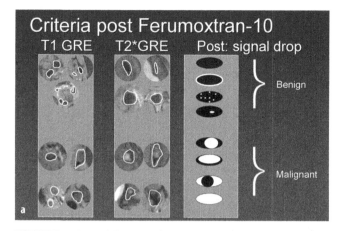

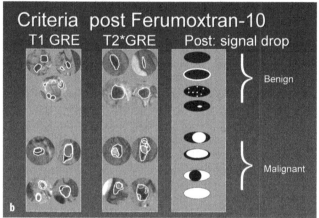

Fig. 7. On post ferumoxtran-10 images, normal nodal tissue is black, and metastatic tissue is either grey (on T1-GRE images) or white (on T2*-GRE images). **b** Nodes are within yellow, and metastatic areas within white lines

Conclusions

Accurate staging of prostate carcinoma is essential for taking treatment decisions. However, pre-operative clinical staging is inaccurate. DRE and PSA can only provide an inexact indication of local extent. Addition of other parameters such as number of positive biopsies and biopsy grade improves clinical staging but is not accurate enough to predict tumour stage in the individual patient. Therefore imaging modalities such as TRUS and MR imaging are needed to increase staging accuracy. Local staging (ECE and SVI) with MRI is at least as good and potentially superior to TRUS [10, 52, 53]. The advantage of MR imaging is that both nodal, bone marrow and local staging can be done in one imaging session, limiting the number of examinations and cost.

In future research, cost-effectiveness should be an important guideline when working with these 'expensive' imaging techniques. In this respect, detection of advanced disease by imaging and thereby the prevention of an unnecessary radical prostatectomy should be weighed against the cost of imaging itself and its value to assess the stage of tumour for the individual patient. In a recent paper,

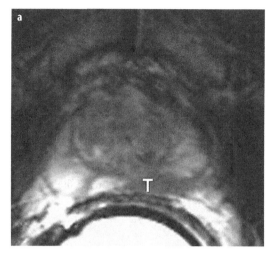

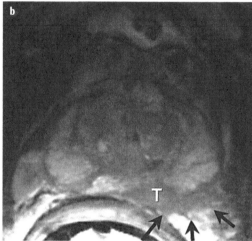

Fig. 8. Stage T3a prostate cancer. **a** ERC T2-weighted MR image at 1.5 T shows tumor (*T*) but no definite capsular penetration. **b** High resolution ERC image obtained at 3T shows clear extra capsular extension (*arrows*)

Jager et al. [54] determined the appropriate use of MR imaging for preoperative staging of prostate cancer. They performed a literature review by using the principles of evidence-based medicine and medical technology assessment. A decision analytic model was used to compare the strategy where radical prostatectomy is performed on the basis of clinical staging with the strategy where extracapsular disease detected at MR imaging contraindicates radical prostatectomy in patients who were considered surgical candidates on the basis of clinical staging. After review of the literature, expert panel opinion did not recommend MR staging. No studies in which therapeutic efficacy was addressed were found. However, the decision analytic model indicated that the strategy including MR staging decreased costs (MR imaging, \$10,568; radical prostatectomy, \$11,669) and resulted in almost equal life expectancy (MR imaging, 12.59 years; radical prostatectomy, 12.60 years) and quality-adjusted life-years ([QUALYs] MR imaging, 12.53; radical prostatectomy, 12.52). Furthermore, results of sensitivity analyses demonstrated that the

MR strategy was both more effective and less costly if the prior probability of extracapsular disease was at least 39% when considering QUALY, and 50% when considering unadjusted life expectancy. It was concluded that it is not yet conclusively determined whether preoperative MR staging is appropriate, but results of decision analysis suggest that MR staging is cost-effective for men with moderate or high prior probability of extracapsular disease.

Thus it remains very important to select appropriate patients for staging with the imaging techniques mentioned above. Finally, it should be mentioned that the role of imaging, especially MR imaging and MRS, is rapidly changing and improving and more research needs to be done to establish its definite role.

Part II: Magnetic Resonance Imaging in the Assessment of Urinary Bladder Carcinoma*

Introduction

Urinary bladder carcinoma is more common in males than females, with a ratio of approximately 4:1, and is predominantly seen in the sixth and seventh decades of life [55, 56].

Determination of local tumor staging and detection of nodal or bone metastases is extremely important [55, 57, 58]. Appropriate use of the different techniques is crucial for accurate assessment of prognosis and for the development of appropriate treatment planning. As clinical staging is not reliable for determining tumor extension beyond the bladder wall, imaging techniques are needed [59].

Among the non-invasive imaging modalities, magnetic resonance imaging (MRI) is the modality of choice for imaging the urinary bladder cancer. Multi-planer capabilities and superior soft tissue make this technique a valuable tool for imaging the urinary bladder. In addition, recent advances, such as high resolution fast imaging sequences and the use of pelvic phased array coils and contrast agents, further improve the imaging quality and thus the diagnostic accuracy for staging urinary bladder carcinoma [55, 60].

In Part II, the general features of urinary bladder cancer, the role of imaging and especially of MRI will be reviewed.

Radiological Examination of Urinary Bladder Carcinoma

Plain Radiography

In a bladder with Bilharzia (schistosomasis) complicated by carcinoma, the plain radiography may suggest the correct diagnosis. The calcification of the wall of the bilharzial bladder usually appears as a continuous curved line of calcification, either smooth or irregular in contour, depending on the state of distension (Fig. 9). If bladder cancer develops, the continuity of the linear calcification is usually interrupted [61].

* J.O. Barentsz, E. Abouh-Bieh

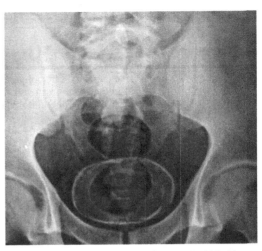

Fig. 9. Plain X-ray of the pelvis showing calcified bladder wall due to bilharzia

Dystrophic calcification may infrequently occur in the necrotic bladder tumor, which is visible on the plain film as a finely speckled collection of calcifications, or as a well circumscribed calcification with a dense or even a calcified nodule in the bladder region [61, 62].

Intravenous Urography (IVU)

Intravenous urography is performed to exclude upper renal tract abnormalities [63]. It is important to take films with the patient both in the prone and supine position. A filling defect is only visible when the lesion is surrounded by opaque urine. Hence, carcinoma of the posterior wall of the bladder is best seen with the patient in the supine position, and carcinoma of the anterior wall with the patient in prone position. Oblique views of the bladder may also be helpful in the detection and localization of lesions [63].

If the tumor is located near the ureteral orifice, there may be incomplete or even complete obstruction, subsequent dilatation of the urinary tract or even decreased excretion of the kidney on that side [64]. When one non-excretory kidney is found in the presence of bladder cancer, an antegrade pyelogram can be helpful. It is important to distinguish between complete obstruction due to the tumor in the bladder itself and tumor extension up into the ureter [64].

Ultrasonography (US)

In Table 2 the TNM system is correlated with ultrasound (US) findings. Non-invasive trans-abdominal ultrasound is seldom used today because it is inaccurate for the assessment of tumor spread beyond the bladder wall. Also, visualization of the tumor is limited in obese patients, and by air containing bowel loops adjacent to the bladder wall. Further problems are related to inaccessibility of US to accurately visualize tumors arising in the region of the bladder neck and to the limitations in evaluating lymph node metastasis [64].

Table 2. Demonstration of TNM and MRI-staging cancer bladder

STNM	AUS	Histological Description	MRI criteria
T_{is}	O	Carcinoma in situ	Not applicable
T_a		Non-invasive papillary carcinoma	
T_1	A	Superficial limited to mucosa and submucosa.	Stage T_1, T_2 are diagnosed when the tumor is confined to
T_2	B_1	Superficial invasion of the muscle layer	bladder wall with the outer bladder wall being of normal low signal intensity on T2-W1
T_{2b}	B_2	Deep invasion of the muscular wall	Interruption of low signal intensity bladder wall on T2-W1
T_{3a-b}	C_1	Perivesical fat invasion: 3a: microscopic, 3b: macroscopic	Trans-mural tumor extension into the perivesical fat
T_4	C2	Invasion of adjacent organs	Direct invasion of adjacent organs
NO	D1	No lymph node involvement	
N_1		Single homo-lateral side	More than 8 mm
N_2		Collateral, bilateral regional nodes	More than 8 mm
N_3		Fixed regional nodes	More than 8 mm
N_4		Common iliac, aortic, or inguinal nodes	More than 8 mm
M_1	D_2	Distant metastasis	Distant metastasis

Bladder tumors appear on US as echogenic lesions. The bladder wall has a more intense echo pattern than tumor tissue, thus permitting distinction of early superficial lesions from those invading the deeper layers of the bladder wall. However tumors involving the superficial muscle cannot be distinguished accurately from tumors involving the deep muscle (Table 2).

Trans-rectal and trans-urethral US carried out with a higher frequency transducer allow better resolution and better staging, but ventral tumors and tumors at the dome are poorly visualized.

Computed Tomography (CT)

The CT appearance of bladder tumors is not specific; it can simulate invasive carcinoma of the prostate or rectal metastasis, pheochromocytoma, Leiomyoma, lymphoma, and malakoplakia [62].

The major role of CT in bladder carcinoma is to stage, rather than to detect the primary tumor. This technique is less accurate in low stage tumors, and its reliability increases with more advanced disease [61] (Table 3).

On CT, bladder neoplasm appears as sessile, pedunculated, soft tissue masses projecting into the bladder lumen (Fig. 10). The tumors have a density similar to that of the bladder wall on enhanced scans and occasionally the intra-luminal surface is encrusted with calcium. However, these tumors may show increased attenuation due to neovascularization. Bladder cancer involving superficial and deep muscles usually produce focal bladder wall thickening and retraction, but CT cannot reliably differentiate between the various layers of the bladder wall and cannot, therefore, distinguish lesions of the lamina propria (stage T1) from those invading the superficial (stage T2a) and deep muscle (stage T2b).

Tumors of the anterior, posterior and lateral walls are easily detected and evaluated, but difficulties arise in showing tumors at the dome and trigone because of the axial plane imaging used routinely in body CT. CT is clinically useful for detecting invasion into perivesical fat

Table 3. Accuracy of different staging techniques

Stage	Clinical staging including transurethral resection	CT	MRI
T0-T+	++	–	+
Tis-Ta	++	–	–
Ta-T1	++	–	–
T1-T2a	++	–	+
T2a-T2b	0	–	+
T2b-T3a	–	–	–
T3a-T3b	–	++	++
T3b-T4a	–	+	++
T4a-T4b	–	+	++
N0-N+	–	+	+
M0-M+	–	0/+	++

M+, bone marrow infiltration; *T0*, no malignancy e.g. scar, fibrosis, granulation tissue, hypertrophy; *T+* malignancy; *++*, highly accurate; *+*, accurate; *0*, not accurate; *–*, not possible

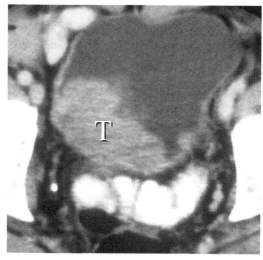

Fig. 10. Stage T2b bladder cancer (*T*). On post contrast CT both bladder wall and tumor have identical signal intensity and cannot be separated

(stages T3a and T3b), as CT can distinguish tumors confined to the bladder wall from those spreading into the fat.

Macroscopic extra-vesical extension (stage T3b) is characterized by poor definition of the outer aspect of the bladder wall with an increase in density of the perivesical fat and often requires 5 mm sections. When no distinct fat planes are present between the bladder and the rectum, uterus, prostate and vagina, early tumor invasion into these neighboring structures may be difficult to exclude.

Tumor invasion of the seminal vesicle should be suspected if a soft tissue mass obliterates the seminal vesicle fat angle. This sign should be interpreted with caution because the normal seminal vesicle angle may be lost if the rectum is over-distended or if the patient is scanned in prone position.

CT can, in addition, evaluate retro-peritoneal pelvic lymph nodes. Nodes greater than 10 mm are suspected to contain metastases.

Magnetic Resonance Imaging (MRI)

MRI is superior to CT for staging urinary bladder carcinoma. The multiplanar capabilities and soft tissue characterization capabilities of MR imaging make it a valuable diagnostic tool for visualizing the urinary bladder [66, 67].

Normal MR Anatomy

On T1-weighted images, the urine has low-signal intensity, and normal bladder wall has an intermediate signal intensity equal to skeletal muscle (Fig. 11a). On these images, the perivesical vessels and vas deferens appear as low signal intensity tubular structures surrounding the bladder base interspersing the perivesical fat. On fat saturation T1-weighted images the bladder wall has a slightly higher signal intensity than urine or perivesical fat [66-69].

On T2-weighted images the urine has a very high, and the bladder a low signal intensity [66-69] (Fig. 11b). The thickness of the bladder wall varies with the degree of the bladder distension. The normal values range from 2.9 to 8.8 mm, with a mean of 5.4 mm. When the bladder is distended, the wall should not exceed 5 mm in thickness.

The peri-vesical fat has a high signal intensity both on T1- and on fast spin-echo T2-weighted images, and an intermediate signal intensity on spin echo T2-weighted images [66-69]. On fat saturation T2-weighted images not only the signal intensity of perivesical fat that is similar to the bladder wall. Therefore on these images the bladder wall can only be delineated if there are adjacent higher signal intensity perivesical venous plexus or seminal vesicles [66-70].

Immediately after injection of Gadolinium (Gd)-contrast, the urinary bladder wall shows rapid enhancement [73]. Differential enhancement between the inner mucosa and submucosa, and the outer muscular layer has been reported on early images. The inner layer is more vascular and shows early enhancement while the less vascular muscular layer enhances later [71, 72]. About 2 minutes

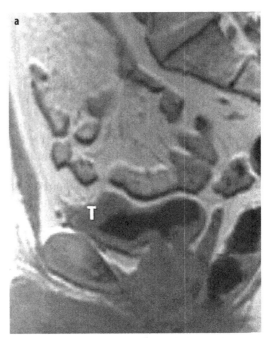

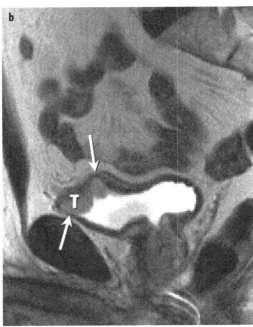

Fig. 11. Stage T2b bladder cancer (*T*). **a** T1-weighted MR-image tumor has the identical signal intensity as the wall. Urine has lower and perivesical fat has higher signal intensity. **b** T2-weighted MR image shows bladder wall with higher signal intensity than wall, and lower than urine. At *arrows* low signal bladder wall is disrupted by tumor, which argues for at least deep muscle invasion (stage T2b)

after contrast injection, the Gd-contrast is excreted into the urine. In order to visualize enhancement within the bladder wall, these images must be acquired within 2 minutes. Within the urinary bladder urine containing concentrated Gd, contrast concentrates by its higher gravity on the dorsal side of the bladder (if the patient is supine) and is seen as a low signal intensity layer. More diluted urine containing contrast material is seen as a middle layer of high signal intensity. Finally, another low intensity layer can be identified anteriorly, representing unenhanced urine. Patent blood vessels with normal flow can be recognized without intravenous contrast by their typical signal void on turbo or fast spin-echo images.

On T1-weighted images, lymph nodes have an intermediate signal intensity (Fig. 12). On T2-weighted images, the signal intensity varies (Fig. 13). It is, however, always higher than that of muscle. T1-weighted images provide the optimal contrast between medium nodes and high signal intensity fat.

In general, axial images should be acquired using T1- and T2-weighted sequences followed by imaging in other planes. The direction of these planes depends on the site of the tumor. For example, coronal images are particularly helpful for visualizing tumors arising from the base, dome and lateral bladder wall, whereas sagittal images can be used to visualize anteriorly and cranially located tumors and tumors at the bladder sphincter. In addition, images should be acquired in a plane perpendicular to the wall at the base of the tumor. This allows better delineation of muscle involvement. Use of multiplanar

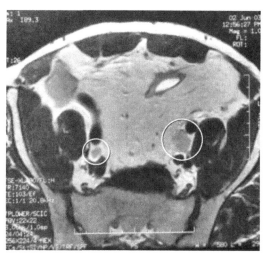

Fig. 13. Metastatic enlarged nodes (*circles*). On T2-weighted image, nodes have higher signal intensity than muscle, and identical signal intensity as bladder cancer

reconstruction with a 3D sequence gives the best results. An important plane direction in evaluating lymph nodes is parallel to the psoas muscle. This so-called 'obturator plane' allows visualization of nodes along their long axis, and can locate them in relation to the iliac vessels and obturator nerve (Fig. 12).

The slice thickness should be 4 mm at the most, with a maximal gap of 1 mm. A thinner slice thickness produces better anatomical details and improved partial volume; however, the signal-to-noise (SNR) then also decreases. The field of view (FOV) usually ranges from 24 to 36 cm in diameter.

Image quality in the pelvis should be improved by using surface coils. Phased array body coils are well suited for pelvic MR imaging. The high SNR obtained with these coils facilitates excellent image quality with superior spatial resolution

Pulse Sequences

Since MRI is a highly flexible and versatile system, many different imaging sequences and imaging planes are used for pelvic scanning. The choice depends largely on the type of the scanner used and its ability to obtain fast images. However, irrespective of the scanner features, T1- and T2-weighted sequences are mandatory.

T1-weighted Imaging

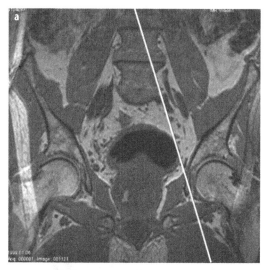

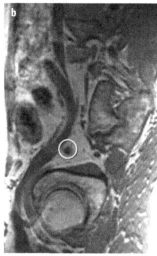

Fig. 12. Normal node. On (**a**) coronal T1-weighted image imaging plane of (**b**), parallel to psoas muscle ('obturator' plane) is indicated by white line. On (**b**) T1-weighted 'obturator' plane a small 3 mm normal node (*circle*) can easily be separated from longitudinal running vessels

For T1-weighted images, turbo or fast spin echo (SE) or gradient recalled echo (GRE) sequences should be used. On these sequences, bladder carcinoma has intermediate signal intensity equal to that of the muscle and can be delineated from fat and urine. T1-weighted images are therefore used to determine tumor infiltration into the perivesical fat. As mentioned before, these sequences are also most suitable for imaging lymph nodes (Fig. 12). In addition, there is a good contrast between the metastasis and surrounding fatty bone marrow. Gradient echo images are susceptible to motion and therefore may cause motion artifacts. They can be helpful for demonstrating pelvic side-wall infiltration, vessels, and for distinguishing these from enlarged lymph nodes. In addition, as these sequences have a short imaging time they can be used for dynamic contrast-enhanced imaging, or for quickly acquiring 3D data. The combined time-saving of turbo or fast SE sequences and excellent image quality has led to the widespread use of this sequence type. With an attempt to trade-off the time-saving for an improvement in image quality at many institutions, fast spin echo (FSE) has replaced conventional SE for T1- and T2-weighted imaging scans.

T2-weighted Imaging

For T2-weighting, turbo or fast SE sequences are considered state-of-the-art. On T2-weighted images, urine has high signal intensity and tumor has an intermediate intensity, higher than bladder wall or fibrosis and lower than the urine (Fig. 11b). The zonal anatomy of the prostate or uterus and vagina can also be easily recognized on these images. The T2-weighting should, however, not be too strong, as then bladder cancer has a low signal intensity that is too low, and results in decreased discrimination from the wall. To obtain this goal, a TE of no longer than 90 ms should be used. These sequences allow high resolution images in a relatively short time, and are used for determining depth of tumor infiltration within the bladder wall, for differentiating tumor from fibrosis, for assessment of invasion into the prostate, uterus or vagina, and for confirming bone marrow metastasis seen on T1-weighted images (Fig. 14a). For last purpose a Short Tou Inversion Recovery (STIR) sequence can also be used can be used (Fig. 15). Metastases have a high, and bone marrow has a low signal intensity on this sequence type (Fig. 14b) [73].

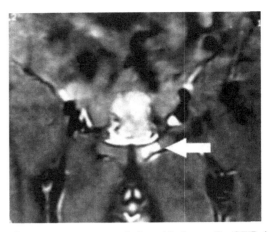

Fig. 15. Bone marrow metastasis in pubic bone. On STIR image bone marrow metastasis has high signal intensity (*arrow*)

Dynamic Contrast Enhanced Sequences

MRI using extra-cellular Gd-based contrast medium can be used to improve visualization of bladder cancer (Fig. 16). The success of dynamic contrast-enhanced MRI depends on its ability to demonstrate intrinsic differences between a variety of tissues that affect contrast medium behavior [64-47]. Gd-contrast is given intravenously as a bolus injection with a power injector in the anticubital vein in a dose of 0.1 mmol/kg. This extracellular contrast agent readily passes from the vasculature into the extravascular, extracellular space and gives rise to enhancement. The contrast medium causes shortening of the T1-relaxation time, and thus causes increased signal intensity on T1-weighted images. The early phase of contrast-enhancement – often referred to as the first pass – includes the arrival of contrast medium. In this phase, the increased signal seen on T1-weighted images arises from both the

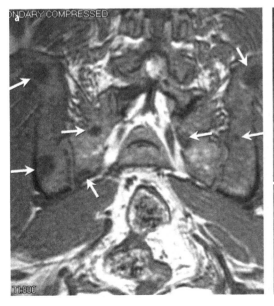

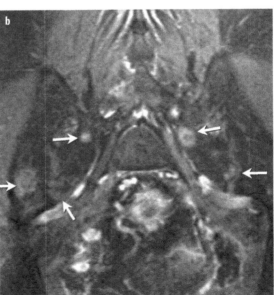

Fig. 14. Bone marrow metastases (*arrows*). **a** T1-weighted MR image shows metastases as low signal intensity round lesions. **b** On the post-Gd fat saturated T1-weighted image, due to enhancement, bone marrow metastases can be recognized as high signal intensity lesions

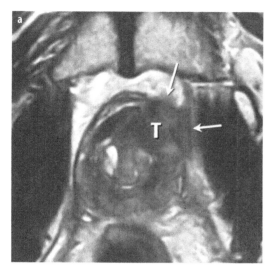

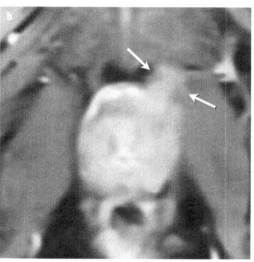

Fig. 16. Stage T4b urinary bladder cancer infiltrating prostate and pelvic sidewall muscle (*arrows*). **a** T2-weighted tSE image shows bladder cancer (*T*) infiltrating in prostate and periprostatic fat (*arrows*). **b** On the post-Gd fat saturated T1-weighted image, enhancing tumor infiltration in muscle of pelvic sidewall (*arrows*) is also visible

be obscured by urine; improved differentiation of bladder tumors from blood clots and other debris; improved detection of muscular and perivesical fat invasion and improved conspicuity of (small) vessels. For contrast-enhanced imaging of bladder cancer, T1-weighted sequences with a time resolution of less than 20 seconds should be used. In the early phase (first pass phase), discrimination between cancer and wall or fibrosis is best visible. Also, this speed avoids the filling of the bladder lumen due to renal excretion. To enhance tumor visualization in the perivesical fat, either subtraction or fat-saturation must be applied. Usually GRE sequences are used for dynamic MRI. The imaging plane can be preselected based on the previously performed T1- and or T2-weighted sequences

Bladder Cancer Staging

Local tumor extension, the degree of lymph node and distant metastases, and histologic tumor type largely determine treatment and prognosis. Therefore, exact staging is imperative. To determine local tumor extension (T), presence of lymph node (N) and distant metastases (M), the International Union against Cancer proposed a uniform clinical staging method (Table 1). In this table, a correlation is also presented between the TNM-system and MRI-findings. Patients with superficial tumors, i.e., tumors without muscle invasion (stages Ta and T1) are treated with local endoscopic resection followed by adjuvant intravesical installations. Patients with a tumor invading the muscle layer of the bladder wall or with minimal perivesical extension (stages T2a to T3a) will be treated by radical cystectomy and lymphadenectomy. However, if the tumor is in a more advanced stage (stages T3b-T4b) or if there are nodal or distant metastases, the patient will have palliative chemo- or radiation therapy.

Local Staging

Bladder tumors demonstrate different patterns of growth: papillary, sessile, infiltrative or mixed. Papillary tumors are usually superficial (stage T1 or less. i.e., with no muscle wall infiltration) and are best demonstrated on T1-weighted images in which the intermediate signal intensity of the intraluminal tumor is outlined by surrounding low signal intensity urine. On T2-weighted images, the signal intensity of both bladder tumor and intravesical urine increase, and intraluminal projections of bladder tumors may be less conspicuous than on T1-weighted images [66-69]. Papillary transitional cell carcinoma of the bladder has a loose connective tissue stalk. On MRI, the stalk is defined as a structure that extends from the bladder wall to the center of the tumor, with signal intensity different from that of the tumor [84]. Most of stalks show lower signal intensity than tumor on T2-weighted images, less enhancement on dynamic images and stronger enhancement on delayed enhanced images (Fig. 17). The

vascular and interstitial component. Also, when a bolus of contrast medium passes through the capillary bed, it produces magnetic field inhomogeneities that result in a decrease in the signal intensity of the surrounding tissues.

Urinary bladder carcinoma develops neovascularization [56, 59, 77-84], therefore after intravenous administration of gadolinium, bladder cancer shows earlier and more enhancement than normal bladder wall or other non-malignant tissues. Urinary bladder cancer starts to enhance 7 seconds after the beginning of arterial enhancement, which is at least 4 seconds earlier than most other structures [56].

Contrast enhancement has many advantages, including improved detection of small bladders tumors, especially those measuring less than 1 cm that may be missed on T2-weighted images because the high signal tumor can

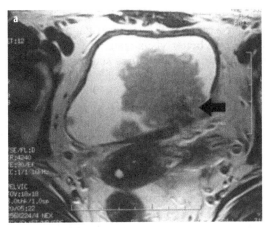

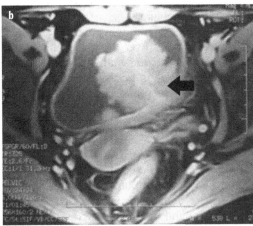

Fig. 17. Papillary stage T1 tumor with stalk (*arrowhead*). **a** On the T2-weighted tSE image, low signal intensity muscle is not disrupted by higher signal intensity tumor. In the center of the papillary tumor a low signal intensity stalk (*arrowhead*) can be seen. **b** Post-Gd fat saturated T1-weighted image shows that the stalk has more enhancement than the rest of the tumor (*arrowhead*)

identification of the stalk of a polypoid tumor may be an important observation to exclude muscle wall invasion of the tumor [84].

Muscle wall infiltrative tumors (stages T2a or above) present as a diffuse or focal thickening of the bladder wall with increased signal intensity on T2-weighted images. This increase is in contrast to the low signal intensity of normal bladder wall. Early contrast enhanced images may help to recognize muscle wall infiltration. Findings suggesting superficial tumors are: smooth muscle layer, tenting of the bladder wall, fern-like vasculature and uninterrupted submucosal enhancement. Findings that suggest muscle invasion are: irregular wall at the base of the tumor, focal wall enhancement or wall thickening around the tumor.

MRI can differentiate between neoplastic infiltration of bladder wall and bladder wall hypertrophy secondary to outlet obstruction. In bladder wall hypertrophy, the wall is diffusely thickened (more than 5 mm), but no alternation of the low signal intensity wall is present on T2-weighted images.

Muscle wall invasion is separated into superficial (stage T2a) and deep (stage T2b). In stages T2b, the low signal intensity layer of the bladder wall is disrupted on T2-weighted images by the higher signal tumor (Fig. 11b). Stage T2b cannot be separated on MRI from stage T3a (microscopic fat infiltration). Macroscopic tumor extension through the bladder wall into the perivesical fat (stage T3b) will cause a focal irregular decrease of signal intensity of the fat on standard T1- or T2-weighted images (Fig. 18a). Contrast-enhanced images with fat saturation also show tumor (enhancement) in the perivesical fat. Invasion of adjacent organs may be inferred from the extension of abnormal tumor signal intensity through fat planes into adjacent structures (Fig. 18b). This is well demonstrated with contrast-enhanced images. Invasion of the seminal vesicles can be demonstrated by an increase in vesicular size, decrease in signal intensity on T2-weighted images and obliteration of angle between the seminal vesicle and the posterior bladder wall (Fig. 19). Invasion of the prostate and rectum is seen as direct tumor extension with an increase of signal intensity. Obliteration of the angle between bladder and prostate also indicates prostate invasion. Invasion of the pelvic side-

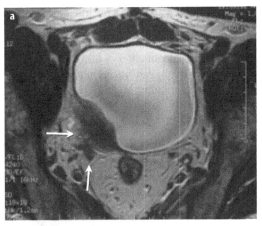

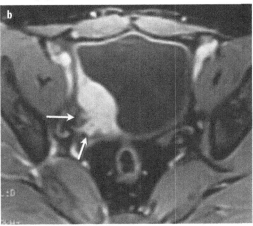

Fig. 18. Stage T3b urinary bladder cancer infiltrating perivesical fat (*arrows*). Both on (**a**) T2-weighted tSE and (**b**) post-Gd fat-saturated T1-weighted image, bladder cancer at right latero-dorsal wall can be seen with macroscopic infiltration of perivesical fat (*arrows*)

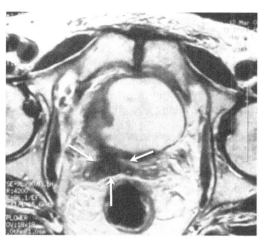

Fig. 19. Stage T4a urinary bladder cancer infiltrating right seminal vesicle (*arrows*). T2-weighted tSE image shows hypointense intravesical mass arising from right lateral wall with obliteration of fat plain between the bladder and right seminal vesicle and abnormal signal intensity of left seminal vesicle denoting invasion by the tumor (*arrows*)

wall (stage T4b) is seen on T1-weighted images as a loss of normal fat plane between bladder wall (tumor) and the vessels or musculature of the sidewall, or on T2-weighted images as invasion of the sidewall musculature in by intermediate to high signal intensity tumor (Fig. 20).

As clinical staging is not reliable to determine tumor extension beyond the bladder wall, other methods are needed. CT is a valuable addition, but since the introduction of pelvic MR imaging in 1983, several reports have shown the superiority of this technique for staging urinary bladder carcinoma [57].

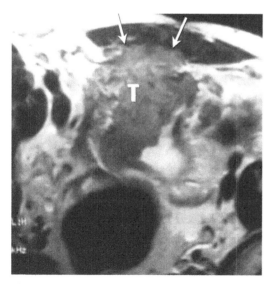

Fig. 20. Stage T4b urinary bladder cancer (T) infiltrating the ventral abdominal wall. T2-weighted tSE image shows large intravesical mass arising from anterior bladder wall with abnormal high signal intensity in muscles of anterior pelvic wall denoting invasion by the tumor (*arrows*)

MR imaging appears to be superior to CT scanning for staging carcinoma of the urinary bladder. Multi-planar imaging allows better visualization of the bladder dome, trigone, and adjacent structures such as the prostate and seminal vesicles. The accuracy of MR imaging in staging bladder cancer varies from 73% to 96%. These values are 10-33% higher than those obtained with CT [61]. Recently, several reports have been published on the staging of urinary bladder carcinoma with the use of IV-Gd contrast. A 9-14% increase in local staging accuracy has been reported using these contrast agents. Furthermore, when using contrast agent, visualization of small tumors (> 7 mm) improves. The most accurate staging results using IV gadolinium contrast material are obtained with very fast T1-weighted sequences [56]. This can be explained by earlier enhancement of tumors compared to surrounding tissues. Although contrast-enhanced MR imaging has advantages over the use of unenhanced T2-weighted sequences, such as higher SNR ratio and shorter acquisition time, it is advised not to skip the T2-weighted images. Large prospective studies in this regard are necessary.

Lymph Node Staging

Normal nodes can be recognized with MRI down to a size of 2 mm. With multiplanar imaging, both the size and shape of the nodes can be assessed. The maximal length (long axis) and the minimal axial size of the node can be determined. Round nodes can be distinguished from oval nodes by using an index that divides the axial size by the long axis. Lymph nodes are considered rounded when this index is in-between 1.0 and 0.8, and spheric or elongated if this index is greater than 0.8. The cut-off value for the minimal axial diameter is 10 mm for a spherical/elongated node and 8 mm for a rounded node. An asymmetric cluster of small lymph nodes is also considered to be pathologic [58].

Lymph node metastasis in patients with superficial tumors (less than stage T2) is rare, but if the deep muscle layer is involved (stages T2a and higher) or if extravesical invasion is seen, the incidence of lymph node metastasis rises to 20-30% and 50-60%, respectively. A non-invasive, reliable method for detecting and staging nodal metastasis would reduce the extent of surgery. Currently, there are five imaging techniques described for nodal staging: lymphangiography, CT, MRI, and [18]FDG positron emission tomography (PET) scanning.

Bipedal lymphangiography is no longer used as an imaging method, although it has the capacity to show micrometastases in normal-sized nodes. Its inability to depict internal iliac nodes and its invasiveness are major drawbacks.

CT and MRI

Detection of lymph node metastases has very important clinical consequences. If metastatic disease is present, usually curative cystectomy will no longer be performed. Current imaging techniques can only show nodal size. Different sensitivities and specificities are acquired depending on the selection of cut-off size for lymph nodes [85]. Recently Jager and co-workers [58] showed that using a three-dimensional (3D) high-resolution technique, not only nodal size, but also nodal shape could be assessed. Using the nodal shape in relation to the cut-off size also improved their results. They obtained an accuracy of 90% and a positive predictive value of 94% [60]. This is clinically relevant as a high positive predictive value in the detection of nodal metastasis can facilitate the indication for (MR-guided) biopsy [86]. In case of a positive biopsy, this can avoid an invasive pelvic lymph node dissection. Cross-sectional imaging modalities like CT and (3D) MR imaging have a low sensitivity (76%) as metastases in normal sized lymph nodes are still missed, since both modalities use the non-specific criterion of size to distinguish between normal and malignant nodes [4, 31]. Although fast dynamic MRI has been shown to improve sensitivity by showing fast and high enhancement in metastatic nodes, specificity decreases. In addition, fast dynamic is further limited by its low resolution and pronounced vascular artifacts [56].

Staging PLND still remains the most sensitive method for assessing lymph node metastases and thus continues to be the first step in the management protocol. Cost-effective analysis performed by Wolf et al. [86] pointed out that imaging should be restricted to patients with a high probability of lymph node metastases. Thus they concluded that imaging was superior to no imaging only when the pretest probability of lymph node metastasis was high, i.e., if tumor infiltration is in or beyond the muscular layer of the bladder wall.

The most important parameter was the sensitivity of cross-sectional imaging for lymph adenopathy. Pelvic imaging combined with fine needle aspiration has also been investigated. The data of Wolf et al. [86] suggest that only a subset of patients at high risk for lymph node metastasis benefits from cross-sectional imaging and pre-operative lymph node sampling.

Bone Marrow Metastases

Currently, the mainstay for the detection of bone metastases is a radionuclide bone scan. However, MR imaging is superior to ^{99m}Tc bone scan in assessment of bone marrow involvement. The high sensitivity of MRI for evaluating bone marrow metastasis makes it an ideal tool for detecting suspected osseous metastatic disease and determining its extent. Osseous metastases are generally hematogenously spread, and the vascular bone marrow is usually the earliest site of involvement. For purposes of screening, T1-weighted and STIR image are adequate to detect foci of abnormal marrow. Therefore, MR imaging can be useful in the evaluation of patients suspected of having vertebral metastases with equivocal or negative bone scans. Thanks to its high spatial resolution, MR

imaging may also guide needle biopsy procedures. Plain radiographs are the least sensitive in evaluating the axial skeleton for metastases. Fifty percent of bone mineral content must be altered before evidence of metastases is visible. However, the limitation of MR imaging is the inability to produce 'whole body' images.

New MRI Techniques

USPIO MRI

Previous reports have shown that the information about lymph nodes on MR images can be improved by pharmaceutical manipulation of tissue proton relaxation times. Ultra small Super Paramagnetic Iron Oxide Particles (USPIO) with a long plasma circulation time have been shown to be suitable as a MR contrast agent for intravenous MR lymphangiography (Fig. 21) [87-90]. In a study performed at UMC in Nijmegen and Mass General

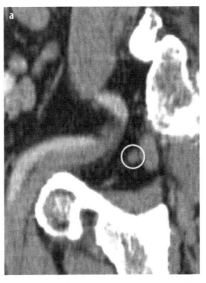

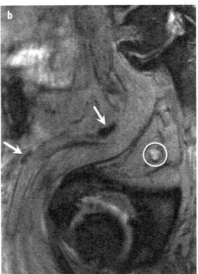

Fig. 21. Normal size (5 mm) metastatic node (*circle*). **a** MDCT reconstruction in 'obturator' plane shows normal size (5 mm) node (*circle*). **b** On T2*-weighted MR image in identical plane obtained 24 hours post-USPIO, this node (*circle*) has high signal intensity which argues for metastasis. Also, two small normal nodes (*arrows*) are visible, which have low signal intensity due to accumulation of iron loaded macrophages in normal nodal tissue. These nodes are not visible on MDCT

in Boston [91], in 80 patients with histologically proven prostate cancer, using high-resolution techniques (at 1.5 T using a body phased-array coil), on post USPIO MRI the rate of detection of small nodal metastases in normal 5-8 mm sized nodes was significantly improved. Sensitivity, accuracy and negative predictive value showed a significant improvement using post-USPIO to 100%, 98% and 100%, respectively. This was due to the detection of small 3-4 mm metastases in normal-sized nodes. In addition, MRI nodes were found outside of the surgical field in 9 out of 80 patients thanks to post USPIO. Similar post US-PIO results – sensitivity, accuracy and negative predictive value, respectively 96%, 95% and 98% – were acquired recently in urinary bladder cancer [93].

Conclusions and Recommendations for Imaging Approach

To summarise, Table 2 (based on published reports and our own experience) offers an overview of the value of the several staging techniques for urinary bladder. MRI is superior to CT for staging, as CT cannot differentiate between the various layers of the bladder wall and cannot, therefore, distinguish lesions of the lamina propria from those invading the superficial and deep muscle wall. There are also difficulties in assessing tumors at the dome and trigone. The multiplanar and soft tissue characterization capabilities of MRI make it a valuable diagnostic tool among the non-invasive imaging modalities. Also, MR imaging is the most promising technique for the detection of nodal and bone marrow metastases. When MR imaging is available, CT is no longer needed. In addition, recent advances in MRI, such as fast imaging, fast dynamic Gd-enhanced techniques, and the use of specific contrast for the assessment of lymph nodes, improve the imaging quality and diagnostic accuracy for staging urinary bladder carcinoma. However, due to limited resources, this technique should only be used to obtain information that directly influences therapeutic management and outcome. To achieve this, both the knowledge of urologists in MR imaging and knowledge of the radiologist in clinical handling is required, therefore, continuous education and communication between these two specialties is a necessity.

Table 3 presents the diagnostic management of urinary bladder cancer. Detection of bladder cancer should be performed by cystoscopy. Once bladder cancer is diagnosed, the following step should be staging. For superficial tumors, clinical staging, which includes transurethral resection, is the best technique. If, however, there is muscle invasion, further staging has to be performed with MR imaging. To avoid post-biopsy over-staging from edema and fibrosis, or the inconvenience of waiting 2-3 weeks after transurethral biopsy, we recommend fast dynamic imaging. Superficial tumors without muscle invasion (stages Ta-T1) are treated with local endoscopic resection with or without adjuvant intravesical installations. If cystoscopy reveals large multiple nodular or papillary

tumors, a MRI examination can be helpful to provide an overview of the tumor prior to the biopsy.

Patients with muscle invasion (stages T2a-b) and with perivesical infiltration (stages T3a-b) or with invasion into prostate, vagina or uterus (stage T4a) will be treated by radical cystectomy and lymphadenectomy.

Part III: Scrotal Imaging*

With the continued evolution of high-resolution linear transducers over the past fifteen years, clinicians, patients, and imagers are able to rely on ultrasound as a tool with near 100% sensitivity for significant intrascrotal pathology. Not only is the technique non-invasive and relatively inexpensive, it is also highly effective for both the detection and characterization of a wide variety of disorders. A comprehensive treatment of these conditions is beyond the scope of this discussion, which instead focuses on diseases that are of interest because of some combination of clinical relevance or characteristic imaging features.

Intratesticular Disorders

Neoplastic

Germ Cell Tumors (GCT) are the most common neoplasms of the testis. The vast majority of these are malignant. Among the various histologic types, seminoma is the most common to occur as a pure tumor. Most tumors (approximately half of all lesions) are of the mixed variety, containing two or more histologic types. Thus, the non-seminomatous tumors typically include one or more of these types: embryonal carcinoma, teratoma, endodermal sinus tumor, or choriocarcinoma – with or without seminoma. Lesions typically present as a palpable mass, although some aggressive tumors may present with metastatic foci to the lung, bone, or nodal masses.

Most lesions are hypoechoic relative to the background homogeneous, medium-high echogenicity of the testis. Calcifications are seen in at least one third of cases, especially in non-seminomatous tumors.

Management nearly always involves orchiectomy for definitive diagnosis and treatment of the local disease. Seminomas are highly radiosensitive, and in most cases prophylactic radiotherapy to the retroperitoneum is offered. The prognosis is generally good unless there is advanced metastatic disease, such as lung nodules, at the time of presentation [94].

For the non-seminomatous tumors, CT is often used to determine if patients need retroperitoneal lymph node dissection. Patients with (1) nodal involvement (either enlarged on CT, or confirmed on pathologic assessment) and/or (2) hematogenous metastasis are generally treated with chemotherapy. The prognosis for non-seminomatous

---

* B.J. Wagner

tumors is more guarded than that for seminoma, although patients with stage I disease (limited to the scrotum) have five year survival rates approaching 90%.

Gonadal stromal tumors are less common (less than 10% of lesions) and are often incidental findings. Both Leydig cell and Sertoli tumors are occasionally the cause of gynecomastia. The vast majority of these tumors are benign, but have non-specific grey scale sonographic features. One study reported characteristic peripheral hypervascularity in these lesions [95], but it is unlikely that orchiectomy could be avoided in most cases because the sonographic features do not allow confident exclusion of malignancy nor absolute differentiation from the more common (and more sinister) germ cell tumors.

Lymphoma of the testis is typically seen in older patients than those affected with GCTs, and it is rarely demonstrated in patients without a known diagnosis of systemic lymphoma. Hypoechoic, multifocal (or geographic), bilateral lesions, which often have increased vascularity compared with GCTs, are seen [96].

While not strictly neoplastic, five entities deserve discussion in this context: simple cysts, tubular ectasia, epidermoid cyst, congenital adrenal rests, and testicular microlithiasis (TML).

Simple cysts are typically peripheral, multiple, and contiguous with the tunica albuginea (more central cysts are usually a manifestation of tubular ectasia). These have no malignant potential and are rarely of clinical significance, although they may be palpable and clinically mimic a germ cell tumor. Rarely, they may be complicated by hemorrhage; most cases are easily diagnosed as simple cysts. Features that raise concern for malignancy (and prompt surgical removal), include solitary lesions complicated by internal soft tissue, calcification, or a thick irregular wall.

Tubular ectasia represents a dilatation of the rete testis as it converges along the mediastinum testis. Patients may have a history of prior epididymitis or vasectomy, but most have no specific symptoms. An ovoid or linear area of decreased echogenicity, contiguous with the epididymis, can usually be differentiated from neoplasm based on the pattern of branching anechoic channels [97]. In occasional cases that may mimic neoplasm, T2-weighted MRI will show a hyperintense focus (in contrast to the hypointensity characteristic of most testicular neoplasms), which is often bilateral.

Epidermoid cyst is not considered to be a neoplasm by most authorities. Instead, it is an inclusion cyst, lined by squamous epithelium and filled with keratinized debris. Although it accounts for less than 10% of intratesticular masses, differentiation of the epidermoid cyst from germ cell neoplasm is important in order to avoid radical surgery for this lesion that can, instead, be effectively diagnosed and treated with a more limited procedure (enu-

cleation, sparing the testis). Epidermoid cyst can be recognized in many instances by an 'onion-skin' appearance: alternating concentric rings of hypo- and hyperechogenicity [98]. A minority of cases will show wall calcification. The absence of Doppler flow may be of some help (the presence of central flow excludes the diagnosis), but one should remember that some neoplasms, especially when small, will not have flow detected sonographically. Additionally, the onion-skin appearance is neither sensitive (it is seen in approximately half of cases) nor entirely specific (some neoplasms, including teratoma, may rarely have the same feature) [99].

Congenital adrenal rest tumors are seen in patients with poorly-controlled congenital adrenal hyperplasia (CAH). Aberrant adrenal cortical cells migrate with gonadal tissue during fetal development, and may hypertrophy at some point during the disease. The sonographic appearance is extremely variable, but is typically distinguished from malignant germ cell tumor by the multiplicity of the lesions, their eccentricity, and their contiguity with the mediastinum testis. Treatment is glucocorticoid replacement or, rarely, surgery (partial orchiectomy) [100].

Testicular microlithiasis (TML) describes the presence of numerous small (1-2 mm) calcifications scattered throughout the testicular parenchyma. This idiopathic condition is associated with oligospermia in a minority of cases; in most patients this is merely an incidental finding. Although somewhat controversial, most published reports conclude that there is an increased risk of testicular germ cell tumors in patients with TML. For this reason, patients should be carefully screened for coexistent tumors, and followed sonographically at annual intervals for interval development of malignancy [101-103].

Non-neoplastic

Infection typically begins in the epididymis. Epididymoorchitis is usually a clinical diagnosis; sonography is sometimes used to rule out torsion or progression to abscess. Sonographic findings are often absent, although some patients will show a hydrocele (with or without complicating elements indicating pyocele). There may also be increased Doppler flow to the epididymis. Progression to involvement of the testis occurs in a minority of cases, and may result in abscess formation or infarction.

Ischemia/infarction may result from torsion or less commonly from a variety of other causes (including vasculitis, diabetes, or orchitis). Patients with torsion typically have an acute clinical presentation with severe unilateral scrotal pain, often following minor trauma or physical exertion. The typical finding is an asymmetric decrease in color or amplitude (power) Doppler signal to the symptomatic side. However, subtle variations of arterial spectral Doppler waveforms may be seen early, including absence of the dicrotic notch and/or increased resistance (decreased or absent diastolic flow) [104]. The latter finding may also be seen in early stages of torsion when venous flow is altered but arterial flow is still seen by color Doppler.

Emergent surgery is indicated to detorse and save the testis; however, when grey scale findings are present, including heterogeneity and decreased echogenicity, the ischemia has almost always progressed to infarction [105]. At this point, testicular salvage is not possible.

Important pitfalls in Doppler evaluation must be recognized in order to avoid misdiagnosis. The examiner must be careful not to alter Doppler settings (gain, scale, etc.) when comparing the normal (asymptomatic) testis to the painful side. One must also remember that paratesticular tissues may show reactive hyperemia, despite the absence (or significant decrease) in Doppler flow to the testis itself. Focal infarction has a variety of causes with a common pathway of microvasculitis and will show regional wedge-shaped areas of decreased perfusion, often with adjacent hyperemia [106].

Sarcoidosis is an unusual cause of a scrotal mass, and may rarely be the presenting site of disease in some patients. The pattern of multiple hypoechoic intratesticular masses associated with epididymal enlargement and heterogeneity is characteristic, although it may also be seen in lymphoma.

Extratesticular Disorders

Neoplastic

In adults, malignant extratesticular neoplasms are rare and have a non-specific appearance [107]. *Mesothelioma* is an uncommon neoplasm, which usually presents as a hydrocele, with soft tissue nodules of the tunica vaginalis. Alternatively, it may present as a large heterogeneous mass, which may be difficult to separate from the testis. Mesotheliomas tend to occur in individuals who are decades older than those typically diagnosed with testicular germ cell tumors.

Lymphoma may occasionally involve the epididymis, although in the majority of patients this does not lead to a diagnostic dilemma as (1) the patient will be known to have lymphoma and (2) there will be coexistent involvement of the testis itself. Very rarely, solid tumors may metastasize to the epididymis. Affected patients almost always have advanced disease elsewhere throughout the body.

The most common extratesticular intrascrotal neoplasm is *lipoma*, which arises from the spermatic cord and can often be diagnosed clinically based on palpation. *Adenomatoid tumors* are nearly as common as lipomas, and account for about one third of extratesticular masses. These are benign, but may be surgically removed either to establish the diagnosis or because of local pain or tenderness. They are solid, well-marginated lesions that are typically less than 20 mm in size. They most frequently arise from the epididymis.

Papillary cystadenomas of the epididymis are seen in about one quarter of patients with von Hippel-Lindau disease (VHL). The lesions are rare in individuals without VHL. They are typically solid, measure between 1 and 5 cm, and may be indistinguishable from adenomatoid tumors [107].

Sarcoidosis is more likely to affect the epididymis than the testis. More than one third of patients will have bilateral disease. Although discrete nodules will occasionally be seen, the appearance is more commonly one of heterogeneous enlargement. A diagnostic pattern that may be of use in a previously undiagnosed patient with hilar adenopathy (which could be either lymphoma or sarcoid), is to compare the testicular and the epididymal involvement: in sarcoidosis, the degree of epididymal disease typically exceeds testis involvement, whereas in lymphoma the converse is expected.

References

1. Landis SH, Murray T, Bolden S, Wingo PA (1998) Cancer statistics. CA Cancer J Clin 48:6-29
2. Imperial Cancer Research Fund (1995) Cancer statistics (online: http:www.icnet uk/research/factsheet/canstats.html)
3. American Cancer Society (1998) Cancer facts and figures. http://www.cancer.org.statistics cff98/graphicaldata.html
4. Catalona WJ (1995) Surgical management of prostate cancer: contemporary results with anatomic radical prostatectomy. Cancer 75:1903-1908
5. Donovan JL, Frankel SJ, Faulkner A et al (1999) Dilemmas in treating early prostate cancer: the evidence and a questionaire survey of consultant urologists in the United Kingdom. BMJ 318:299-300
6. Jewett HJ (1956) Significance of the palpable prostatic nodule. JAMA 160:838-939
7. Smith DS, Catalona WJ (1995) Interexaminer variability of digital rectal examination in detecting prostate cancer. Urology 45:70-74
8. Voges GE, McNeal JE, Redwine E et al (1992) Morphologic analysis of surgical margins with positive findings in prostatectomy for adenocarcinoma of the prostate. Cancer 69:520-526
9. Epstein JI, Pizov G, Walsh PC (1993) Correlation of pathologic findings with progression after radical retropubic prostatectomy. Cancer 71:3582-3593
10. Partin AW, Yoo J, Ballentine Carter JY et al (1993) The use of prostate specific antigen, clinical stage and gleason score to predict pathological stage in men with localized prostate cancer. J Urol 150:110-115
11. Kleer E, Oesterling JE (1993) PSA and staging of localized prostate cancer. Urol Clin North Am 20:695-704
12. Jager GJ, Barentsz JO (1998) Prostate cancer. In: Husband J (ed) Oncology imaging. Isis Medical Media, Oxford, pp 239-257
13. Langlotz CP (1996) Benefits and costs of MR imaging of prostate cancer. MR Clin Nort Am 4:533-545
14. Schiebler ML, Schnall MD, Pollack HM et al (1993) Current role of MR imaging in the staging of adenocarcinoma of the prostate. Radiology 189:339-352
15. Chernoff DM, Hricak H, Higgins CB, Hricak H (1997) The Male pelvis: prostate and seminal vesicles. In: Hricak H (ed)

Magnetic resonance imaging of the body, 3rd edn. Lippincott-Raven Press, New York, pp 875-900

16. Ramchandani P, Schnall MD, LiVolsi VA et al (1993) Senile amyloidosis of the seminal vesicles mimicking metastatic spread of prostatic carcinoma on MR images. AJR Am J Roentgenol 161:99-100

17. Jager G, Ruijter E, de la Rosette J, van de Kaa CA (1997) Amyloidosis of the seminal vesicles simulating tumor invasion of prostatic carcinoma on endorectal MR images. Eur J Radiol 7:552-554

18. Langlotz CP, Schnall MD, Pollack H (1995) Staging of prostatic cancer: accuracy of MR imaging. Radiology 194:645-646

19. Jager GJ, Thornbury J, Barentsz JO et al (1998) MR staging in prostate cancer (pc): influence on patient outcome and effective analysis. Abstract, RSNA 181

20. Rifkin MD, Zerhouni EA, Gatsonis CA et al (1990) Comparison of magnetic resonance imaging and ultrasonography in staging early prostate cancer. Results of a multi-institutional cooperative trial. N Engl J Med 323:621-626

21. Rørvik J, Halvorsen OJ, Albrektsen G et al (1999) MR imaging with an endorectal coil for staging of clinically localised prostate cancer prior to radical prostatectomy. Eur Radiol 9:29-34

22. Schnall MD, Imai Y, Tomaszewski JE et al (1991) Prostate cancer: local staging with endorectal surface coil MR imaging. Radiology 178:797-802

23. Hricak H, White S, Vigneron DB et al (1994) Carcinoma of the prostate gland: MR imaging with pelvic phased-array coils versus integrated endorectal-pelvic phased-array coils. Radiology 193:703-709

24. Bartolozzi C, Menchi I, Lencioni R et al (1996) Local staging of prostate carcinoma with endorectal coil MR imaging: correlation with whole mount radical prostatectomy specimens. Eur Radiol 6:339-345

25. Langlotz CP, Schnall MD, Malkowicz SB, Schwartz JS (1996) Cost-effectiveness of endorectal magnetic resonance imaging for the staging of prostate cancer. Acad Radiol 3:24-27

26. Chelsky MJ, Schnall MD, Seidmon EJ, Pollack HM (1993) Use of endorectal surface coil magnetic resonance imaging for local staging of prostate cancer. J Urol 150:391-395

27. Outwater E, Petersen RO, Siegelman ES et al (1994) Prostate carcinoma: assessment of diagnostic criteria for capsular penetration on endorectal coil MR images. Radiology 193:333-339

28. White S, Hricak H, Forstner R et al (1995) Prostate cancer: effect of postbiopsy hemorrhage on interpretation of MR images. Radiology 195:385-390

29. Kedar RP, Kier R, Viner N (1999) Proceedings of the International Society of Magnetic Resonance in Medicine (poster ISMRM, Philadelphia) nr. 1106

30. Scheidler J, Hricak H, Yu KK et al (1997) Radiological Evaluation of lymph node metastases in patients with cervical cancer. JAMA 278:1096-1101

31. Jager GJ, Barentsz JO, Oosterhof G, Ruijs JHJ (1996) 3D dimensional MR imaging in nodal staging of bladder and prostate cancer. AJR Am J Roentgenol 1503-1507

32. Barentsz JO (1997) MR-intervention in the pelvis: an overview and first experiences in MR-guided biopsy in nodal metastases in urinary bladder cancer. Abdominal Radiology 22:524-530

33. Vinnicombe SJ, Norman AR, Nicolson V, Husband JE (1995) Normal pelvic lymph nodes: evaluation by CT scanning after bipedal lymphangiography. Radiology 194:349-355

34. Oyen RH, Van Poppel HP, Ameye FE et al (1994) Lymph node staging of localized prostatic carcinoma with CT and CT-guided fine-needle aspiration biopsy: prospective study of 285 patients. Radiology 190:315-322

35. Wolf JS, Cher M, Dall'era M et al (1995) The use and accuracy of cross-sectional imaging and fine needle aspiration cytol-ogy for detection of pelvic lymph node metastases before radical prostatectomy. J Urol 153:993-999

36. Haukaas S, Rørvik J, Halvorsen OJ, Foellings M (1997) When is bone scintigraphy necessary in the assessment of newly diagnosed, untreated prostate cancer. Br J Urol 79:770-776

37. Algra PR, Bloem JL, Tissing H et al (1991) Detection of vertebral metastases: comparison between MR imaging and bone scintigraphy. Radiographics 11:219-323

38. Delorme S, Knopp MV (1998) Non-invasive vascular imaging: assessing tumour vascularity Eur J Radiol 4:517-527

39. Jager G, Ruijter E, Kaa van de C et al (1997) Dynamic turbo-flash subtraction technique for contrast-enhanced MR images of the prostate: correlation with histopathology. Radiology 203:645-652

40. Fütterer JJ, Engelbrecht MR, Huisman HJ et al (2005) Staging prostate cancer with dynamic contrast-enhanced endorectal MR imaging prior to radical prostatectomy: experienced versus less experienced readers. Radiology 237:541-547

41. Padhani AR, MacVicar AD, Gapinski CJ et al (2001) Effects of androgen deprivation on prostatic morphology and vascular permeability evaluated with MR imaging. Radiology 218:365-374

42. Engelbrecht MR, Huisman HJ, Laheij RJ et al (2003), Discrimination of prostate cancer from normal peripheral zone and central gland tissue by using dynamic contrast-enhanced MR imaging. Radiology 229:248-254

43. Kurhanewicz J, Males R, Sokolov D (1998) Combined endorectal/phased-array MR imaging and 3-D H-MR Spectroscopic imaging for improved diagnosis of extracapsular extension in prostate cancer. Proceedings of the International Society of Magnetic Resonance in Medicine (abstract ISMRM, Philadelphia)

44. Heerschap A, Jager GJ, van der Graaf M et al (1997) In vivo proton MR spectroscopy reveals altered metabolite content in malignant prostate tissue. Anticancer Res 17:1455-1460

45. Kurhanewicz J, Vigneron DB, Hricak H et al (1998) Three-dimensional H-1 MR spectroscopic imaging of the in situ human prostate with high (0.24-0.77-cm^3) spatial resolution. Radiology 198:795-805

46. Vigneron DB, Males R, Noworolski S (1998) 3D MRSI of prostate cancer: correlations with histologic grade. Proceedings of the International Society of Magnetic Resonance in Medicine (abstract ISMRM, Philadelphia)

47. Males R, Vigneron DB, Nelson AD (1998) Addition of MR spectroscopic imaging to MRI significantly improves detection and localization of prostate cancer. Proceedings of the International Society of Magnetic Resonance in Medicine (abstract ISMRM, Philadelphia)

48. Weissleder R, Elizondo G, Wittenberg J et al (1990) Ultrasmall superparamagnetic iron oxide: an intravenous contrast agent for assessing lymphnodes with MR imaging. Radiology 175:494-498

49. Harisinghani MG, Barentsz J, Hahn PF et al (2003) Noninvasive detection of clinically occult lymph-node metastases in prostate cancer. N Engl J Med 348:2491-2499

50. Fütterer JJ, Scheenen TW, Huisman HJ et al (2004) Initial experience of 3 tesla endorectal coil magnetic resonance imaging and 1H-spectroscopic imaging of the prostate. Invest Radiol 39:671-680

51. Fütterer J, Heijmink S, Scheenen T et al (2006) Local staging of prostate cancer using 3T endorectal coil MR imaging – Early Experience. Radiology 238:184-191

52. Presti JC, Hricak H, Narayan P et al (1996) Local staging of prostatic carcinoma: comparison of transrectal sonography and endorectal MR imaging. AJR Am J Roentgenol 166:103-108

53. Yu KK, Hricak H, Alagappan R et al (1997) Detection of extracapsular extension of prostate carcinoma with endorectal and phased-array coil MR imaging: multivariate feature analysis. Radiology 202:697-702

54. Jager GJ, Severens JL, Thornbury JR et al (2000) Prostate cancer staging: should MR imaging be used? A decision analytic approach. Radiology 215:445-451

55. Barentsz JO, Debruyne FMJ, Ruijs SHJ (eds) (1990) Magnetic resonance imaging of carcinoma of the urinary bladder. Kluwer Academic Publishers, Dordracht, London, Boston

56. Barentsz JO, Jager GJ, van Vierzen PB et al (1996) Staging urinary bladder cancer after transurethral biopsy: value of fast dynamic contrast-enhanced MR imaging. Radiology 201:185-193

57. Barentsz JO, Jager GJ, Mugler JP et al (1995) Staging urinary bladder cancer, value of T1weighted three-dimensional magnetization prepared-rapid gradient-echo two-dimensional spin-echo sequences. AJR Am J Roentgenal 164:109-115

58. Jager GJ, Barentsz JO, Oosterhof GO et al (1996) Pelvic adenopathy in prostatic and urinary bladder carcinoma: MR imaging with a three-dimensional TI-weighted magnetization-prepared-rapid gradient-echo sequence. AJR Am J Roentgenol. 167:1503-1507

59. Barentsz JO, Berger-Hartog O, Witjes JA et al (1998) Evaluation of chemotherapy in advanced urinary bladder cancer with fast dynamic contrast-enhanced MR imaging. Radiology 207:791-7

60. Maeda H, Kinukawa T, Hottori R et al (1995) Detection of muscle layer invasion with submillmeter pixel MRI: Staging of bladder carcinoma. Magn Reson Imaging 13:9-19

61. Hricak H, White S (1997) Radiological evaluation of the urinary bladder and prostate. In: Grainger RG, Allison D (eds) Grainger and Allison's diagnostic radiology: a textbook of medical imaging, Vol. 2, 3rd edn. Churchill Livingstone, New York, pp 1427-1438

62. Sherwood T (1980) Bladder and urethra. In: Sherwood T, Davidson AJ, Talner LB (eds) Uro-Radiology, 1st edn, Part 4, Division 3. Blackwell Scientific, Oxford, pp 255-312

63. Hatch TR, Barry JM (1986) The value of excretory urography in staging bladder cancer. J Urol 135:49-54

64. Richards D, Jones S (1998) The bladder and prostate. In: Sutton D (ed) Textbook of radiology and imaging. 6th British Library cataloguing in publication data. Longman Asia, Hong Kong , pp 1167-1187

65. Dershow PD, Scher HI (1987) Sonography in the evaluation of carcinoma of the bladder urology 29:454-457

66. Barentsz JO, Jager GJ, Witjes JA, Ruijs JHJ (1996) Primary staging of urinary bladder carcinoma: the role of MR imaging and a comparison with CT. Eur Radiol 6:134-139

67. Barentsz JO, Witjes JA, Ruijs JH (1997) What is new in bladder cancer imaging. Urol Clin North Am 24:583-602

68. Takeda K, Kawaguchi T, Shiraishi T et al (1998) Normal bladder wall morphology in Gd-DTPA-enhanced clinical MR imaging using an endo-rectal surface coil and histological assessment of submucosal linear enhancement using, Gd- DTPA auto-radiography in an animal model. Eur J Radiol 26:290-296

69. Barentsz JO (1998) Magnetic resonance imaging of urinary bladder carcinoma. In: Jafri SH, Diokno AC, Amendola MA (eds) Lower genitourinary radiology, imaging and intervention. Springer-Verlag, New York, pp 138-158

70. Barentsz JO, Ruijs JHJ, Strijk SP (1993) The role of MR imaging in carcinoma of the urinary bladder. AJR Am J Roentgenol 160:937-947

71. Siegelman ES, Schnall MD (1996) Contrast-enhanced MR imaging of the bladder and prostate. Magn Reson Imaging Clin N Am 4:153-169

72. Narumi Y, Kadota T, Inoue E et al (1993) Bladder tumors: staging with gadolinium-enhanced oblique MR imaging. Radiology 187:145-50

73. Eustace S, Tello R, De Carvalho V et al (1997) A comparison of whole body turbo short tau inversion recovery MR imaging and planar technetium 99m methylene diphosphonate scintigraphy in the evaluation of patients with suspected skeletal metastases. AJR Am J Roentgenol 169:1655-1661

74. Padhani AR, Husband JE (2001) Dynamic contrast enhanced MRI studies in oncology with an emphasis on quantification, validation human studies. Clin Radiol 56:607-620

75. Lin W, Hoacke EM, Smith AS et al (1992) Gadolinium enhanced high resolution MRA with adaptive vessel tracking: preliminary results in the intracranial circulation. Magn Reson Imaging 2:227-284

76. Vens S, Hosten N, Ilg J et al (1996) Pre-operative staging of bladder carcinomas with Gd-DTPA-supported dynamic magnetic resonance tomography. Comparison with plain and Gd-DTTA-supported spin-echo sequences. Rofo 164:218-225

77. Hamm P, Laniado M, Saini S (1990) Contrast-enhanced magnetic resonance imaging of the abdomen and pelvis. Magn Reson 6:108-135

78. El-Diasty T, EI-Sobky E, Abou EI-Ghar M et al (2002) Triphasic helical CT of urinary bladder carcinomas correlation with tumour angiogenesis and pathologic types. Eur Radol 12:D1-D25 (abs)

79. Nicolas V, Spielmann R, Mass R et al (1991) The diagnostic value of MRI tomography following gadolinium-DTPA compared to computed-tomography in bladder tumors [German]. Rofo 154:357-363

80. Braun RD, Lanzen JL, Dewhirst NW (1999) Fourier analysis of fluctuations of oxygen tension and blood flow in R3230Ac tumors and muscle of rats. Am J Physiol 277:551-568

81. Dovark HF, Nagy JA, Feng D et al (1999) Vascular permeability factor/vascular endothelial growth factor and the significance of micro-vascular hyper-permeability in angiogenesis. Curr Top Microbiol Immunol 237:97-132

82. Dewhirst M (1993) Angiogenesis and blood flow in solid tumors. In: Teicher B (ed) Drug resistance in oncology. New York, NY, USA, pp 3-24

83. Neeman M, Provenzale JP, Dewhirst MW (2001) MRI application in evaluation of tumor angiogenesis. Semin Radiol Oncol 11:70-82

84. Saito W, Amanuma M, Tanaka J et al (2000) Histopathological analysis of bladder cancer stalk observed on MRI. Magn Reson Imaging 18:411 (abs)

85. Husband JE (1992) Review of staging bladder cancer. Clin Radiol 46:153-159

86. Wolf JS, Cher M, Dall'era M et al (1995) The use and accuracy of cross-sectional imaging and fine needle aspiration cytology for detection of pelvic lymph node metastases before radical prostatectomy. J Urol 153:993-999

87. Vassallo P, Matei C, Heston WDW et al (1994) AMI-227-enhanced MR Lymphography: usefulness for differentiating reactive from tumor bearing lymph nodes. Radiology 193:501-506

88. Weissleder R, Elizondo G, Wittenberg J et al (1990) Ultrasmall paramagnetic iron oxide: an intravenous contrast agent for assessing lymph nodes with MR imaging. Radiology 175:494-498

89. Gerlowski LE, Jain RK (1986) Microvascular permeability of normal and neoplastic tissues. Microvasc Res 31:288-305

90. Bellin MF, Roy C, Kinkel K et al (1998) Lymph node metastases: safety and effectiveness of MRI with ultrasmall superparamanetic iron oxide particles - initial clinical experience. Radiology 207:799-808

91. Harisinghani MG, Saini S, Slater GJ et al (1997) MR imaging of pelvic lymph nodes in primary pelvic carcinoma with ultrasmall superparamagnetic iron oxide (Combidex): preliminary observations. J Magn Reson Imaging 7:161-163

92. Harisinghani MG, Barentsz J, Hahn PF et al (2003) Noninvasive detection of clinically occult lymph-node metastases in prostate cancer. N Engl J Med 348:2491-2499

93. Deserno WM, Harisinghani MG, Taupitz M et al (2004) Urinary bladder cancer: preoperative nodal staging with feromoxtran-10- enhanced MR imaging. Radiology 233:449-456

94. Woodward PJ, Sohaey R, O'Donoghue MJ, Green DE (2002) Tumors and tumorlike lesions of the testis: radiologic-pathologic correlation. Radiographics 22:189-216

95. Maizlin ZV, Belenky A, Kunichezky M et al (2004) Leydig cell tumors of the testis: gray scale and color Doppler sonographic appearance. J Ultrasound Med 23:959-964

96. Mazzu D, Jeffrey RB, Ralls PW (1995) Lymphoma and leukemia involving the testicles: findings on gray-scale and color Doppler sonography. AJR Am J Roentgen 164:645-647

97. Tartar VM, Trambert MA, Balsara ZN, Mattrey RF (1993) Tubular ectasia of the testicle: sonographic and MR imaging appearance. AJR Am J Roentgenol 160:539-542

98. Cho J-H, Chang J-C, Park B-H et al (2002) Sonographic and MR imaging findings of testicular epidermoid cysts. AMJ Am J Roentgenol 178:743-748

99. Maizlin ZV, Belenky A, Baniel J et al (2005) Epidermoid cyst and teratoma of the testis: sonographic and histologic similarities. J Ultrasound Med 24:1403-1409

100. Nagamine WH, Mehta SV, Vade A (2005) Testicular adrenal rest tumors in a patient with congenital adrenal hyperplasia: sonographic and magnetic resonance imaging findings. J Ultrasound Med 24:1717-1720

101. Peterson AC, Bauman JM, Light DE et al (2001) The prevalence of testicular microlithiasis in an asymptomatic population of men 18 to 35 years old. J Urol 166:2061-2064

102. Bach AM, Hann LE, Shi W et al (2003) Is there an increased incidence of contralateral testicular cancer in patients with intratesticular microlithiasis? AJR Am J Roentgen 180:497-500

103. Cast JEI, Nelson WM, Early AS et al (2000) Testicular microlithiasis: prevalence and tumor risk in a population referred for scrotal sonography. AJR Am J Roentgen 175:1703-1706

104. Dogra VS, Rubens DJ, Gottlieb RH, Bhatt S (2004) Torsion and beyond: new twists in spectral Doppler evaluation of the scrotum. J Ultrasound Med 23:1077-1085

105. Middleton WD, Middleton MA, Dierks M et al (1997) Sonographic prediction of viability in testicular torsion: preliminary observations. J Ultrasound Med 16:23-27

106. Fernández-Pérez GC, Tardáguila FM, Velasco M et al (2005) Radiologic findings of segmental testicular infarction. AJR Am J Roentgenol 184:1587-1593

107. Woodward PJ, Schwab CM, Sesterhenn IA (2003) Extratesticular scrotal masses: radiologic-pathologic correlation. Radiographics 23:215-240

Spread of Metastatic Disease in the Abdomen

J.A. Brink[1], T. Hany[2]

[1] Department of Diagnostic Radiology, Yale University School of Medicine, New Haven, CT, USA
[2] Nuclear Medicine, Zurich University Hospital, Zurich, Switzerland

Neoplastic disease may spread within the abdomen by embolic metastasis, lymphatic extension, direct invasion, and intraperitoneal seeding. Direct invasion may occur from contiguous primary tumors and usually implies that a locally aggressive tumor has broken through fascial planes. Direct invasion from non-contiguous primary tumors typically occurs via spread along the peritoneal ligaments and mesenteries. Intraperitoneal spread of malignancy occurs initially through seeding of the peritoneal cavity with metastatic cells. Tumor spread occurs via the natural flow of ascitic fluid within the peritoneal spaces, which, in turn, are defined by the peritoneal ligaments and mesenteries.

Tumors that arise within the abdominal cavity have the propensity to spread via the peritoneal ligaments and mesenteries that suspend their organs of origin, either by lymphatic extension or direct invasion, or via seeding of the peritoneal spaces in which they reside. Although the anatomy of the peritoneal ligaments, mesenteries, and spaces is complex, a working knowledge of this anatomy permits one to narrow the diagnostic possibilities when metastatic disease is recognized [1].

Metastatic Spread via the Peritoneal Ligaments

The major ligamentous attachments of the upper abdomen include the lesser omentum, the gastrosplenic ligament, and the splenorenal ligament. The lesser omentum is subdivided into the gastrohepatic ligament and the hepatoduodenal ligament. In the embryo, the gastrosplenic ligament gives rise to the gastrocolic ligament (also known as the greater omentum) and the transverse mesocolon.

Gastrohepatic Ligament

The gastrohepatic ligament can be recognized on computed tomography (CT) scanning as a fatty plane, which joins the lesser curvature of the stomach to the liver. It extends from the fissure for the ligamentum venosum to the porta hepatis and contains the left gastric artery, the coronary vein, and associated lymphatics. The criterion for nodal enlargement in this region is somewhat smaller than for elsewhere in the abdomen; nodes in the gastrohepatic ligament are generally considered abnormal when they exceed 8 mm in diameter [2]. On occasion, pathology in the gastrohepatic ligament may be mimicked by unopacified bowel loops, the pancreatic neck, or the papillary process of the caudate lobe of the liver projecting into the expected plane of the gastrohepatic ligament [3, 4].

The gastrohepatic ligament provides an important conduit of disease from the stomach to the liver, in that the subperitoneal areolar tissue within the ligament is continuous with the Glisson capsule (the perivascular fibrous capsule within the liver). Thus, gastric malignancy can spread via this pathway directly into the left lobe of the liver and vice-versa. Common neoplasms spreading via the gastrohepatic ligament include nodal metastases from gastric, esophageal, breast, pancreatic, and lung cancer as well as nodal involvement of lymphoma. Gastric and esophageal cancer can directly invade this ligament and spread into the left hepatic lobe [2].

Hepatoduodenal Ligament

The hepatoduodenal ligament is the free edge of the gastrohepatic ligament along its rightward aspect. It contains important structures of the porta hepatis including the common bile duct, the hepatic artery, and the portal vein. The hepatoduodenal ligament extends from the flexure between the first and second duodenum to the porta hepatis; the foramen of Winslow is immediately posterior to this ligament, permitting communication between the greater and lesser sacs [5]. Nodes of the foramen of Winslow, or portocaval space, have an unusual morphology such that their transverse dimension is greater than their antero-posterior (AP) dimension. Generally, the upper limits of normal for the AP dimension is 1.0-1.3 cm, whereas the transverse dimension can be up to 2.0 cm in width. Size criteria are somewhat less helpful than in other lymph nodes. In the absence of frank enlargement, a more spherical shape or central necrosis suggests the presence of tumor within these nodes (Fig. 1) [6, 7].

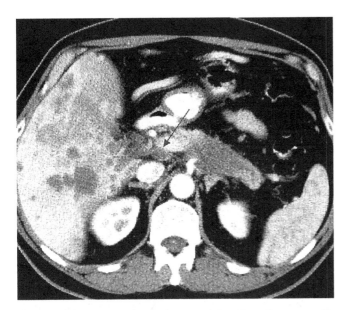

Fig. 1. Invasive pancreatic carcinoma arising from the pancreatic tail with numerous hematogenous metastases to the liver. A porto-caval lymph node at the base of the hepato-duodenal ligament (*arrow*) is not enlarged by size criteria but contains metastatic disease as evidenced by its central necrosis

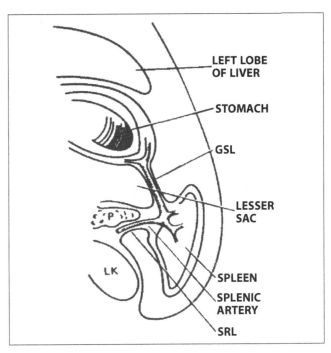

Fig. 2. The gastrosplenic ligament (*GSL*) and splenorenal ligament (*SRL*) comprise the left wall of the lesser sac and provide a conduit for the spread of metastatic disease from the greater curvature of the stomach to the retroperitonium and vice versa. *LK*, left kidney (Reprinted with permission from [8])

A broad range of tumors may spread via the hepato-duodenal ligament. Liver or biliary cancer, whether primary or metastatic, may spread in an antegrade fashion through lymphatics in the hepatoduodenal ligament to deposit in periduodenal or peripancreatic lymph nodes. Similarly, malignant disease in the nodes about the superior mesenteric artery (commonly involved with pancreatic and colon cancer) can spread in a retrograde fashion up the lymphatics in the hepatoduodenal ligament. Lymphoma can involve these nodes as well. Primary gastric cancer arising in the lesser curvature of the stomach can directly spread through the gastrohepatic ligament to the hepatoduodenal ligament and then to peripancreatic and periduodenal nodes. Vascular complications related to the portal vein and hepatic artery can result; portal venous thrombosis and hepatic arterial pseudoaneurysms can occur in advanced cases owing to their coexistence in the hepatoduodenal ligament [1, 5].

Gastrosplenic and Splenorenal Ligaments

In the embryo, the gastrosplenic ligament is a long ligamentous attachment between the stomach and the retroperitoneum which gives rise to the gastrocolic ligament (greater omentum) and the transverse mesocolon. In the adult, the gastrosplenic ligament is a thin ligamentous attachment between the greater curvature of the stomach and the splenic hilus (Fig. 2). It contains the left gastroepiploic and short gastric vessels, as well as associated lymphatics. The gastrosplenic ligament is continuous with the gastrocolic ligament inferiorly and medially and is continuous with the splenorenal ligament posteriorly

and medially [9, 10]. As such, it provides an important pathway of communication between the stomach, the spleen, and the retroperitoneum. Gastric malignancies commonly spread through this ligament (Fig. 3). Such diseases can involve the spleen and ultimately result in disease about the tail of the pancreas. Conversely, pancreatic neoplasms may spread via the splenorenal ligament to the gastrosplenic ligament and involve the greater curvature of the stomach [1].

Gastrocolic Ligament

The gastrocolic ligament (or greater omentum) joins the greater curvature of the stomach to the transverse colon. On the left it is continuous with the gastrosplenic ligament, and on the right it ends at the gastroduodenal junction near the hepatoduodenal ligament. It results from fusion of the anterior and posterior leaves of the gastrosplenic ligament in the embryo, therefore it contains the four layers of peritoneum that invest the stomach, and has a potential space within it (Fig. 4). The gastrocolic ligament contains the gastroepiploic vessels and associated lymphatics. It provides an important conduit of malignant disease from the greater curvature of the stomach to the transverse colon and vice versa. When viewed in concert with the transverse mesocolon, a conduit exists between the greater curvature of the stomach and the retroperitoneum. In addition to direct spread of disease between

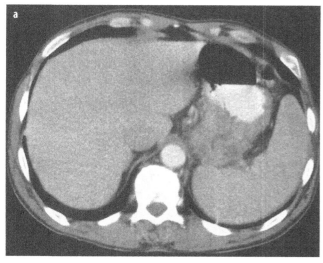

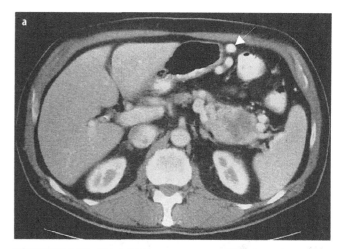

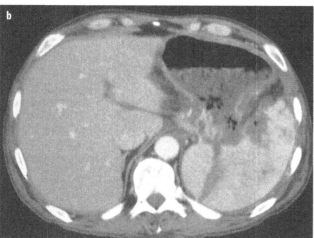

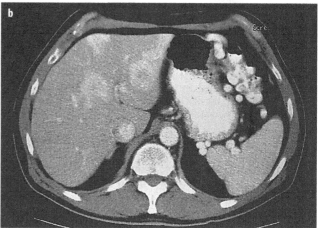

Fig. 5. Pancreatic islet-cell tumor arising in the pancreatic tail (**a**) and metastatic to liver (**b**) has resulted in splenic vein thrombosis with secondary short gastric venous collaterals in the gastrosplenic and splenorenal ligaments (**b**) and gastroepiploic venous collaterals (*arrow*) in the gastrocolic ligament (**a**)

Fig. 3. Gastric adenocarcinoma invading the spleen via the gastrosplenic ligament. **a** Initial contrast-enhanced CT scan reveals circumferential tumor involving the gastric fundus. **b** Six months later, a repeat CT scan shows invasion and dissection of the spleen secondary to tumor spread via the gastrosplenic ligament

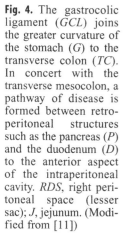

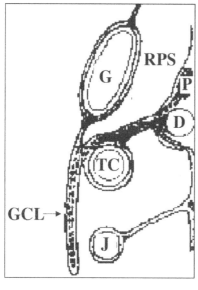

Fig. 4. The gastrocolic ligament (*GCL*) joins the greater curvature of the stomach (*G*) to the transverse colon (*TC*). In concert with the transverse mesocolon, a pathway of disease is formed between retroperitoneal structures such as the pancreas (*P*) and the duodenum (*D*) to the anterior aspect of the intraperitoneal cavity. *RDS*, right peritoneal space (lesser sac); *J*, jejunum. (Modified from [11])

the stomach, transverse colon, and pancreas, the gastrocolic ligament serves as an important nidus for the peritoneal metastases that commonly occur with ovarian, gastric, colon, and pancreatic cancer [12, 13]. Finally, dilated veins within this ligament may represent gastroepiploic collaterals resulting from splenic venous compromise that might occur in the setting of invasive pancreatic tumors, or intraperitoneal tumors, which spread to the retroperitoneum via the transverse mesocolon (Fig. 5).

Transverse Mesocolon

The transverse mesocolon serves as a broad conduit of disease across the mid-abdomen; bare areas link the pancreas to the transverse colon, the spleen, and the small bowel. On the right, the transverse mesocolon is continuous with the duodenocolic ligament; in the middle, it is continuous with the small bowel mesentery; and on the left, it is continuous with the phrenicocolic and splenorenal ligaments (Fig. 6). It contains the middle colic vessels and associat-

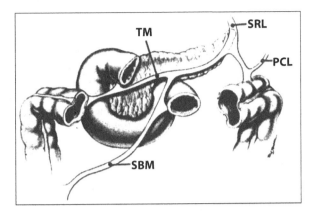

Fig. 6. The transverse mesocolon (*TM*) provides an important conduit for the spread of disease across the mid-abdomen. It is continuous with the splenorenal ligament (*SRL*) and phrenicocolic ligament (*PCL*) on the left and with the duodenocolic ligament on the right. In its mid-portion, it is continuous with the small bowel mesentery (*SBM*). (Reprinted with permission from [8])

ed lymphatics. On CT, it may be recognized as a fatty plane at the level of the uncinate process. Pancreatic tumors often spread ventrally into the transverse mesocolon to involve the transverse colon. In addition, they have the propensity to continue through the gastrocolic ligament to involve the stomach (Fig. 7). Alternatively, they may spread through the transverse mesocolon to involve

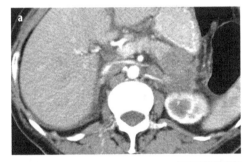

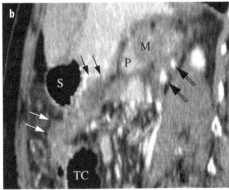

Fig. 7. Invasive pancreatic carcinoma invading the retroperitoneum, transverse mesocolon, and greater omentum. **a** Transaxial image. **b** Parasagittal reformation (*M*, mass; *P*, normal pancreas; *S*, stomach; *TC*, transverse colon). The transverse mesocolon (*black arrows*) provides a pathway for the spread of metastatic disease to the greater omentum (*white arrows*). Also noted is encasement of the left renal artery and ovarian vein (*double arrows*)

the proximal jejunum just beyond the ligament of Treitz (Fig. 8). Like the gastrocolic ligament, a potential space exists within the transverse mesocolon, due to embryologic fusion of the gastrosplenic ligament with the embryologic transverse mesocolon [9]. A less common but important route of spread also exists between the right colon and the periduodenal and peripancreatic nodes via the rightward aspect of the transverse mesocolon (duodenocolic ligament). This is important because lymphadenopathy in the periduodenal and peripancreatic region may herald a right colon cancer when other more common causes of lymphadenopathy in this region are excluded [1].

Three routes of spread between the intraperitoneal viscera and the retroperitoneum are thus provided by three pairs of ligaments. The gastrohepatic and hepatoduodenal

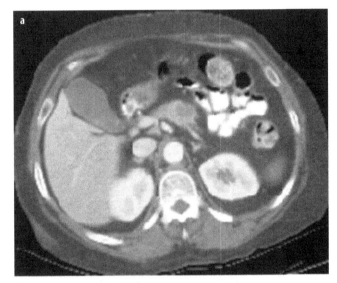

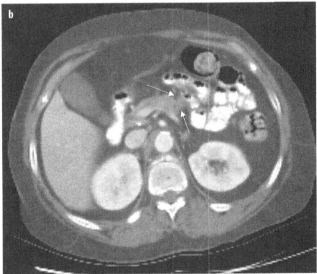

Fig. 8. Incidental pancreatic adenocarcinoma involving the splenic vein (**a**) was thought to be resectable owing to the lack of extrapancreatic involvement. At surgery, upon elevation of the transverse colon, the tumor was found to have penetrated the base of the transverse mesocolon and involved the proximal jejunum just beyond the ligament of Treitz (seen in retrospect in (**b**), *arrows*)

ligaments link the liver and lesser curvature of the stomach to the retroperitoneum; the gastrosplenic and splenorenal ligaments link the superior greater curvature of the stomach and spleen to the retroperitoneum and the gastrocolic and transverse mesocolon link the inferior greater curvature of the stomach and transverse colon to the retroperitoneum. The ligamentous pair in which metastatic disease is recognized can suggest the organ of origin, and, in the case of gastric cancer, the location of the primary tumor within the stomach.

Metastatic Spread via the Peritoneal Spaces

The initiation and growth of seeded metastases on the peritoneal surfaces depend on the natural flow of ascites through the peritoneal spaces. Primary abdominal malignancies and secondary nodal metastases can break through the visceral peritoneum and shed cells into the peritoneal cavity. Once intraperitoneal, such cells propagate through the peritoneal spaces along predictable routes. A thorough understanding of the anatomy of the peritoneal spaces may help refine differential diagnoses for the source of intra-abdominal metastases. By recognizing that a process is intraperitoneal, one may better predict its organ of origin and likely routes of spread (Fig. 9).

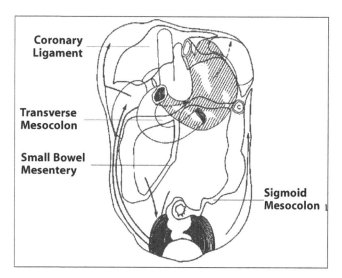

Fig. 9. Posterior peritoneal reflections and recesses. Intraperitoneal fluid flows naturally from the pelvis to the upper abdomen. Flow occurs preferentially through the right rather than left paracolic gutters owing to the broader diameter of the right gutter. In addition, flow in the left paracolic gutter is cut off from reaching the left subphrenic space by the phrenicocolic ligament. The transverse mesocolon divides the abdomen into supra- and inframesocolic spaces. In the right inframesocolic space, fluid is impeded from draining into the pelvis via the small bowel mesentery. Owing to natural holdup of fluid at the root of the small bowel mesentery and sigmoid mesocolon, these structures are naturally predisposed to involvement with serosal-based metastases in the setting of peritoneal carcinomatosis. (Reprinted with permission from [8])

Left Peritoneal Space

The left peritoneal space can be subdivided into four compartments. Although these compartments freely communicate with each other, the inflammatory nature of exudative fluid collections within them predisposes to fibrous adhesions, which may seal off one or more portions of the left peritoneal space from the others.

The *left anterior perihepatic space* is limited on the right by the falciform ligament and on the left by the anterior wall of the stomach. It follows the posterior curve of the diaphragm, and is limited posteriorly by the left coronary ligament (Fig. 10a).

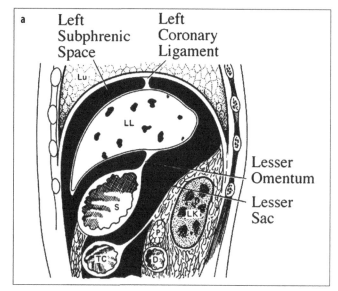

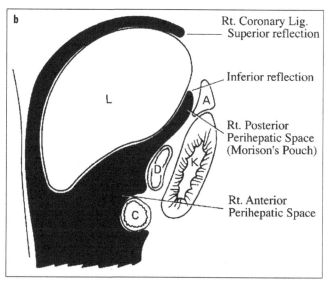

Fig. 10. Left (**a**) and right (**b**) perihepatic spaces. The left and right perihepatic spaces are bordered posteriorly by the coronary ligaments. The reflections of the coronary ligaments mark the site of the nonperitonealized 'bare area' of the liver (*LL*, left lobe of the liver; *LK*, left kidney; *S*, stomach; *TC*, transverse colon; *P*, pancreas; *D*, duodenum; *Lu*, lung; *L*, liver [right lobe]; *A*, adrenal; *K*, kidney; *C*, colon) (Reprinted with permission from [8])

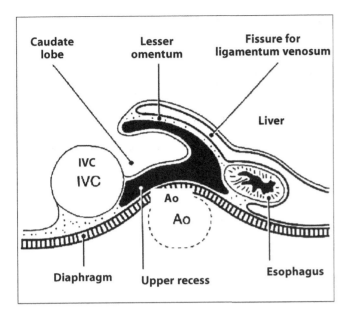

Fig. 11. The boundaries of the superior recess of the lesser sac may be recognized when fluid engulfs the caudate lobe. The lesser omentum separates this fluid from fluid in fissure for the ligamentum venosum, which is in continuity with the left posterior periheptatic space (gastrohepatic recess) (*IVC*, inferior vena cava; *Ao*, aorta) (Reprinted with permission from [8])

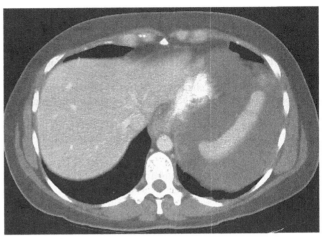

Fig. 12. Cystic mesothelioma. Cystic and solid lesions are seen filling the left anterior and posterior subphrenic spaces

The *left posterior perihepatic space (gastrohepatic recess)* is limited on the left by the lateral wall of the stomach. This space follows the posterior margin of the left hepatic lobe deep into the fissure for the ligamentum venosum to form the posterior margin of the left hepatic lobe. Thus, it is in close proximity to the lesser curve of the stomach, the anterior wall of the duodenal bulb, and the anterior wall of the gallbladder [9].

Although the gastrohepatic recess is close to the lesser sac (divided from it by the lesser omentum), it is a portion of the left peritoneal space, while the lesser sac is a portion of the right peritoneal space (Fig. 11). This distinction is important in that lesser sac collections are very difficult to approach percutaneously, whereas gastrohepatic recess collections are usually accessible by guiding a catheter along the inferior margin of the left hepatic lobe.

The *anterior left subphrenic space* is in direct continuity with the left anterior perihepatic space, which forms its right boundary. Far to the left, on the anterolateral surface of the stomach, this space is limited by the greater omentum. This is a common site for fluid loculation in the setting of malignant ascites [14].

The *posterior left subphrenic (perisplenic)* space is the posterior continuation of the anterior subphrenic space and generally surrounds the lateral and superior margins of the spleen. The 'bare areas' of the spleen are reliably observed in perisplenic fluid collections [15-17]. Superiorly, the perisplenic space is entirely subphrenic and surrounds the top of the spleen (Fig. 12) [18].

Right Peritoneal Space

There are three major subdivisions of the right peritoneal space: the right subphrenic space, the hepatorenal recess, and the lesser sac (Figs. 10, 11). The *right subphrenic space* occupies the smoothly contoured area between the superolateral margin of the liver and the right hemidiaphragm. The medial extension of this compartment is limited by the right coronary ligament, which is simply the right lateral margin of the liver's bare area [19]. The *hepatorenal recess* (or Morrison's pouch) is the posteromedial extension of the subphrenic space, inferior to the coronary ligament. As its name implies, it extends between the right hepatic lobe and the anterior border of the right kidney.

The *lesser sac* has two major components [10, 20]: a small *superior recess* is immediately posterior to the hepatoduodenal ligament. The caudate lobe of the liver is enveloped by this peritoneal reflection (Fig. 11). The larger *inferior recess* occupies the space behind the stomach, anterior to the transverse mesocolon and medial to the gastrosplenic ligament. As both portions of the lesser sac are surrounded by abdominal viscera, percutaneous drainage of collections within this space is difficult. Inferiorly, the superior recess communicates with the right perihepatic space through the foramen of Winslow. A potential extension may exist caudally behind the duodenum and pancreatic head, which may be responsible for peritoneal fluid collections behind the pancreatic head in some cases [8].

References

1. Meyers MA, Oliphant M, Berne AS, Feldberg MAM (1987) The peritoneal ligaments and mesenteries: pathways of intraabdominal spread of disease. Radiology 163:593-604
2. Balfe DM, Mauro MA, Koehler RE et al (1984) Gastrohepatic ligament: normal and pathologic CT anatomy. Radiology 150:485-490

3. Auh YH, Rosen A, Rubenstein WA et al (1984) CT of the papillary process of the caudate lobe of the liver. AJR Am J Roentgenol 142:535-538

4. Donoso L, Martinez-Noguera A, Zidan A, Lora F (1989) Papillary process of the caudate lobe of the liver: sonographic appearance. Radiology 173:631-633

5. Weinstein JB, Heiken JP, Lee JKT et al (1986). High resolution CT of the porta hepatis and hepatoduodenal ligament. Radiographics 6:55-74

6. Zirinsky K, Auh YH, Rubenstein WA et al (1985) The portacaval space: CT with MR correlation. Radiology 156:453-460

7. Ito K, Choji T, Fujita T et al (1993) Imaging of the portacaval space. AJR Am J Roentgenol 161:329-334

8. Meyers MA (1994) Dynamic Radiology of the Abdomen: Normal and Pathologic Anatomy. (4th edn) Springer, New York

9. Vincent LM, Mauro MA, Mittelstaedt CA (1984) The lesser sac and gastrohepatic recess: sonographic appearance and differentiation of fluid collections. Radiology 150:515-519

10. Dodds WJ, Foley WD, Lawson TL et al (1985) Anatomy and imaging of the lesser peritoneal sac. AJR Am J Roentgenol 144:567-575

11. Longman J (1971) Medical embriology. Saunders, Philadelphia

12. Cooper C, Jeffrey RB, Silverman PM et al (1986) Computed tomography of omental pathology. J Comput Assist Tomogr 10:62-66

13. Rubesin SE, Levine MS, Glick SN (1986) Gastric involvement by omental cakes: radiographic findings. Gastrointest Radiol 11:223-228

14. Halvorsen RA, Jones MA, Rice RP, Thompson WM (1982) Anterior left subphrenic abscess: characteristic plain film and CT appearance. AJR Am J Roentgenol 139:283-289

15. Vibhakar SD, Bellon EM (1984) The bare area of the spleen: a constant CT feature of the ascitic abdomen. AJR Am J Roentgenol 141:953-955

16. Rubenstein WA, Auh YH, Zirinsky K et al (1985) Posterior peritoneal recesses: assessment using CT. Radiology 156:461-468

17. Love L, Demos TC, Posniak H (1985) CT of retrorenal fluid collections. AJR Am J Roentgenol 145:87-91

18. Crass JR, Maile CW, Frick MP (1985) Catheter drainage of the left posterior subphrenic space: a reliable percutaneous approach. Gastrointest Radiol 10:397-398

19. Rubenstein WA, Auh TH, Whalen JP, Kazem E (1983) The perihepatic spaces: computed tomographic and ultrasound imaging. Radiology 149:231-239

20. Jeffrey RB, Federle MP, Goodman PC (1981) Computed tomography of the lesser peritoneal sac. Radiology 141:117-122

Abdominal Vascular MRA

T.M. Grist

Departments of Radiology and Medical Physics, University of Wisconsin, Madison, WI, USA

Introduction

Following the development of breath-hold, contrast-enhanced techniques, magnetic resonance angiography (MRA) has become an important tool for the evaluation of patients with abdominal vascular pathology. Specifically, the lack of ionizing radiation, lack of nephrotoxic contrast media and the non-invasive nature of MRA make it a useful modality for abdominal vascular pathology. The objective of this work is to describe the acquisition techniques, relevant anatomy, and pathologic conditions for accurate application of MRA in the abdomen.

MRA Technique

General techniques for MRA in the abdomen include localizer images, a fast T2 scan, a dose-timing acquisition, and breath-hold three-dimensional gradient recalled echo images acquired before, during, and following the intravenous administration of gadolinium contrast agent. In addition, delayed, post-contrast T1-weighted gradient echo imaging with fat suppression is helpful. Additional optional scans include two-dimensional cardiac-gated phase contrast images, as well as three-dimensional phase contrast imaging.

Localizer images are typically obtained using a three-plane localizer acquisition, therefore allowing the visualization of the aorta along its long axis, as well the position of the kidneys posteriorly and the mesenteric circulation anteriorly. Subsequently, a fast, breath-hold T2-weighted image is very useful to evaluate masses incidentally found on the MRA portion of the exam. A fat-suppressed single-shot fast spin echo image is highly desirable (HASTE, single-shot fast spin echo). Using these techniques, T2-weighted images can be obtained throughout the abdomen in a single breath-hold, therefore speeding the examination. The heavily T2-weighted single-shot methods are sensitive to fluid, however, it should be cautioned that subtle differences in T2 may be masked due to magnetization transfer effects occurring within the fast spin echo sequence. Therefore, these techniques are most useful for confirming cystic fluid collections, rather than complete characterization of all abdominal masses.

Subsequently, the arrival time of contrast agent in the region-of-interest must be determined. Several options for determining the arrival time of contrast media are available. These include first, a dose-timing scan, in which a small test dose of contrast agent (1-2 cc) is administered, and serial gradient recalled images are obtained at 1-2 second intervals. The arrival time of contrast can be determined by measuring a region of interest in the serial images [1]. Second, fluoroscopically-triggered MRA, in which serial gradient recalled images are obtained and rapidly reconstructed so that the individual performing the exam can detect the arrival of contrast agent within the region-of-interest [2]. Third, automatically triggered techniques, where a sampling volume is placed over the aorta, and the MRI scanner detects the arrival of contrast agent within the sampling volume automatically, triggering the three-dimensional acquisition [3].

For the contrast-enhanced scan, meticulous attention to detail is important to ensure diagnostic studies. Typically, a three-dimensional T1-weighted spoiled-gradient recalled echo acquisition is acquired. Fast gradients are important in order to ensure that a short repetition time (TR) and echo time (TE) are achieved, therefore maximizing spatial resolution per unit time. Images are acquired prior to contrast agent in order to verify that the location of the three-dimensional volume covers the anatomic region-of-interest. In addition, the pre-contrast image set is used as a mask, if mask subtraction is necessary. An image volume is then acquired during the arterial phase of contrast enhancement, followed by an additional volume during the venous phase.

Following the three-dimensional volume acquisition, delayed post-contrast T1-weighted gradient echo imaging with fat suppression is performed. These images are very useful for determining the true size of aortic aneurysms, evaluating venous contrast enhancement patterns for parenchymal lesions that are detected on the three-dimensional contrast MRA, as well for evaluating venous abnormalities including venous thrombosis. These images are typically obtained using an interleaved gradient echo technique in order to optimize signal-to-noise ratio and contrast resolution.

Finally, optional supportive sequences include two-dimensional phase contrast methods for measuring the direction of blood flow, and the volumetric flow rate in selected vessels of interest. Typically, a segmented k-space gradient recalled echo acquisition is used, and is acquired during a single breath-hold. Accurate flow measurements may be obtained if high spatial resolution studies are acquired to limit partial volume errors associated with flow measurement. Three-dimensional phase contrast acquisitions are also helpful, especially in the renal arteries, where the presence of signal void at, or distal to, a stenosis implies a hemodynamically significant stenosis.

The dose of gadolinium contrast agent required for abdominal vascular imaging is dependent on the resolution that is acquired during the examination. Many studies have been performed demonstrating that a single dose (20 cc) is satisfactory for aortic and renal artery imaging [1]. For high-resolution examinations, it may be necessary to increase the dose to 30, or even 40 cc, gadolinium contrast agent. The rationale for the increased dose is that it is necessary to provide consistent arterial enhancement throughout the acquisition technique. Typically, the gadolinium contrast is injected at a rate of 3 cc per second. The contrast administration is followed immediately by a saline flush of at least 20 cc in order to clear the line and flush the contrast agent through the venous system. It should be noted that a saline flush as large as possible should be used, because large saline flushes have been shown to provide greater arterial signal.

Aorta

Technical Considerations

The general MRA techniques are described above. However, it is important to note the need for a delayed image acquisition in patients with abdominal aortic pathology. Many of these patients have delayed filling of vessels distal to the aneurysm or occlusion, or delayed filling of a false lumen in dissection. Therefore, it is important to review at least a two-phase exam, one phase timed to the arterial arrival of contrast, and one phase immediately following arterial enhancement. Several groups have demonstrated the utility of a time-resolved exam in this setting [4, 5]. Finally, in the case of aortic aneurysm, it is important to note that the delayed two-dimensional fat-suppressed T1-weighted gradient echo exams provide a better estimate of the true aortic diameter, including the thrombosed lumen.

Anatomy

The normal caliber of the abdominal aorta at the renal arteries measures from 1.5 cm in adult woman, to 2.1 cm in adult men [6]. The celiac artery arises at the T12/L1 level, the small mesenteric artery (SMA) at the L1 level, and the intermediate mesenteric artery (IMA) at the L3 level. The renal arteries typically arise at the L1/2 level. The four paired lumbar arteries arise from the aorta posterio-laterally, and they create important collateral pathways with the intercostal arteries, the ilio-lumbar vessels, and the gluteal arteries in the setting of aortic occlusive disease.

Pathologic Conditions

Aortic Aneurysm

Abdominal aortic aneurysms are defined as localized enlargement of the aorta by 50% of its diameter or more [7]. Most abdominal aortic aneurysms are infrarenal; an estimated 10% are either supra- or juxtarenal. While an infrarenal abdominal aortic aneurysm is considered present when the diameter exceeds 3 cm, the risk of significant morbidity and mortality increases as the size increases, with an estimated five-year risk of rupture of 25% if the aneurysm exceeds 5 cm in diameter [8].

MRA has been shown to be accurate for the detection and delineation of abdominal aortic aneurysms (Fig. 1) [9]. In addition, MRA is useful for delineation of branch vessel involvement with aneurysm or stenosis. The delayed images on contrast-enhanced exams are also helpful for determining the relationship of the venous anatomy to the aneurysm.

Mycotic aneurysms typically are eccentric and saccular in location, which is atypical for atherosclerotic aneurysms. Common organisms include salmonella and staphylococcus, and inflammatory abdominal aneurysms are seen more commonly in immunosuppressed patients, intravenous drug abusers, and patients with bacterial endocarditis. Magnetic resonance angiography demonstrates the lumen of the aneurysm in mycotic aneurysms. However, the delayed images on MRA techniques also demonstrate marked enhancement of a thickened rind of aorta in cases of inflammatory aortic aneurysm. However, the enhancing aortic wall can also be seen in noninfected aortic aneurysms.

Inflammatory abdominal aortic aneurysms comprise approximately 5% of all abdominal aneurysms [10]. Retroperitoneal fibrosis is a special case of inflammatory aortic aneurysmal disease felt to be due to an immune reaction that results in leakage of antigen across the aortic wall, which then triggers a fibrotic immune response to the antigen [10]. This results in extensive retroperitoneal fibrosis associated with the aneurysm. MRA, due to its sensitivity to extraluminal soft tissue anatomy, can be useful for following the response of patients to treatment for retroperitoneal fibrosis. The progression and regression of the retroperitoneal fibrotic process can be monitored on serial exams.

Fig. 1. Abdominal aortic aneurysm. **a** Sagittal and (**b**) coronal subvolume MIP displays demonstrate Crawford Type IV infrarenal abdominal aortic aneurysm with extensive thrombosed lumen (*arrow*). The subvolume MIP in (**b**) demonstrates multiple left renal arteries

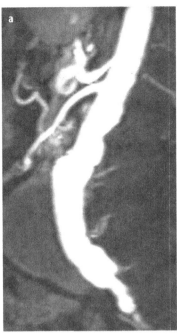

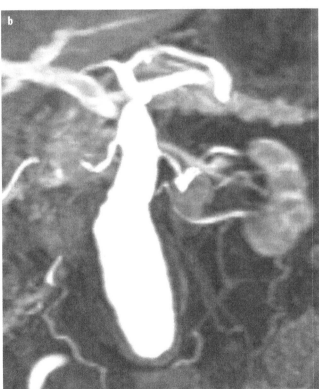

Aortic Occlusion

Aortic occlusion typically occurs in the infrarenal abdominal aorta [11]. The majority of aortic occlusions occur due to embolization, often a cardiac source, although thrombosis superimposed on aortic atherosclerotic disease is not an uncommon cause. Other causes of aortic occlusion include thrombosis of an abdominal aortic aneurysm, trauma, dissection, and extrinsic compression

of the aorta. In most of these cases, a distal aortic occlusion propagates back to the level of the origin of the renal arteries.

MRA techniques are ideally suited for the evaluation of infrarenal abdominal aortic occlusion (Fig. 2). Many of these patients have superimposed renal insufficiency, and the relative lack of nephrotoxicity associated with the gadolinium dyes reduces the risk of renal failure in these patients. In addition, the intravenous injection eliminates the need for intra-arterial access, which in the case of aortic occlusive disease must occur from an approach in the arm, with a small but significant increase in morbidity associated with catheter-induced complications. It is possible to visualize the common femoral and distal vascular run-off in patients with aortic occlusion using MRA due to the complete opacification of blood during the intravenous injection.

Abdominal aortic coarctation is an uncommon disease found in children and young adults that can present with claudication, renal vascular hypertension, and symptoms of mesenteric ischemia. Congenital causes of abdominal aortic coarctation include William's syndrome, congenital rubella, and neurofibromatosis. Acquired cases, seen in young adults, are often due to Takayasu's arteritis, fibromuscular dysplasia (FMD), and radiation therapy. As opposed to abdominal aortic occlusion, the abdominal aortic narrowing in coarctation usually involves the renal arteries [12]. The inferior mesenteric artery serves as a major collateral pathway in the setting of abdominal aor-

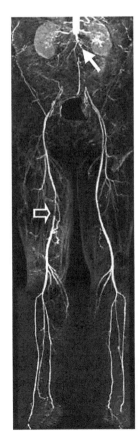

Fig. 2. Aortic occlusion with Leriche syndrome. Coronal image depicting the entire abdominal and lower extremity circulation. The image is a combination of the MIP images from the pelvis and thigh station and the below-knee time-resolved (TRICKS) acquisition. Occlusion of the infra-renal abdominal aorta is shown with collateralization (*white arrow*), and right superficial femoral artery occlusion or high-grade stenosis (*open arrow*). Three-vessel run-off is shown bilaterally

tic coarctation, and can often enlarge to several centimeters in diameter.

MRA is suitable for evaluating patients with abdominal aortic coarctation. In particular, MRA as a noninvasive technique, with a non-nephrotoxic contrast agent is suitable for following these patients to assess the need for medical or surgical intervention. Typical findings are seen on MRA exams, including diffuse attenuation of the aorta, with extensive collateral filling of the distal vessels via intracostal, internal iliac, and mesenteric collaterals.

Postoperative Aorta

Surgical repair of abdominal aortic aneurysm remains the mainstay of operative treatment to reduce the risk of rupture [7]. Two grafts are used primarily for abdominal aortic aneurysm repair that do not involve the iliac arteries. Bifurcation grafts are used in settings of abdominal aortic aneurysm with aortoiliac occlusive disease.

Two types of aortic bifurcation grafts are commonly used. In the aortic onlay graft, the proximal end of the graft is anastomosed to the ventral wall of the aorta, and the distal limbs of the graft are anastomosed to both common femoral arteries. The abrupt angle at the distal aorta to proximal graft interface results in a slightly higher incidence of graft occlusion in these patients. For the end-to-end Y-graft, the proximal graft is anastomosed in an end-to-end fashion to the distal aorta. The distal bifurcated graft is anastomosed to each common femoral artery. The end-to-end Y-graft is felt to provide a more physiologic flow state at the proximal and distal anastomoses.

MRA is useful for evaluating complications associated with surgical graft placement. Complications include perigraft infection, anastomotic pseudoaneurysm, graft occlusion, and aortoenteric fistula (Fig. 3). In particular, delayed, contrast-enhanced images and T2 fast spin echo images are useful for evaluating perigraft infection, which is characterized by a thick rind of enhancing tissue around the graft, as well as increased signal intensity associated with fluid collection within the thick rind of tissue.

Recently, aortic stent grafts have provided a less invasive alternative to standard surgical repair of aortic aneurysms. MRA may be used for the preoperative assessment of features of the aorta that are important to measure prior to stent graft placement. These features include the diameter of the proximal landing zone, diameter of the distal landing zone, length of the aneurysm, length of the proximal landing zone, length of the distal landing zone, and status of the aortic branch vessels.

MRA can be used postoperatively to assess the presence of endoleak associated with endovascular stents for abdominal aortic aneurysm. However, it should be noted that the artifact associated with the metallic cage requires the use of slightly different parameters for the MRA acquisitions. Specifically, a minimum echo is

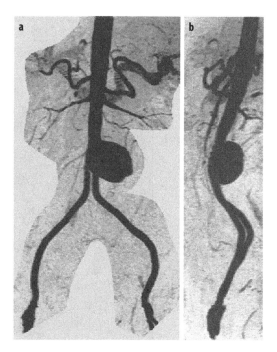

Fig. 3. Aortic graft pseudoaneurysm. **a** Coronal and **b** Sagittal MIP display in patient with aorto-bifemoral graft and pseudoaneurysm at graft anastamosis. The location and eccentric origin of the aortic sac suggests pseudoaneurysm, which was confirmed upon surgery

used in order to reduce the susceptibility-induced signal use associated with the metallic portion of the cage. In addition, the cage itself creates a radiofrequency shield that can limit radiofrequency energy deposition within the stent graft. This limitation can be overcome by increasing the flip angle of the MRA acquisition to ensure penetration of radiofrequency energy within the stent graft. A flip angle of 70 degrees will often demonstrate the lumen of the vessel within the stent graft, despite the radiofrequency shielding that occurs due to the stent graft itself.

Renal Arteries

Technical Considerations

The renal arteries typically measure 4-5 mm in diameter. Therefore, high-resolution techniques are necessary for accurate characterization of renal artery stenosis. In addition, it is necessary to use a breath-hold acquisition sequence in order to limit the effects of respiratory motion on spatial resolution.

Two approaches are possible for obtaining high-resolution images of the renal arteries. One approach uses a small field of view (FOV) localized to the renal arteries only, which is used in conjunction with a 256 × 192 acquisition matrix, for example, over a 24 cm FOV. The other approach takes account of the fact that it is often desirable to image the iliofemoral arteries at the same time that the renal arteries are imaged, in order to provide a road map for a possible percutaneous catheter placement if renal artery angioplasty is contemplated. In this approach, a 36 cm FOV is desirable, with a high-resolution acquisition matrix along the superior inferior direction (e.g., 512 imaging matrix). For these scans, it is also desirable to use an oblique three-dimensional acquisition in order to include the renal arteries as well as the iliacs and common femoral arteries as they move anteriorly in the distal part of the imaging FOV.

Pathologic Conditions

The clinical consequences of renal artery stenosis include renal vascular hypertension and ischemic nephropathy. Renal artery stenosis is the cause of hypertension in an estimated 1-5% of patients with elevated blood pressure. In addition, bilateral renal artery stenosis, or unilateral renal artery stenosis in a single kidney, is a cause of chronic renal ischemia, and can result in end stage renal disease. An estimated 16% of patients with end stage renal disease have ischemic nephropathy.

Causes of renal artery stenosis include atherosclerotic disease in approximately 75%, and fibromuscular dysplasia in approximately 25% of patients. The clinical features of the two diseases are distinct; atherosclerotic disease affects older individuals, and causes proximal renal artery disease (Fig. 4). In contrast, fibromuscular dyspla-

sia tends to cause renal artery stenosis involving the more distal renal artery and its branches, and is found in individuals at a younger age.

Renal MRA has been shown to be accurate for depicting proximal renal artery stenoses associated with atherosclerotic vascular disease. High-grade stenoses are often depicted with a small focus of signal loss at the site of the stenosis. For mild to moderate stenoses, it is often helpful to acquire an additional three-dimensional phase contrast exam, which is more sensitive to the signal loss associated with turbulent flow distal to the stenosis.

As discussed above, FMD is known to cause more focal web-like stenosis, often involving the distal main renal artery or its segmental branches (Fig. 5). The accuracy of renal MRA in this situation is unknown at this time. It is clear that some cases of FMD can clearly be demonstrated using MRA, however it is necessary to carefully review the MIPs as well as the source images to identify the beaded, irregular appearance of the renal artery. It should be noted, however, that visualization of the segmental renal artery is obscured by enhancement of the renal parenchyma by the gadolinium contrast agent. Therefore, small focal segmental artery stenoses are difficult to identify on renal MRA.

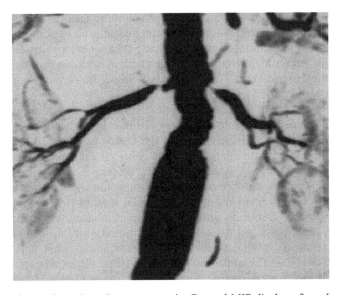

Fig. 4. Bilateral renal artery stenosis. Coronal MIP display of renal arteries during IV infusion of 30 cc gadolinium contrast agent demonstrates bilateral renal artery stenosis, high exceeding 80% diameter. The patient presented with renal failure, edema, and congestive heart failure. The symptoms reversed after renal endarterectomy. The lack of nephrotoxic contrast agent makes MRA an ideal diagnostic study in patients with renal insufficiency and suspected renal artery stenosis

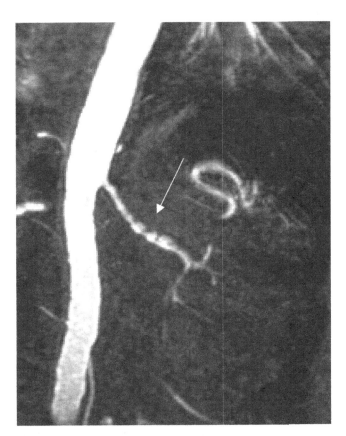

Fig. 5. Renal fibromuscular dysplasia. Oblique coronal MIP display demonstrates classic string-of-pearls appearance of FMD (*arrow*), indicating medial fibrodysplasia subtype

Mesenteric Arteries

Technical Considerations

In suspected cases of mesenteric ischemia, it is important to maintain high spatial resolution in the anterior/posterior direction, therefore either a coronal acquisition with thin slices or a sagittal acquisition is often chosen. In addition, the use of fat suppression improves the contrast between the opacified vessels and the surrounding mesenteric fat. Likewise, visualization of the distal mesenteric vessels can be improved by administering a meal, since mesenteric flow increases substantially following a meal, therefore improving opacification of the distal vessels.

Anatomy

Mesenteric Anatomy

The celiac axis arises from the aorta at the T12/L1 level, and classically gives off three branches including the left gastric, the splenic, and the common hepatic artery [13]. Variations in the branching pattern are seen in up to 40% of individuals; most commonly (in 15% of individuals) the right hepatic artery arises from the superior mesenteric artery. The left hepatic artery arises from the left gastric artery in an additional 10% of individuals, and an estimated 5% of individuals have an accessory left hepatic artery arising from the left gastric artery or an accessory right hepatic artery arising the superior mesenteric artery [13].

The SMA arises at the L1 level, while the IMA typically arises from the anterior aorta at the level of L3. Mesenteric collateral pathways form important anastomotic pathways for blood flow in cases of mesenteric ischemia or aortic occlusion. Collateral pathways from the celiac artery to the SMA are commonly seen via the pancreaticoduodenal arcade and the arc of Buehler, which is an embryonic ventricle communication of the celiac artery to the SMA. Collateral pathways from the SMA to the IMA including the arc of Riolan, which are short SMA to IMA collaterals centrally, and the marginal artery of Drummond, which is the arcade along the mesenteric border of the colon. Finally, collaterals exist between the IMA and the internal iliac arteries via the superior hemorrhoidal arteries.

Pathologic Conditions

Mesenteric Ischemia

Mesenteric ischemia may either be acute or chronic in etiology. Chronic ischemia occurs when there is progressive atherosclerotic occlusive disease of all three mesenteric arteries, and patients typically present with weight loss and chronic abdominal angina (Fig. 6).

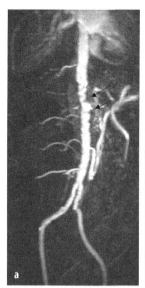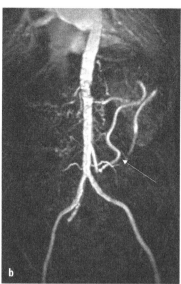

Fig. 6. Chronic mesenteric ischemia. **a** Oblique and **b** coronal MIP demonstrating occlusion of the celiac and superior mesenteric arteries (*arrows*). A large inferior mesenteric artery supplies blood flow to the gut via collateral pathways (arc of Riolan, *white arrow*)

Patients with acute mesenteric ischemia, in contrast, usually present with an acute abdomen and are not suitable candidates for MR due to their altered metabolic and septic status. Chronic mesenteric ischemia is most commonly caused by atherosclerosis with stenotic involvement at the origin of the three mesenteric vessels. Acute mesenteric ischemia is most often caused by embolization, and therefore MRA or CTA may be used to detect the presence of an acute thrombus within the mesenteric artery. Additional causes of acute mesenteric occlusion include aortic dissection with sudden occlusion of the mesenteric vessels due to branch vessel involvement of the flap and vasculitis.

A median arcuate ligament syndrome is an additional, somewhat controversial syndrome, whereby there is compression of the origin of the celiac axis due to the median arcuate ligament, which connects the crura of the diaphragm [14]. The angiographic diagnosis is classically seen as compression of the superior aspect of the artery, and this finding is most often seen in young, thin women. Some patients complain of abdominal pain, weight loss, and nausea, however the relationship of the celiac narrowing to these symptoms is somewhat controversial. The apparent stenosis is often worse on expiration abuse.

The finding is not infrequently seen on MRA examinations of the abdomen. Repeat imaging during inspiration and expiration may be useful to further characterize whether the lesion is fixed or not. In addition, it is possible to measure blood flow velocity increases at the site of the stenosis, although the role of these flow measurements is currently unclear.

References

1. Earls J, Rofsky NM, De Corato DR et al (1996) Breath-hold single-dose gadolinium enhanced MR aortography: usefulness of a timing examination and a power injector. Radiology 201:705-710
2. Riederer SJ, Tasciyan T, Farzaneh F et al (1988) MR fluoroscopy: technical feasibility. Magn Res Med 8:1-7
3. Foo T, Manojkumar S, Prince M, Chenevert T (1996) MR Smart Prep: an automated method for detecting the bolus arrival time and initiating data acquisition in fast 3D gadolinium-enhanced MRA. Proceedings of the International Society for Magnetic Resonance in Medicine. New York.
4. Grist T (1998) Renal magnetic resonance angiography: an update. Current Opinion in Urology 8:105-109
5. Korosec F, Frayne R, Grist TM, Mistretta CA (1996) Time-resolved contrast-enhanced 3D MR angiography. Magn Reson Med 36:345-351
6. Horejs D, Gilbert PM, Burstein S, Vogelzang RL (1988) Normal aortoiliac diameters by CT. J Comput Assist Tomogr 12:602-603
7. Ernst C (1993) Abdominal aortic aneurysm. N Engl J Med 328:1167-1172
8. Cronenwett J, Sargent S, Wall M (1990) Variables that affect the expansion rate and outcome of small abdominal aortic aneurysms. J Vasc Surg 11:260-268
9. Kaufman J et al (1994) MR imaging (including MR angiography) of abdominal aortic aneurysms: comparison with conventional angiography. AJR Am J Roentgenol 163:203-210
10. Amis EJ (1991) Retroperitoneal fibrosis. AJR Am J Roentgenol 157:321-329
11. Dossa C, Shepard AD, Reddy DJ et al (1994) Acute aortic occlusion: a 40-year experience. Arch Surg 129:603-607
12. Yamato M et al (1986) Takayasu arteritis: radiographic and angiographic findings in 59 patients. Radiology 161:329
13. Kornblith P, Boley S, Whitehouse B (1992) Anatomy of the splanchnic circulation. Surg Clin North Am 72:1-30
14. Bech F (1997) Celiac artery compression syndromes. Surg Clin North Am 77:409-424

Abdominal Vascular Imaging Including Mesenteric Ischemia

M. Prokop

Department of Radiology, University Medical Center Utrecht, Utrecht, The Netherlands

Abdominal vascular imaging is moving away from catheter angiography towards computed tomographic angiography (CTA), and to a lesser degree, magnetic resonance angiography (MRA) or ultrasound. Ultrasound used to be performed mainly in young patients and in acute settings, but computed tomography (CT) is starting to take over most of the work in patients with acute abdomen. MRA remains a good technique for follow-up of stented aortic aneurysms and for the detection of renal artery stenoses. Its ease and speed has led to CT becoming the technique of choice for the vast majority of indications in abdominal vascular imaging.

Abdominal Aorta

Abdominal Aortic Aneurysms

Abdominal aortic aneurysms (AAA) become more common with severe atherosclerosis and old age. They are mainly located in the infrarenal aorta, which makes them amenable to endoluminal repair by stent graft placement. Extensive disease, however, may involve most of the thoracoabdominal aorta. More frequently, AAAs extend distally into the iliac arteries. Most aneurysms are fusiform, a minority are saccular. Rupture is the main cause of death, although a substantial number of patients die from other causes related to their atherosclerosis.

The most important information that imaging should provide is listed in Table 1. In addition to spatial information for treatment planning, it is important to detect complications, such as (contained) rupture, perianeurysmatic fibrosis, fistulation or compression of abdominal structures. CTA and, to a lesser degree, gadolinium (Gd)-enhanced MRA are the imaging procedures of choice for the diagnosis of abdominal aortic aneurysms. If information is needed about the spinal blood flow, the coronary arteries, or cerebral or peripheral blood flow, catheter angiography may remain necessary. 64-slice CT has the ability to provide this information in many cases, if necessary in combination with electrocardiogram (ECG) gating. Longitudinal curved planar reformats (CPR), maximum intensity projections (MIP) or volume-rendered images are necessary for optimum evaluation (Fig. 1). Volume rendering is able to simultaneously display calcifications, vessel lumen and thrombus, and is particularly useful for surgical planning. CPR are most important for measurements prior to stent graft placement. The involvement of vessel origins in the aneurysm complicates surgical treatment. It is therefore important to determine the precise location of the abdominal side branches in relation to an aneurysm of the abdominal aorta.

Mural thrombus is a frequent finding and causes underestimation of the size of an aneurysm on three dimensional (3D) representations unless there is calcification of the aneurysm wall. The thrombus itself may partially calcify. Irregularities and ulceration of the mural thrombus may indicate an increased risk of distal emboli, in particular during angiographic procedures.

Penetrating ulcers are a consequence of ulcerative aortic plaques [1, 2]. They develop after destruction of the intima and may form saccular aneurysms with a high propensity for acute hemorrhage or may progress to aortic dissection (Fig. 1). A penetrating ulcer can be suspected if the aneurysm has overhanging edges or a focal dissection.

Table 1. Checklist for AAA and suspected aortic rupture

AAA workup
- Diameter
- Signs of rupture (confined perforation is not uncommon)
- Penetrating ulcer?
- Inflammatory aneurysm (perianeurysmal fibrosis)
- Length
- Distance from the aneurysm to the origin of the renal arteries (proximal neck?)
- Involvement or stenosis of splanchnic arteries
- Involvement of aortic bifurcation and iliac arteries
- Retroaortic left renal vein

Signs of perforation
- Stranding of para-aortic tissue
- Para-aortic hematoma
- Hyperattenuating ascites

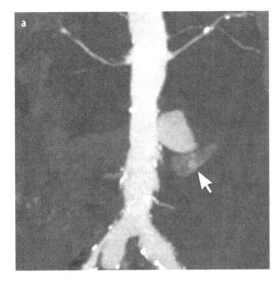

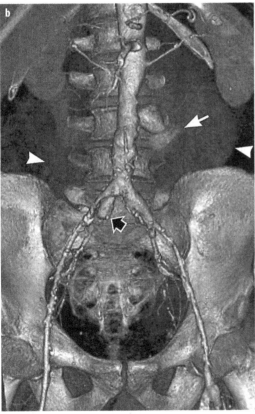

Fig. 1. Maximum intensity projection (MIP) (**a**) and volume rendered display (**b**) of a 64-detector-row CT angiography of a saccular infrarenal aortic aneurysms, probably caused by a penetrating ulcer. Note the location of an acute extravasation (*arrow*), the retroperitoneal hematoma (*arrowheads*) and another penetrating ulcer in the right common iliac artery (*black arrow*)

Inflammatory aneurysms are characterized by perianeurysmal inflammatory tissue and fibrosis, similar to retroperitoneal fibrosis [3]. No infectious organism is found. Possible secondary effects are ureteral obstruction or the involvement of intestinal loops. Characteristically, three distinct layers surround the perfused lumen: mural thrombus, aortic wall with calcifications, and perianeurysmal soft tissue. The soft-tissue rim surrounding the aorta shows contrast enhancement that increases on late scans (> 90 s) after contrast injection.

Fistulation into adjacent organs is a rare but severe complication. Aorto-enteric fistula may cause hyperattenuating clots in the bowel lumen, as well as direct contrast extravasation into the affected bowel segment, which is often the horizontal portion of the duodenum. If there is mural thrombus, fistulation may cause air bubbles in the wall.

Concomitant vascular disease is quite frequent. Concomitant aneurysms are found in the visceral and renal arteries, and the iliac arteries. AAA are associated with stenoses of various side branches. Therefore it is important to evaluate the main branching vessels for the presence of stenoses or aneurysms. In patients with stenosis of the superior mesenteric artery and collateralization via the inferior mesenteric artery, left colonic ischemia may develop as a complication of surgery, if no reimplantation of this artery is performed. Involvement of the iliac arteries (aneurysms, stenoses) is an important factor in deciding whether to implant a tubular or Y-shaped prosthesis. Accessory renal arteries are present in 25% of the population. They may only be sacrificed during implantation of stent grafts if they are small.

Aortic Rupture

The most important complication of aortic aneurysms is rupture, which is defined as seepage of blood through clefts in the aortic wall. The larger the diameter of the aneurysm, the greater is the likelihood of eventual rupture. In the abdomen, the life-time risk for rupture grows from 10% in aneurysms smaller than 4 cm to 60% in aneurysms larger than 10 cm. Elective surgical or endoluminal repair is usually indicated if the aneurysmal diameter exceeds 5 cm in the descending and abdominal aorta. Saccular aneurysms have a higher risk of rupture, and there is no absolute size limit that governs the decision to intervene. Surgical mortality rises substantially in patients with ruptured aneurysms.

CT is indicated for suspected aortic rupture, provided the patient is not referred for immediate surgery based on ultrasound findings. Non-contrast CT is no longer indicated. CTA is the present technique of choice. CTA is able to define whether insertion of a bifurcated prosthesis or reimplantation of the renal arteries is required. Scan delay has to be determined individually, because the circulation time may be substantially prolonged (to beyond 60 s) in patients with shock. The patient can be taken off the CT table as soon as it is clear that contrast enhancement of CTA is sufficient. To speed up evaluation, it may be advisable to reconstruct fewer images first with larger spacing to determine the major findings. Later an overlapping data set can be reconstructed, from which 3D representations for fine-tuning of the surgical procedure can be derived.

Impending rupture may be indicated by freshly clotted blood within the aortic wall or a mural thrombus. Hyperdense portions within a pre-existing hypodense mural thrombus on CT are an indicator of fresh thrombus formation and thus recent growth of an aneurysm. Furthermore, nose-like protrusions of perfused lumen into a clotted region suggest a higher risk for rupture. Small amounts of stranding around an aneurysm indicate minor hemorrhage and can be the precursor to aortic rupture.

Contained rupture occurs mainly in the abdominal aorta in a posterior-lateral location and is characterized by local hemorrhage or acute pseudoaneurysm formation. Sometimes interruption of a wall calcification may be detected at the site of the pseudoaneurysm.

AAA commonly rupture into the retroperitoneum, which contains the hemorrhage to a certain degree. If the peritoneum itself ruptures, the blood may freely flow into the peritoneal cavity, leading to a high risk of sudden death. Rarely, an aneurysm can rupture into the gastrointestinal tract, causing massive gastrointestinal hemorrhage (aortoduodenal fistula), or into the inferior vena cava, leading to rapid cardiac decompensation. Acute rupture leads to stranding of the retroperitoneal fat surrounding the aorta. Free intraperitoneal fluid is rare, but its presence signals a very unstable situation in which the rupture is no longer confined by the peritoneum. Acute hemorrhage need not be hyperattenuating, but may be isoattenuating relative to muscle because of a lack of clotting or separation between blood cells and serum. It may even be hypoattenuating if the hematocrit is low because of plasma expanders. Active bleeding is present if contrast extravasation can be observed.

Dissection of the Abdominal Aorta

Isolated dissection of the abdominal aorta is rare and is usually caused by a penetrating ulcer. Abdominal malperfusion as a consequence of a thoracic dissection of the aorta is not uncommon. Compression or occlusion of major aortic branches may lead to renal failure, mesenteric ischemia, or acute claudication. The false channel has a propensity to dilate and to compress the true lumen or the orifice of a side branch vessel.

CTA has almost completely substituted for angiography in the diagnosis and evaluation of abdominal complications in patients with suspected aortic dissection. MRA is a good alternative in patients with chronic dissection, but patient monitoring is problematic in the acute stage and makes MRA not very convenient for this patient group.

Imaging is used to evaluate whether there is compression of the true or false channel, thrombosis of one channel, or stenosis of a side branch. The risk of malperfusion becomes higher if there is no distal reentry but imbalance between blood velocities, inflow and outflow from the false channel, as well as compression of one channel or obstruction of the branch vessel by intimal flaps can all cause clinically relevant organ malperfusion. Some pat-

terns may look quite harmless because CT will display opacification of all vascular beds that are perfused, despite high-grade obstruction of the blood flow. Differences between left and right-sided enhancement of the kidneys or markedly reduced organ perfusion may be readily apparent on CT. Malperfusion of the bowel may occur with involvement of one or more splanchnic arteries, especially when combined with pre-existing stenoses.

The *true lumen and false channel* can be distinguished by tracing the true lumen from the beginning of the dissection in the ascending aorta (type A), or following the continuity of the normal aorta (type B), but this requires a combined for thoraco-abdominal evaluation, which is always suggested in an acute situation [4].

Aortic dissection at unusual locations should raise the suspicion of a *penetrating aortic ulcer* as the etiology. Initially, such dissections are localized, but can dissect in an antegrade or retrograde fashion and involve large portions of the aorta.

Aortic Stenosis and Aortic Occlusion

Aortic stenosis may occur in older patients as a consequence of severe atherosclerosis. In young patients it is caused by *congenital hypoplasia* or *midaortic syndrome*. The latter has an unknown etiology but is probably related to fibromuscular hyperplasia. In midaortic syndrome it is common to find involvement of the renal arteries and splanchnic vessels [5]. Extensive collateralization with a hypertrophic artery of Riolan is present if the splanchnic vessels are involved. The stenoses are most pronounced in the proximal vessel segments. Inflammatory para-aortic changes are not observed.

Leriche syndrome includes an acute occlusion of the aortic bifurcation, usually caused by acute thrombosis at a pre-existing site of atherosclerotic stenosis. An embolic pathogenesis is less common. The terminal aortic occlusion in acute Leriche syndrome is usually located just above the bifurcation. In chronic cases the aorta becomes filled with clot to the level of the renal arteries. Concomitant renal artery stenosis has to be excluded. Thrombotic and embolic occlusions can be distinguished by detecting an intraluminal embolus, which appears as a partially occlusive filling defect. Embolic occlusions are typically associated with a milder grade of aortic sclerosis.

CTA and MRA provide excellent information about the vascular lumen. In addition, CTA is able to detect large calcified plaques or other wall changes in atherosclerotic stenosis. CTA can diagnose Leriche syndrome, but only multislice scanning can exclude concomitant renal artery stenosis and assess the peripheral arteries. Gd-enhanced MRA requires modern equipment to assess multiple levels from the aorta to the peripheral arteries. Only under these conditions is MRA a diagnostic alternative.

Endovascular Aortic Repair

Endovascular aortic prostheses (stent grafts) are used for minimally invasive treatment of abdominal aortic aneurysms and penetrating aortic ulcers. CTA has an essential role in the preinterventional planning and postinterventional follow-up of these procedures, but MRA is assuming an increasingly important role for follow-up because superior for the detection of endoleaks (Table 2).

After successful endovascular repair, associated abnormalities affecting the aneurysm wall or periaortic fat tissue (e.g., stranding in covered perforation) should disappear. Even the periaortic reaction in inflammatory aneurysms has been reported to decrease over time.

Fracture of stent material can best be appreciated on conventional plain radiographs of the stent area, but MIP or volume-rendered displays from multislice CT data may also demonstrate such events. *Stenoses* of the stent lumen may occur in aortoiliac grafts, especially at juncture sites between the various components of the graft. *Dissection* of the access vessel during graft placement is usually associated with excessive vascular tortuosity. Thrombosis of the stent lumen is most frequently caused by mechanical obstruction, either by the stent itself or by dislocated coating material. In very large aneurysms, the stent graft may migrate to the anterior portion of the aortic lumen, especially when the distal anchoring site is not stable. Such a migration may cause massive type I endoleaks and has an increased risk of aneurysm rupture.

The *diameter* of the aneurysm (lumen including thrombus) is measured at follow-up, and serial measurements should not show an increase in size. Successfully treated aneurysms or dissections should thrombose completely and shrink in size over a period of months to years. An increase in size should prompt the search for an endoleak [6], which may be treated interventionally. If no leak is detected despite a growth over time (endotension), an occult leak must be suspected. Gd-enhanced MRA is more sensitive to small amounts of contrast material in the aneurysmal sac than CTA.

Aortitis / Arteritis

If there is clinical suspicion of aortitis, MRA is preferred over CTA because patients are frequently younger. Both techniques sensitively detect the wall changes even in the initial stage of the disease.

Takayasu arteritis is a rare disorder that leads to progressive occlusion of the thoracic and abdominal aortic branch vessels. In the acute inflammatory stage, a granulomatous infiltration of the vessel wall occurs that leads to nonspecific signs of fever, weight loss, myalgia, and arthralgia. In the later fibrotic stage, constriction of the vessel wall with stenosis, occlusion (lack of pulse) or aneurysm formation may occur. Type II and III involve the abdomen: type II in the descending and abdominal aorta and its side branches, type III has also the aortic arch and supra-aortic arteries [7]. In the acute stage, there is thickening and enhancement of the vessel wall. The vessel wall takes up contrast substantially, which can already be seen in the arterial phase, but is more prominent in later phases (which also allows for a better differentiation from atherosclerotic wall thickening). Inflammatory wall changes may be detected even if the digital subtraction angiography (DSA) is normal.

Granulomatous arteritis cannot be distinguished morphologically from Takayasu arteritis, but it can be suspected if the arteries involved are ones that are rarely affected by Takayasu disease. It is commonly bilateral and symmetric, and there is a lack of atherosclerotic changes to account for the vascular narrowing.

Polyarteritis nodosa is characterized by small saccular aneurysms of 1-5 mm size, which can sometimes be detected by thin-section CTA but are best displayed on DSA. Aneurysms can be found in the intrarenal or intrahepatic branches and the mesenteric side branches. Additional luminal irregularities and stenoses of small arteries are typical. In the kidneys, multiple cortical infarcts may be present.

Abdominal Arteries

Anatomic Variants

Anatomic variants are incidental findings in examinations of the abdomen. They assume importance when they cause symptoms or have a bearing on planning of surgery or interventional radiological procedures.

Table 2. Types of endoleaks after stent graft placement (from [6])

Type	Description
Type I	Attachment site leaks
IA	proximal end of endograft
IB	distal end of endograft
IC	iliac occluder (plug)
Type II	Branch leaks (without attachment site connection)
IIA	simple or to-and-fro (from one patent branch)
IIB	complex or flow-through (two or more patent branches)
Type III	Graft defect
IIIA	junctional leak or modular disconnect
IIIB	fabric disruption – midgraft hole: minor ($<$ 2 mm) or major ($\geq$ 2 mm)
Type IV	Graft wall porosity (within 30 days of placement)
Endotension increased intrasac pressure without visualized endoleak at delayed CT	
Type A	with no endoleak
Type B	with sealed endoleak
Type C	with type I or III endoleak
Type D	with type II endoleak

Anatomic variants of the arterial supply to the liver are found in up to 50% of patients [8]. They are typical incidental findings in arterial phase CT examinations of the abdomen but can also be picked up on MR. They become diagnostically relevant for planning partial liver resection or interventional radiological procedures. The following signs suggest a variant:

- Branches of the celiac trunk arising separately from the aorta.
- A vessel running posterior to the portal vein may be an accessory right hepatic artery, a replaced right hepatic artery, or a replaced proper hepatic artery. Accurate identification requires tracing the vessel into the liver and toward its origin.
- A vessel coursing between the caudate and left lobes of the liver superior to the porta hepatis may be an accessory or replaced left hepatic artery arising directly from the left gastric artery.
- An accessory right hepatic artery that arises from the gastroduodenal artery presents as a second vessel just below the right hepatic artery. Such vessels are easily missed and require thin-section imaging. They are best seen on thin-slab MIP (1-2 cm thickness) parallel to the course of the proper hepatic artery.

Superior mesenteric artery syndrome is caused by compression of the duodenum by the superior mesenteric artery (SMA) in thin individuals [9]. The *nutcracker syndrome* is due to compression of the left renal vein and may present as painless hematuria in slim patients.

Accessory renal arteries occur in up to 25% of individuals. Usually one vessel is dominant on either side. However, multiple small vessels may be present, and accessory arteries may originate even above the SMA (exceedingly rare) or the iliac vessels (some 1% of cases). Main renal arteries enter the kidney via the hilum, while polar arteries enter the renal parenchyma directly. Such variants are important for interventional radiological dilatation of renal artery stenosis and for the work-up of *living renal donors* [10]. The gonadal arteries usually arise from the aorta just below the level of the kidneys but may also rarely originate from the renal artery (more common on the right). Early branching of a normal sized artery or multiple or abnormal arteries or veins may make harvesting a kidney from a living renal donor difficult.

Renal Artery Stenosis

Renal artery stenosis (RAS) is an uncommon cause of arterial hypertension (approximately 5%). The commonest cause of RAS is atherosclerotic disease (65-70%). Angioplasty has been considered the treatment of choice for these hypertensive patients, but newer longer-term studies suggest that optimum medical treatment is equally effective [11]. There is also an ongoing discussion about the positive effects of angioplasty or stenting on the preservation of renal function in these patients. Thus, the

final role of noninvasive techniques (CTA, MRA, ultrasound) for diagnosis of renal artery stenosis will depend on whether or not interventional therapy is considered.

The *sensitivity and specificity* of all imaging methods are well above 90% for the detection of significant stenoses if imaging is performed by experienced radiologists [12]. However, substantially lower numbers have been reported as well.

Indirect signs can already be appreciated on standard examinations. Differences in size (right kidney 2 cm smaller than left kidney, or left kidney 1.5 cm smaller than right kidney), cortical thickness (on corticomedullary phase images), level of enhancement, and time to excretion between the two kidneys all suggest unilateral significant renal artery stenosis.

Effective *interpretation* of CTA or MRA examinations is based primarily on 3D views such as volume-rendered displays (VRT) or curved thin-slab MIP. In order not to miss eccentric plaques, anteroposterior (AP) views as well as caudocranial views should be used. Whenever a suspicious finding is encountered, it should be confirmed by cross-sectional images. This can either be done by interactive analysis of cross-sectional images, or by generating CPR through the vessel segment of interest.

Fibromuscular dysplasia is the next most common cause of renal artery stenosis (25%). It affects younger patients and is more prevalent in women (3:1). Angioplasty is usually a very effective treatment. Fibromuscular dysplasia may present as a unifocal stenosis in the middle and distal third of the main renal artery, multifocal stenosis with string-of-pearls appearance, or aneurysm formation. The right renal artery is most commonly affected, but bilateral disease is seen in up to two thirds of cases. It is characteristic that the proximal third of the main renal artery is spared (in over 95% of cases). Renal artery branches are rarely affected without concomitant disease in the extrarenal arteries. Such cases of isolated intrarenal fibromuscular dysplasia are extremely hard to detect with cross-sectional imaging techniques.

Celiac and Mesenteric Stenosis

Abdominal angina is a postprandial abdominal pain that occurs some 15-20 minutes after food ingestion. It is considered to be due to gastric steal, which diverts blood from the intestine. Patients have a food aversion, complain of weight loss, and can develop malabsorption or bowel strictures. This intermittent mesenteric ischemia is caused by severe stenosis of splanchnic arteries without adequate collateralization: combined severe stenoses of at least two of the three vessels supplying the bowel (celiac, superior, and inferior mesenteric artery) are present. More rarely, successive proximal and peripheral stenoses may be found in such patients. A lateral MIP or VRT (the width of the volume of interest [VOI] covers only the aorta) is best for demonstrating proximal stenoses of the celiac trunk and superior mesenteric artery. Coronal thin-slab MIP parallel but anterior to the aorta provide the best anatomic overview. Volume-rendered views are a good alternative to demonstrate more peripheral stenoses as well as collateralization via the arc of Riolan [13]. Dilated collaterals display a typical pattern on axial sections.

Isolated *stenosis of the celiac artery* is a common incidental finding that is usually caused by a transverse ligament spanning the left and right crus of the diaphragm, just below the level of the thoracoabdominal junction. This stenosis is typically exacerbated by inspiration and causes no symptoms. Association with an increased rate of pancreatitis or complications of the liver transplantation has been discussed. Stenoses due to *diaphragmatic trapping* can be diagnosed in a celiac trunk running straight downward from its aortic origin with an elliptical distortion of the normally round cross-section of the artery. The trunk displays a normal diameter in the AP projection but shows marked narrowing on lateral projections.

Stenosis of the superior or inferior mesenteric artery are also relatively frequent incidental findings in patients with severe arteriosclerosis. They are asymptomatic unless adequate collateral supply can no longer be maintained between the superior and inferior mesenteric arteries through the Riolan anastomosis or between the superior mesenteric artery and celiac artery through gastroduodenal vessels.

Ultrasound is well suited for the detection of proximal stenosis, but CTA and MRA are superior when it comes to display of collateral pathways. CTA and MRA are effective imaging procedures prior to surgical revascularization of patients with chronic mesenteric ischemia. For CTA, however, is important to use a negative contrast agent such as water for bowel distension.

Acute Mesenteric Ischemia

Acute mesenteric ischemia is responsible for 8% of cases of acute abdomen. It is a life-threatening event with a mortality that varies between 50 and 90%, depending on comorbidity and age of patients. Prognosis depends on the time of diagnosis, the extent of ischemia (mucosal versus transmural), secondary damage due to infection and pre-existent illnesses. Due to the unspecific symptoms in multimorbid patients, diagnosis is frequently delayed. Acute mesenteric ischemia can be caused by:

- An arterial occlusion (60-70%)
- Nonocclusive mesenteric insufficiency (NOMI, 20-30%) or
- A venous occlusion (5-10%).

Acute mesenteric ischemia remains a diagnostic challenge because of a large list of potential etiologies. Mesenteric angiography used to be the first-line technique for demonstrating suspected acute mesenteric ischemia, but the increased spatial resolution and its ability to detect alternative *diagnoses* has made multislice CTA the current technique of choice [14, 15].

The most frequent direct imaging sign is a perfusion defect, most frequently approximately 3-10 cm distal from the origin of the SMA (due to acute embolism). Next frequent is an acute thrombotic *occlusion*, usually on the basis of an atherosclerotic plaque. Proximal occlusions can be more easily compensated via collateral perfusion than distal occlusions that are closer to the bowel wall. Imaging shows the site of obstruction and any residual perfusion distal to the obstructing lesion. One should search for signs that might indicate the etiology, such as embolic disease, thrombosis of a stenosed vessel segment in atherosclerosis, aortic dissection, vasculitis, direct trauma, intravascular coagulation, hypoperfusion due to shock, hypovolemia, or endotoxins.

Associated findings include thickened bowel wall due to edema, reduced bowel opacification as compared to other segments, and gas within the bowel wall (pneumatosis) or in the mesenteric or portal veins indicating infarction. Ascites may be present in the region of the affected bowel. Focal or diffuse bowel dilation is a nonspecific sign.

NOMI can be the consequence of hypovolemic shock, protracted bradycardia, sepsis, heart failure or digitalis intoxication. In these cases, the mesenteric vessels are exceedingly thin without apparent occlusion or focal stenosis, although secondary signs of ischemia are present. Distension ischemia is a form of NOMI: it occurs in a prestenotically dilated colon if the intraluminal pressure exceeds 50 mm Hg, thus causing a nonocclusive critical reduction of colonic microcirculation.

Acute mesenteric thrombosis can be caused by portal hypertension, acute inflammatory processes (e.g., diverticulitis, appendicitis), tumor compression, trauma, surgery (especially in young individuals), or by a paraneoplastic syndrome or as the consequence of coagulopathies. Strangulation of the mesenteric vessels by volvulus and various other conditions also has to be considered. The superior mesenteric vein is most commonly affected, hampering the venous drainage of the small bowel and right-sided colon. Massive bowel edema and hyperemia are the most frequent secondary signs. Local hemorrhage into the bowel wall is possible. Prognosis is generally better than that of arterial ischemia.

Arterial Bleeding

Arterial injury leads to substantial bleeding at the site of injury, with large hematoma formation that can extend into accompanying structures. Complete transection or the presence of an intimal flap may lead to occlusion of the affected vessel. Long-term sequelae are pseudoaneurysm formation or arteriovenous shunts in cases with simultaneous trauma to arteries and veins. The latter is particularly frequent after cardio-angiographic procedures at the site of arterial and venous access in the groin.

Cross-sectional imaging allows for demonstration of the hematoma, accompanying injuries to the skeletal system or to internal organs, as well as the site of active bleeding. In patients with a continuing blood loss, however, angiography with subsequent embolization of the affected artery will be a better choice. CTA is the technique of choice because it is both sensitive and fast. CTA may be helpful in the detection of occult gastrointestinal hemorrhage as well [16], but MRA with blood-pool agents is a good alternative in patients with occult bleeding.

As opposed to venous bleeding, the hematoma in arterial bleeding is usually extensive and often has a convex outer contour. The site of active bleeding should be searched for in the region of the hematoma. A small spot of brightly enhanced blood outside the vessel lumen is indicative of the site of bleeding. The size of the paravasation indicates the amount of active bleeding. This spot will enlarge if a second scan is added in a venous phase. Such venous phase images are especially helpful to rule out injuries to abdominal organs in patients with blunt abdominal trauma.

References

1. Levy JR, Heiken J, Gutierrez FR (1999) Imaging of penetrating atherosclerotic ulcers of the aorta. AJR Am J Roentgenol 173:151-154
2. Hayashi H, Matsuoka Y, Sakamoto I et al (2000) Penetrating atherosclerotic ulcer of the aorta: imaging features and disease concept. Radiographics 20:995-1005
3. Iino M, Kuribayashi S, Imakita S et al (2002) Sensitivity and specificity of CT in the diagnosis of inflammatory abdominal aortic aneurysms. J Comput Assist Tomogr 26:1006-1012
4. LePage MA, Quint LE, Sonnad SS et al (2001) Aortic dissection: CT features that distinguish true lumen from false lumen. AJR Am J Roentgenol 177:207-211
5. Lewis III VD, Meranze SG, McLean GK et al (1988) The midaortic syndrome: diagnosis and treatment. Radiology 167:111-113
6. Veith FJ, Baum RA, Ohki T et al (2002) Nature and significance of endoleaks and endotension: summary of opinions expressed at an international conference. J Vasc Surg 35:1029-1035
7. Sueyoshi E, Sakamoto I, Hayashi K (2000) Aortic aneurysms in patients with Takayasu's arteritis: CT evaluation. AJR Am J Roentgenol 175:1727-1734
8. Covey AM, Brody LA, Maluccio MA, et al Variant hepatic arterial anatomy revisited: digital subtraction angiography performed in 600 patients. Radiology 224:542-547
9. Konen E, Amitai M, Apter S et al (1998) CT angiography of superior mesenteric artery syndrome. AJR Am J Roentgenol 171:1279-1281
10. Kawamoto S, Montgomery RA, Lawler LP et al (2003) Multidetector CT angiography for preoperative evaluation of living laparoscopic renal donors. AJR Am J Roentgenol 180:1633-1638
11. van Jaarsveld BC, Krijnen P, Pieterman H et al (2000) The effect of balloon angioplasty on hypertension in atherosclerotic renal-artery stenosis. Dutch Renal Artery Stenosis Intervention Cooperative Study Group. N Engl J Med 342:1007-1014
12. Willmann JK, Wildermuth S, Pfammatter T et al (2003) Aortoiliac and renal arteries: prospective intraindividual comparison of contrast-enhanced three-dimensional MR angiography and multi-detector row CT angiography. Radiology 226:798-811
13. Cognet F, Ben Salem D, Dranssart M et al (2002) Chronic mesenteric ischemia: imaging and percutaneous treatment. Radiographics 22:863-880
14. Horton KM, Fishman EK (2001) Multidetector row CT of mesenteric ischemia: can it be done? Radiographics 21:1463-1474
15. Urban BA, Ratner LE, Fishman EK (2001) Three-dimensional volume-rendered CT angiography of the renal arteries and veins: normal anatomy, variants, and clinical applications. Radiographics 21:373-386
16. Kim JK, Ha HK, Byun JY et al (2001) CT differentiation of mesenteric ischemia due to vasculitis and thromboembolic disease. J Comput Assist Tomogr 25:604-611

Abdominal Interventions

J. Lammer[1], D. Vorwerk[2]

[1] Department of Cardiovascular and Interventional Radiology, AKH – University Clinics, Vienna, Austria
[2] Department of Diagnostic and Interventional Radiology, Klinikum Ingolstadt, Ingolstadt, Germany

Nonvascular Interventions

Percutaneous biopsies and drainages of abdominal fluid collections are standard procedures that are mainly performed under ultrasound (US) and computed tomography (CT) guidance.

Abdominal Biopsy and Drainage

Organ biopsy is usually performed for lesions of the pancreas, liver and kidney, as well as retroperitoneal masses. Less common indications are lesions of the spleen, which are prone to bleeding complications.

Both fine needle aspiration as for cytology, as well as miniaturized cutting needles for histology, not exceeding 18-20G, can be used for abdominal biopsies. However, automated biopsy guns are preferred because they offer an excellent sampling quality and the possibility to perform repeated biopsies with a single access. Fine needle aspiration is recommended in order to avoid major bleeding complications if an object for biopsy is located close to central and vascular structures. Fine needle aspiration biopsy (Fig. 1) allows bowel structures to be transversed in order to reach the lesion of interest, whereas this must be avoided when performing cutting needle biopsy. A frontal approach to lesions deep in the abdomen is usually performed using fine needle aspiration.

Obviously, access for drainage needs to avoid making both a pathway through the pleural space, as well as traversing through bowel structures.

Depending on their location, abscesses (Fig. 2) within organs or in the peritoneal or retroperitoneal cavity are approached by a trocar technique for a well exposed location, while a difficult approach requires an over-the-wire placement of drainage catheters. It is important to place sufficiently large bore drainage catheters (12-16F) to evacuate highly viscous fluid collections. The drain should be left in place until the abscess cavity has collapsed completely and less than 20 cc of fluid is collected per day.

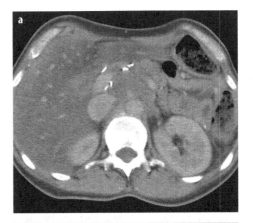

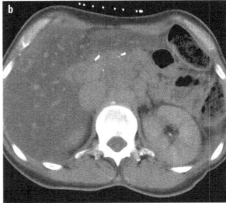

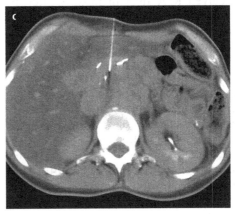

Fig. 1. Biopsy of a pancreatic lesion. **a** 42-year-old female patient after subtotal pancreatoduodenectomy for pancreatic cancer and recurrent symptoms showing a mass in the retroperitoneal space. **b** A usable position was chosen and a grid was placed to plan and mark the potential pathway for biopsy. **c** A 22 G needle was advanced into the lesion and an aspiration biopsy was performed. Cytologic examination proved recurrent pancreatic cancer

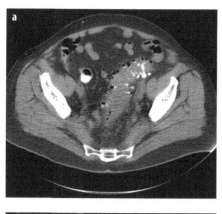
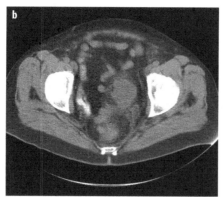
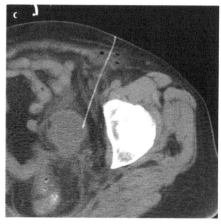
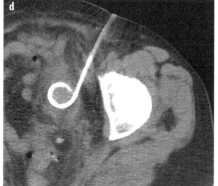
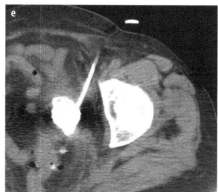

Fig. 2. Abscess drainage in 65-year-old patient with diverticulitis. **a** Massive swelling of the sigmoid due to inflammation and diverticula. **b** A nonseptated collection close to the sigmoid is seen. **c** After needle puncture of the collection that proved abscess formation, a guidewire was inserted into the abscess. **d** In an over-the-wire technique, a 12 F draining catheter was inserted into the abscess. **e** After evacuation of pus and debris, the collection was refilled by diluted contrast medium to test the stability of the cavity and to exclude extravasation

Tumor Ablation

Many tumor ablation techniques are currently performed in liver lesions using lasers, radiofrequency ablation (RFA) and ethanol. They are applied to primary hepatic malignancies and metastatic disease. In patients with hepatocellular carcinoma (HCC), percutaneous ablation is considered the best treatment option when surgical resection or liver transplantation is not suitable for patients with Child-Pugh class A or B; cirrhosis; a single, nodular-type HCC smaller than 5 cm; or as many as three HCC lesions, each smaller than 3 cm. Recent studies have shown that RFA can achieve more effective local tumor control than ethanol injection and with fewer treatment sessions. In a randomized trial, local recurrence-free survival rates were significantly higher in patients who received RFA than in those treated by ethanol injection (one, two, and three year survival rates were 93%, 81%, and 74% in the RFTA group, 88%, 66%, and 51% in the PEI group; one- and two-year local recurrence-free survival rates were 98% and 96% in the RF group and 83% and 62% in the PEI group, respectively [univariate $p = .002$]). In a univariate analysis, tumor-dependent factors with significantly less local recurrences were smaller size, neuroendocrine metastases, nonsubcapsular location, and location away from large vessels. Treatment allocation was confirmed as an independent prognostic factor by multivariate analysis. In the multivariate analysis, significantly less local recurrences were observed for small size ($p <$

0.001) tumors. Preliminary reports have shown that RFA performed after balloon catheter occlusion of the hepatic artery, transarterial embolization, or chemoembolization results in increased volumes of coagulation necrosis, thus enabling successful destruction of large HCC lesions. However, for the time being, laser and radiofrequency therapy can be used to treat only lesions with a maximum diameter of 5 cm. However, these techniques are developing rapidly. There is little experience in ablation of renal tumors. Ablation of renal cell carcinoma has been performed either in patients with a single kidney or with serious contraindications to surgery. Percutaneous ablation needs to be balanced against other minimally invasive techniques such as laparoscopic kidney removal or partial nephrectomy.

Both in renal and hepatic tumor ablation, some patients, especially those with hypervascularized tumors, may profit from a combined approach with both ablation and transarterial embolization.

Biliary Interventions

As an alternative to endoscopic procedures, percutaneous drainage and stenting of biliary ducts can be performed. The indication is obstructive jaundice due to bile duct tumors, metastatic disease to lymph nodes in the hepatoduodenal ligament or pancreatic tumors. In Klatzkin type tumors at the hepatic duct bifurcation, drainage and stenting of both lobes of the liver is required (Fig. 3). Self-expanding metal stents have proven in randomized trials to

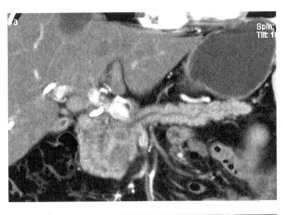

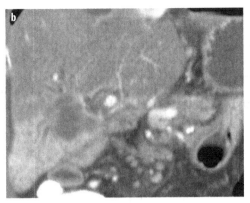

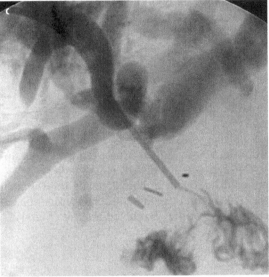

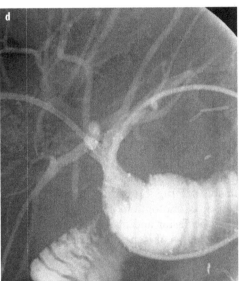

Fig. 3. Biliary obstruction due to metastases of pancreatic carcinoma. **a** CT of pancreatic carcinoma before surgery. **b** CT one year after surgery (tumor resection) demonstrating obstructed common hepatic duct due to tumor recurrence at the liver hilum. **c** PTCD showing obstruction of the bilioenteric anastomosis. **d** Bilateral stenting of the obstructed hepatojejunostomy

show longer patency rates than plastic tubes. Drainage of the gallbladder is rarely performed, but sometimes helpful in multimorbid patients.

Gastrointestinal and Colonic Stent Placement

As a palliative approach or a temporary solution in patients with obstructing tumors of the duodenum or the colon, metallic stents are placed as an alternative to surgical decompression.

Percutaneous Gastrostomy/Ileostomy

Several kits exist that enable radiologists to perform gastrostomy and ileostomy using a percutaneous approach. Indications are in patients with long-term swallowing disorders due to tumors or neurological deficiencies.

Newer Procedures

As a palliative approach to treat ascites, either percutaneous creation of a Denver shunt or percutaneous port-catheter placement – to allow repeat and ease paracentesis have been described.

Vascular Interventions

Acute Arterial Occlusion

If acute occlusion of the abdominal aorta or branch vessels occurs, two causes have to be considered:
- Embolization
- Dissection.

Embolization

Embolization is most common in elderly patients with atrial fibrilation, a history of myocardial infarction and aortic aneurysm. Embolization from the heart or thoracic aorta may cause acute subtotal or total occlusion of the celiac, superior mesenteric (SMA), inferior mesenteric artery (IMA) or the renal arteries. The most common causes of embolization are:
- Atrial fibrillation
- Thoracic aortic aneurysm
- Myocardial infarction with mural thrombus formation
- Advanced aortic arteriosclerosis
- Perforating arteriosclerotic ulcer
- Hypercoagulability syndrome.

The symptoms of acute ischemia are dependent on the involved vascular territory. Embolization to the liver or spleen may cause acute right or left upper abdominal pain. Acute mesenteric ischemia typically causes severe abdominal pain and bowel paralysis. Embolization to the kidney causes flank pain, hematuria and hypertension. In any case, severe elevation of lactose dehydrogenase (LDH) points to the ischemic nature of the acute pain. In case of complete ischemia without a sufficient collateral circulation, the warm ischemic time tolerated by the abdominal organs is less than six hours. Therefore, acute diagnosis and therapy are mandatory.

The primary diagnosis is performed by CT with contrast enhancement (CM 300 mgJ/ml; 4 ml/sec; total bolus volume 80-120 ml; bolus care technique with 20-40 second delay; 2 mm collimation; pitch 2; reconstruction interval 1 mm). The obstructing embolus and the ischemic territory can be visualized in the arterial phase. In the delayed phase, a residual perfusion through collateral arteries may be demonstrated.

Interventional treatment with a thrombectomy device and/or local intra-arterial fibrinolysis with recombinant tissue plasminogen activator (rt-PA) (10 mg loading dose, 5 mg/hr infusion dose) or urokinase (250 000 IU loading dose, 100 000 IU/hr infusion dose) together with a G IIb/IIIa antagonist (Aciximab: 0.25 mg/kg loading dose, 0.125 mg/kg/hr infusion dose) is one option. The other option is surgery, which may be faster and also enables inspection and, if necessary, resection of ischemic organs.

Dissection

Dissection is most common if there is a history of trauma, chronic severe hypertension, or a connective tissue disease such as Marfan syndrome or Ehlers-Danlos syndrome. Acute type A and B aortic dissection may cause dynamic compression of the original lumen of the aorta by the pressurized false lumen. This can cause acute ischemia of liver/spleen, bowel and kidneys. The dissection plane may also run into one of the organ arteries causing obstruction of the true lumen. There are a number of interventional treatment options. In case of a dynamic compression of the true aortic lumen, occlusion of the proximal entry into the false lumen with an aortic stentgraft will cause decompression of the false lumen and results in reopening of the true lumen of the aorta and the side branches. In case of a static compression due to a side-branch dissection, stent placement in the true lumen of the organ artery will cause reconstitution of organ perfusion. In case of organ perfusion through the false lumen, balloon fenestration of the intimal flap will re-establish flow into the malperfused territory.

Chronic Arterial Occlusive Disease

In young patients, causes of chronic arterial occlusion include:
• Fibromuscular disease (FMD)

• Takayasu arteritis
• Recklinghausen neurofibromatosis.

The primary cause of chronic arterial occlusive disease in elderly patients is arteriosclerosis.

Mesenteric Artery Stenosis

Between the three large mesenteric arteries (celiac artery, SMA, IMA), there are many collateral pathways, including:
• Pancreatico-duodenal arteries
• Arc of Buehler between celiac artery and SMA
• Arc of Riolan
• Marginal artery Drummond between SMA and IMA.

Therefore, an obstruction of at least two mesenteric arteries is necessary to cause ischemic symptoms. The typical clinical symptom is the angina abdominalis with:
• Abdominal pain (94% of cases)
• Post prandial cramps (86%)
• Weight loss (74%)
• Abdominal bruit (70%)
• Diarrhea.

The primary diagnosis is made by aortic arteriography in a lateral projection by either intra-arterial catheter angiography, CT angiography, or MR angiography.

Interventional treatment is percutaneous transluminal angioplasty (PTA) with or without secondary stent placement of at least one of the obstructed arteries (Fig. 4).

Celiac Trunk Stenosis

Chronic obstruction may remain asymptomatic because of the collateral pathways through gastroduodenal and pancreatic arteries from the superior mesenteric artery. Causes are arteriosclerotic plaque, compression by the arcuate ligament or carcinoma of the pancreas.

Superior Mesenteric Artery Stenosis

Post prandial abdominal pain, called 'angina abdominalis' occurs only if two or all three gastrointestinal arteries are obstructed. Causes for SMA obstruction are arteriosclerosis, fibromuscular disease (FMD), Takayasu arteritis, pancreatic carcinoma or chronic pancreatitis.

Inferior Mesenteric Artery Stenosis

Obstruction of the IMA is most commonly observed in patients with advanced atheromatosis or partially thrombosed abdominal aortic aneurysm. Due to the collateral circulation through the arc of Riolan and the marginal artery, IMA obstruction normally remains asymptomatic.

Renal Artery Stenosis

Renal artery stenosis (RAS) may cause hypertension and/or renal insufficiency. Acute onset of the clinical

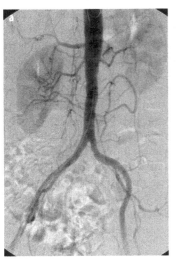
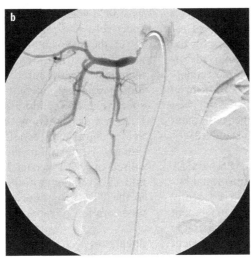
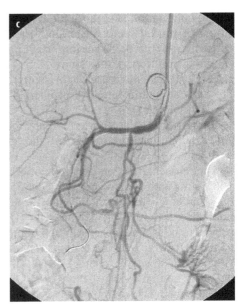

Fig. 4. Balloon angioplasty and stenting in a patient with mesenteric angina. A 77-year-old female patient with recurrent and constant pain after eating. **a** Aortic angiography shows absence of superior mesenteric artery and small inferior mesenteric with a not well-developed Riolan's arch. The celiac artery, however, is present. **b** Selective angiography shows tight stenosis of the common hepatic artery. **c** After stent placement patency was restored. The symptoms disappeared the next day

symptoms and repeated flash pulmonary edema are suggestive for a renal artery stenosis. The etiology can be:

- Arteriosclerosis in 65-75% of cases
  - patients > 50 years
  - male > female
  - proximal 2 cm of renal artery
  - atherosclerotic changes of aorta
  - bilateral in 30%
- FMD in 20-30% of cases
  - patients of 15-30 years
  - female : male ratio 5 : 1
  - middle to distal renal artery including branches
  - bilateral involvement in 50-70%
  - 'string of beads' appearance, aneurysms, dissections
  - no aortic disease
- Takayasu arteritis
- Mid aortic syndrome
- Morbus Recklinghausen
- Post radiation therapy.

The correct algorithm for the diagnosis of a renal artery stenosis is not established.

Color duplex ultrasound is a noninvasive test but is a complex examination and requires an experienced operator. An increased peak systolic velocity of more than 200 cm/s, a renal-to-aortic ratio of peak systolic velocity of more than 3.5, an intrastenotic turbulence and a flattened pulse wave in the periphery (pulsus tardus) are diagnostic criteria for a renal artery stenosis. The sensitivity of color duplex sonography for detection of RAS of more than 70% is 72-92%. Color duplex US with an angiotensin-converting enzyme (ACE) inhibitor provides a positive predictive value of 67-95% for cure or improvement after revascularization.

A nuclear scan (renal scintigraphy with technetium-99m mercaptoacetyltriglycine (MAG3) or Tc-99m diethy-

lenetriaminepentaacetic acid [DTPA]) with an ACE inhibitor (captopril 25 mg) shows a delayed wash-out of the tracer within the post stenotic kidney. However, in bilateral disease and in chronic ischemic nephropathy, the lateralization of the tracer is less evident. In a selected population with a clinical high risk for RAS, the sensitivity for detection of a unilateral RAS of more than 70% is 51-96% (mean 82%). Its positive predictive value for a RAS with improvement of hypertension after revascularization is 51-100% (mean 85%). However, scintigraphy is much less sensitive in patients who are unselected, or have bilateral disease, impaired renal function, urinary obstruction or chronic ACE inhibitor intake.

Newer tests are gadolinium-enhanced magnetic resonance angiography (MRA) and spiral CT angiography (CTA). For a state-of-art MRA, high field-strength systems with high performance gradients are necessary for breath-hold 3D spoiled gradient-echo imaging with short repetition time (TR) and echo time (TE). Intravenous administration of gadolinium contrast material in a double dose (0.2 mmol/kg; 2 ml/sec flow rate), a central k-space readout and background subtraction are additional techniques to improve signal-to-noise ratio and spatial resolution. The sensitivity to detect a RAS of more than 50% is more than 95% with MRA. The main limitations of renal MRA are evaluation of small, accessory renal arteries and branch vessels, the presence of stents and a tendency to overestimate moderate stenoses.

CTA of the renal arteries has a sensitivity of more than 95% to detect RAS and accessory renal arteries. For a high quality opacification of the renal arteries and to avoid renal vein overlap, a correct bolus planning is mandatory (density measurement during bolus rise, flow 4 ml/s, total volume 80-120 ml – multidetector scanners need less contrast). A short breath-hold acquisition, collimation (1-2 mm), pitch (1.5-6, depending on single or multidetector technology) and overlap of reconstruction (0.5-0.75) are important parameters for the spatial resolution of the study. Curved planar reconstruction (CPR, most useful for stents), volume rendering and maximum intensity projection (MIP) are used for 3D imaging (Fig. 5).

Intra-arterial catheter arteriography together with pressure gradient measurement is still the 'gold standard' for evaluation of a RAS.

The revascularization technique of choice is renal PTA without or with stent placement (Fig. 5). Aorto-renal bypass surgery is indicated only if PTA fails. In a recently published meta-analysis, renal arterial stent placement proved to be technical superior and clinically comparable to renal PTA alone. The technical success rate of stent versus PTA was 98% versus 77% and the restenosis rate was 17% and 26%, respectively ($p < 0.001$). In hypertension the cure rate of PTA stent versus was 10% versus 20%, the rate of improvement was 53% and 49%, respectively. In renal insufficiency, the rate of improvement

was 38% versus 30%, of stabilization 41% and 38%, respectively. The complication rate was 11-13% (95% CI 6-19%), the in-hospital mortality rate, 1%. In a randomized study comparing stents to PTA in ostial stenoses, the technical success rate was 88% versus 57% and the six month primary patency rate was 75% versus 29%, respectively. Two randomized trials comparing the effect of PTA and drug therapy on renal hypertension did not reveal a significant benefit of PTA over continuous drug therapy. However, in the Dutch study, PTA patients required only 2.1 versus 3.2 daily drug doses ($p < 0.001$) and 22/53 patients in the drug group had to be switched to the PTA group because of persistent hypertension or deterioration of renal function.

Aneurysms

Abdominal Aortic Aneurysm (AAA)

The incidence of AAA in European adults 60 years and older is 2.5%. Up to 10% of patients with symptomatic

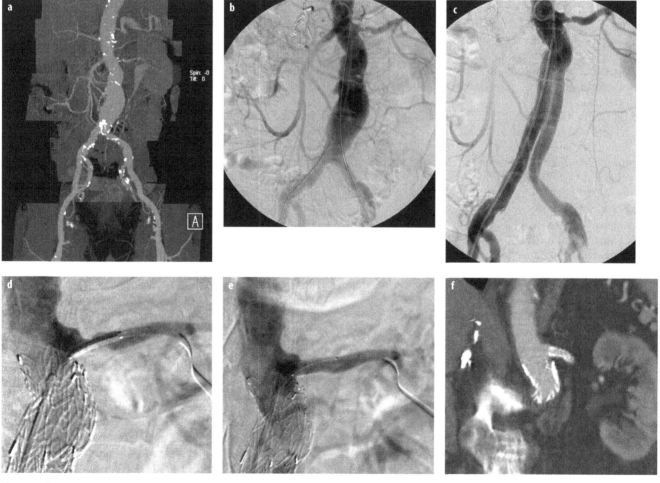

Fig. 5. Patient with abdominal aortic aneurysm and renal artery stenosis. **a** CTA with MIP reconstruction. **b** Aortography before stentgraft placement. **c** After stentgraft implantation. **d** Renal artery stenting after stentgraft implantation. **e** After renal stenting. **f** Control CTA after renal artery stent and AAA stentgraft

peripheral arterial disease (PAD) die from rupture of aneurysm disease.

Currently, the standard treatment is open surgery. However, endovascular implantation of stentgrafts is a new, emerging technique which may replace open surgery in the future. Since the first clinical implant of a tube stentgraft in 1990, many different stentgraft designs have been developed and tested in feasibility studies. Most recently, randomized studies (EVAR 1 Trial, Dream Trial) compared the results of open versus endovascular repair. In the EVAR Trial the 30 day mortality in the EVAR group was 1.7% (9/531) versus 4.7% (24/516) in the open repair group ($p = 0.009$). Four years after randomization, all-cause mortality was similar in the two groups (about 28%; $p = 0.46$), although there was a persistent reduction in aneurysm-related deaths in the EVAR group (4% versus 7%; $p = 0.04$).

Indications

The indications for endovascular treatment of AAA are currently the same as for open surgery:
• Diameter of the aneurysm > 5 cm (Fig. 5)
• Documented growth > 0.5 mm/year
• Symptomatic aneurysm (i.e., embolization, pain, ureteral compression)
• Rupture.
Specific clinical indications for the endovascular approach may be:
• Patients > 75-years-old
• ASA 3 and 4
• Hostile abdomen
• Inflammatory aneurysm, horse-shoe kidney.
The anatomic indications for stentgraft treatment are:
• Infrarenal neck > 15 mm in length
• Infrarenal neck without thrombus or severe calcification
• Angulation of the infrarenal neck < 65°
• Patent celiac trunk and SMA
• Stent graft diameter 10% more than neck diameter
• Iliac artery angulation < 90°
• Iliac artery without thrombus or severe calcification
• More than 15 mm overlap within the iliac arteries.
Endovascular implantation of stentgrafts can be performed under general, epidural or local anesthesia. The use of epidural anesthesia is a major advantage in elderly and high-risk patients.

Stentgraft Designs

Stentgrafts have a self-expandable stent structure covered by an ultrathin polyester or ePTFE fabric. Currently, only bifurcated stentgrafts are used for the treatment of AAA.

Imaging Before Stentgraft Implantation

Contrast-enhanced spiral CT with multiplanar reconstruction (MPR) or MIP reconstruction is the most important examination before stentgraft implantation (Fig.

5). The diameter of the landing zones (infrarenal neck, iliac arteries), the maximum diameter of the aneurysm, thrombus, and calcifications can be well depicted by CT.

Complications

The most common complication of stentgraft implantation is incomplete exclusion of the aneurysm with remaining pressurization of the aneurysm sack through an endoleak. White and May proposed a classification of primary (< 30 days) and secondary (> 30 days) endoleaks:
• Type 1: direct perfusion through the proximal (infrarenal) or distal (iliac) anastomosis
• Type 2: retrograde perfusion through branch vessels (lumbar arteries, IMA, accessory renal artery)
• Type 3: midgraft leak due to disintegration of the stentgraft (disconnection of the second iliac limb, fabric erosion)
• Type 4: fabric porosity
• Type 5: endotension.

Results

The largest database currently available is the Eurostar registry, which has more than 7000 patients. At completion angiography, endoleaks were demonstrated in 15.8% of patients. Type 1 endoleaks were observed in 4.1%, type 2 reperfusion endoleaks were observed in 9.8% and type 3 leaks in 1.9% of patients. Technically successful stentgraft placement was achieved in 99% of patients. Conversion to open surgery was required in 0.7%. The in-hospital mortality rate was 2.6%.

Life-table analysis revealed a survival rate of 92%, 84%, and 77% at 1, 3, and 5 years, respectively. The freedom from persistent endoleaks was 84%, 75%, and 69% at 1, 3, and 5 years, respectively. However, type 2 endoleaks turned out to be rather benign, not causing rupture in the vast majority of cases. 98% of the patients were free from aneurysm rupture at 5 years.

Visceral Artery Aneurysm

Aneurysms of the celiac trunk, splenic artery, hepatic artery, gastroduodenal artery and superior mesenteric artery are caused by arteriosclerosis, arteritis, periarterial inflammation such as pancreatitis, trauma and soft tissue diseases such as Marfan and Ehlers-Danlos syndrome. An aneurysm more than 2.5 cm in diameter should be considered to prevent rupture. Meticulous imaging, including selective catheter angiography and 3D imaging with CTA or MRA is necessary before surgery or endovascular treatment. The endovascular options are embolization and exclusion with a stentgraft.

Renal Artery Aneurysm

The causes of renal artery aneurysm are arteriosclerosis, systemic vasculitis such as polyarteritis nodosa or lupus erythematosus, FMD, soft tissue disorders and trauma. Arteriosclerotic and large aneurysms are usually calcified. Potential rupture and chronic embolization are the indications for treatment. Bypass surgery, coil embolization and stentgraft implantation are the therapeutic options.

Tumor Embolization

Tumor embolization techniques vary from palliative embolization in bleeding genitoureteral tumors, chemoembolization techniques in hypervascularized hepatic neoplasms (in particular HCC), to definite treatment of benign lesions such as uterine fibroids. In the liver, tumor embolization is mainly used for inoperable HCC with still acceptable liver function (Child-Pugh A and B). The classical treatment is chemoembolization with doxorubicine mixed with lipiodol sometimes in combination with a temporary blockade of the hepatic artery by Gelfoam or other embolization particles. In randomized trials, chemoembolization of unresectable HCC has shown to be superior to supportive treatment only. New techniques include doxorubicine-loaded particles as an alternative embolization agent for HCC, chemoperfusion with different cytotoxic agents for metastatic disease and intrahepatic radiation by radioactive particles directly injected into the hepatic arteries.

Treatment for Bleeding Complications

Bleeding in the abdomen may occur due to iatrogenic causes, particularly in the kidneys and the liver after percutaneous interventions, trauma and tumor.

Frequent and typical locations are renal arteriovenous fistulas due to nephrostomy (Fig. 6) or biopsy, laceration

of the hepatic arteries by percutaneous manipulations, psoas and pelvic bleeding due to traumatic arterial injury and also post partum. Temporary occlusion of the uterine artery can then be a valid alternative to emergency hysterectomy in patients with intractable bleeding due to an atonic uterus.

In other locations, type, source and location of the bleeding determine the method that is used to safely interrupt extravasations.

Venous Interventions

Transjugular Intrahepatic Portocaval Shunt (TIPS)

TIPS was introduced into clinical medicine at the end of the eighties. In the meantime, a standardized technique has become available that allows safe application of this artificial connection. The introduction of stentgrafts instead of bare stents led to an improved patency of the shunt tract. Stentgrafts are indicated in acute and chronic bleeders, in patients with liver cirrhosis and esophageal varices, and patients with intractable ascites. Its risks are liver failure from shunted blood volume, and encephalopathy. Endoscopic techniques to treat varices are competitive techniques in bleeders, but in some patients with ascites there are few alternatives. In patients with acute or subacute Budd-Chiari syndrome, TIPS can be a life-saving procedure and help to overcome the acute phase, but is burdened by a relatively high rethrombosis rate.

Tract reobstruction requires a number of different techniques for debulking the stenosed or thrombosed stents, including mechanical thrombectomy, atherectomy, PTA, re-stenting or stent graft implantation.

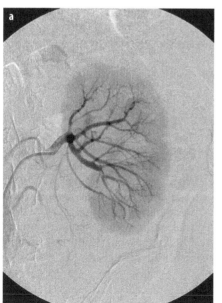
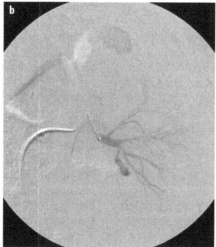
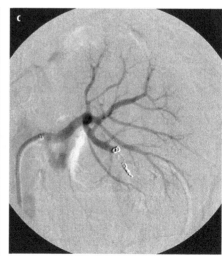

Fig. 6. Iatrogenic perirenal bleeding after percutaneous nephrostomy. **a** Selective left renal angiography in a 73-year-old male who suffered from massive bleeding from a nephrostomy catheter that was placed the same day. Angiographically, laceration of the lower pole artery is seen at a relatively central location. **b** Superselective angiography of the segmental artery clearly shows the bleeding site. **c** After combination of coil placement and glue embolization, the leakage stopped. Due to the central position, a part of the kidney had to be sacrificed

Interventions in the Portal and Mesenteric Veins

Besides TIPS application, a transjugular approach can be used for transjugular liver biopsy in patients with ascites or bleeding disorders, or as an entrance to the portal system, for example, to treat segmental hypertension due to stenoses that are located proximally to the portal vein, such as the mesenteric or splenic vein. Also recanalization of thrombotic portal occlusions may be treated via the transjugular approach to create a conduit that allows outflow from the recanalized vein.

The portal vein may also be accessed in a transhepatic fashion for selective blood sampling or venous recanalization. An intervention of increasing importance is preoperative embolization of the right portal vein in order to induce hypertrophy of the left hepatic lobe prior to extended right hemihepatectomy.

Suggested Reading

Blankensteijn JD, de Jong SE, Prinssen M (2005) Dutch Randomized Endovascular Aneurysm Management (DREAM) Trial Group. Two-year outcomes after conventional or endovascular repair of abdominal aortic aneurysms. N Engl J Med 352:2398-2405

Blum U, Voshage G, Lammer J et al (1997) Endoluminal stent-grafts for infrarenal abdominal aortic aneurysms. N Engl J Med 336:13-20

Covey AM, Tuorto S, Brody LA et al (2005) Safety and efficacy of preoperative portal vein embolization with polyvinyl alcohol in 58 patients with liver metastases. AJR Am J Roentgenol 185:1620-1626

D'Amico G, Luca A, Morabito A et al (2005) Uncovered transjugular intrahepatic portosystemic shunt for refractory ascites: a metaanalysis. Gastroenterology 129:1282-1293

EVAR trial participants (2005) Endovascular aneurysm repair versus open repair in patients with abdominal aortic aneurysm (EVAR trial 1): randomised controlled trial. Lancet 365:2179-2186

Galandi D, Antes G (2004) Radiofrequency thermal ablation versus other interventions for hepatocellular carcinoma. Cochrane Database Syst Rev 2:CD003046

Gorriz E, Reyes R, Lobrano MB et al (1996) Transjugular liver biopsy: a review of 77 biopsies using a spring-propelled cutting needle (biopsy gun). Cardiovasc Intervent Radiol 19:442-445

Greenhalgh RM, Brown LC, Kwong GP et al (2004) EVAR trial participants. Comparison of endovascular aneurysm repair with open repair in patients with abdominal aortic aneurysm (EVAR trial 1), 30-day operative mortality results: randomised controlled trial. Lancet 364:843-838

Kaatee R, Beek FJ, de Lange EE et al (1997) Renal artery stenosis: detection and quantification with spiral CT angiography versus optimized digital subtraction angiography. Radiology 205:121-127

Kasirajan K, O'Hara PJ, Gray BH et al (2001) Chronic mesenteric ischemia: open surgery versus percutaneous angioplasty and stenting. J Vasc Surg 33:63-71

Khuroo MS, Al-Suhabani H, Al-Sebayel M et al (2005) Budd-Chiari syndrome: long-term effect on outcome with transjugular intrahepatic portosystemic shunt. J Gastroenterol Hepatol 20:1494-1502

Laheij RJF, J Buth (2000) for the European Collaborators. Participants report. Overview of the overall patients cohort of the EUROSTAR data registry

Lammer J, Hausegger KA, Fluckiger F et al (1996) Common bile duct obstruction due to malignancy: treatment with plastic versus metal stents. Radiology 201:167-172

Lee BH, Choe DH, Lee JH et al (1997) Metallic stents in malignant biliary obstruction: prospective long-term clinical results. AJR Am J Roentgenol 168:741-745

Leertouwer TC, Gussenhoven EJ, Bosch JL et al (2000) Stent placement for renal artery stenosis: where do we stand? A metaanalysis. Radiology 216:78-85

Lencioni RA, Allgaier HP, Cioni D et al (2003) Small hepatocellular carcinoma in cirrhosis: randomized comparison of radiofrequency thermal ablation versus percutaneous ethanol injection. Radiology 228:235-240

Lin SM, Lin CJ, Lin CC et al (2005) Randomised controlled trial comparing percutaneous radiofrequency thermal ablation, percutaneous ethanol injection, and percutaneous acetic acid injection to treat hepatocellular carcinoma of 3 cm or less. Gut 54:1151-1156

Mann SJ, Pickering TG (1992) Detection of renovascular hypertension: state of the art 1992. Ann Intern Med 117:845-853

Perler AB, Becker GJ (1998) Vascular intervention – a clinical approach. Visceral vascular disease. Thieme, New York Stuttgart, pp 517-637

Prinssen M, Verhoeven EL, Buth J et al (2004) Dutch Randomized Endovascular Aneurysm Management (DREAM) Trial Group. A randomized trial comparing conventional and endovascular repair of abdominal aortic aneurysms. N Engl J Med 351:1607-1618

Rose SC, Quigley TM, Raker EJ (1995) Revascularization for chronic mesenteric ischemia: comparison of operative arterial bypass grafting and percutaneous transluminal angioplasty. J Vasc Interv Radiol 6:339-349

Shankar S, vanSonnenberg E, Silverman SG et al (2004) Imaging and percutaneous management of acute complicated pancreatitis. Cardiovasc Intervent Radiol 27:567-580

Shiina S, Teratani T, Obi S et al (2005) A randomized controlled trial of radiofrequency ablation with ethanol injection for small hepatocellular carcinoma. Gastroenterology 129:122-130

Soulez G, Oliva VL, Turpin S et al (2000) Imaging of renovascular hypertension: respective values of renal scintigraphy, renal Doppler US, and MR angiography. Radiographics 20:1355-1368

van de Ven PJ, Kaatee R, Beutler JJ et al (1999) Arterial stenting and balloon angioplasty in ostial arteriosclerotic renovascular disease: a randomized trial. Lancet 353:282-286

Van Jaarsveld BC, Krijen P, Pieterman H et al (2000) The effect of balloon angioplasty on hypertension in atherosclerotic renal-artery stenosis. Dutch Renal Artery Stenosis Intervention Cooperative Study Group. N Engl J Med 342:1007-1014

Webster J, Marshall F, Abdalla M et al (1998) Randomized comparison of percutaneous angioplasty vs continued medical therapy for hypertensive patients with atheromatous renal artery stenosis. Scottish and Newcastle Renal Artery Stenosis Collaborative Group. J Hum Hypertens 12:329-335

Williams DM, Lee DY (1997) Dissected aorta, parts I-III. Radiology 203:23-44

PEDIATRIC SATELLITE COURSE
"KANGAROO"

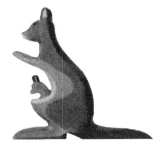

The Fetal Abdomen: From Normal to Abnormal. From Ultrasound to MR Imaging

F.E. Avni, M. Cassart, A. Massez

Department of Medical Imaging, University Clinics of Brussels – Erasme Hospital, Brussels, Belgium

Thanks to improving technology and experience, sonographic surveying of fetal development is now more accurate and precise. Further, more anomalies are detected, allowing the adaptation of postnatal management, if necessary.

Another striking evolution in perinatal imaging has been the increased use of fetal magnetic resonance (MR) imaging for the assessment of various fetal abdominal diseases. Faster sequences and better understanding of the normal appearances of the fetal abdomen on MR imaging have greatly facilitated its use [1-8].

Normal Sonographic Anatomy

In each trimester of the pregnancy, specific landmarks of normal fetal anatomy should be verified by obstetric ultrasound (US) [1, 2].

During the First Trimester

The stomach appears as a cystic structure in the left hypochondrium. It should be constantly visible at around 11-12 weeks.

The small bowel herniates physiologically through the umbilical cord at around 8-9 weeks. The herniation should have resolved by 11-12 weeks.

The rest of the digestive tract is not visible at this stage.

The bladder is the other cystic structure that should be visible during the first trimester. It is located medially in the fetal pelvis and is visible around 8-9 weeks.

The kidneys are visible around the end of the first trimester and appear as hyperechoic bean-shaped structures in each perilumbar area.

At this stage, the amniotic fluid is produced by the placenta and does not reflect the renal function.

During the Second Trimester

The stomach is globally unchanged. The small bowel gets progressively filled with meconium. It will be visible as small parallel tubular echogenic structures, mainly in the left flank. The colon is not visible until the end of the second trimester.

The bladder should always be visible during the mid trimester examination. It should show normal cycles of filling and emptying (during a single examination).

The kidneys now appear more obvious, since their global echogenicity decreases and since cortico-medullary differentiation begins (and should be constantly present by 17-18 weeks).

The rest of the abdomen is 'filled' with the liver and the spleen, both appearing as homogenous triangular structures. The adrenals are triangular hypoechoic masses located on the top of the kidney. The pancreas and the abdominal vessels complete the evaluation of the fetal abdomen.

During the Third Trimester

The esophagus is visible when distended by amniotic fluid.

The stomach shows obvious peristaltic waves. It may be filled with echogenic material (gastric pseudomass) corresponding to swallowed debris.

The small bowel is now filled with swallowed amniotic fluid and appears as small cystic structures of variable sizes due to normal peristalsis.

The colon is progressively visible as it fills with hypoechoic meconium and by 27-28 weeks it can be followed from the cecum to the recto-sigmoid. Its diameter widens progressively (it should be less than 2 cm).

The appearance of the bladder and kidneys should be stable. The kidneys grow progressively with gestational age. Their length measures around 3 cm at 30 weeks.

The adrenals are large and display a corticomedullary differentiation [1, 2].

The liver occupies a large part of the fetal upper abdomen. The gallbladder is almost always visible.

Normal MR Imaging Anatomy

Fetal MR is mainly performed in the second half of the pregnancy. T1- and T2-weighted sequences can be used in order to characterize fetal abdominal anatomy.

The bladder appears as a hypersignal on T2- and a hyposignal on T1-weighted sequences. The normal kidneys are mainly visualized on T2 sequences.

The small bowel is best analyzed on T2 sequence, as the loops appear as a hypersignal, being filled with amniotic fluid. The colon is best analyzed on T1, as it appears as a hypersignal, probably due to the proteic content of the meconium. It appears as a hyposignal on T2 sequences.

The rectum should be identified in all fetuses after 23 weeks. Its cul-de-sac should be localized 10 mm below the bladder neck on a sagittal scan. It should be possible to identify the entire colon after 30 weeks [3-8].

Abnormal Findings and the Complementary Role of US and MR Imaging

Several abnormal conditions observed on US will be discussed:
- The stomach is small or not visualized
- The stomach is too large
- The stomach is in the midline
- The digestive tract is dilated
- The bladder is dilated
- The bladder is not visible
- The kidneys are (is) not visible
- The urinary tract is dilated
- The kidneys are too echogenic
- There is a cyst on the kidneys
- There are inter-abdominal calcifications
- There is an abdominal mass.

The Stomach Is Small or Not Visualized (Second or Third Trimester)

As mentioned above, the stomach should always be visualized during sonographic examination, especially during the second and third trimester examinations.

Its absence or small size raises the suspicion of an abnormality (the first step should be a control examination of the fetus in order to confirm the anomaly).

The most common 'pathological' cause is an esophageal atresia (EA). US is not very effective for an accurate diagnosis of EA unless a pharyngeal pouch is distended. On the contrary, MR imaging can provide important information and improve the detection rate of this diagnosis by easily demonstrating the dilated pouch or by excluding the diagnosis thanks to the visualization of an entire esophagus. The other possibility is the presence of intra-uterine growth retardation with associated oligohydramnios. In this case, no abnormality of the digestive tract would be detected [9, 10].

The Stomach Is Too Big (Third Trimester)

Once again, the first step should be to confirm the anomaly.

The main cause is a duodenal atresia leading to the so-called 'double-bubble' sign. It is associated with aneuploidy in 30% of patients (Trisomy 21).

The differential diagnosis should include duodenal stenosis. US is sufficient for this diagnosis; no complementary imaging modality is necessary [11].

The Stomach Lies on the Midline

The midline position of the stomach could correspond to intestinal malrotation with or without obstruction and should prompt a postnatal work-up [12].

The Digestive Tract Is Dilated (Mainly Third Trimester)

The presence of dilated intestinal loops on US (over 1 cm diameter in the second trimester, over 2 cm diameter during third trimester) suggests intestinal obstruction. Although the technique is very sensitive, it is not specific for the detection of an obstruction and it cannot differentiate between small and large bowel obstructions.

With such a presentation, MR imaging can improve the diagnostic accuracy by demonstrating the colon. If the latter appears normal on T1 sequence, the obstruction most probably affects the small bowel. Conversely, if the colon is not visible, it is more difficult to assess the level of obstruction unless a specific part of it appears dilated. Noteworthy, the diagnosis of Hirschsprung disease or of isolated anal atresia is difficult or even impossible [5, 13].

The Bladder Is Too Large (Any Trimester)

During the first trimester a bladder larger than 3 cm is abnormal. If it persists, a bladder outlet obstruction (BOO) is probable and the prognosis is poor.

During the second trimester, a bladder larger than 5 cm is abnormal. The presence of an oligohydramnios suggests a BOO and again, the prognosis is poor.

During the third trimester, a large bladder can correspond to several diagnoses. The differential should include bladder obstruction related to posterior urethral valve, massive vesico-ureteric reflux and 'megacystis microcolon-hypoperistalsis' syndrome.

Fetal MR imaging may clearly help in this differential diagnosis by demonstrating a normal or abnormal colon [11, 14].

The Bladder Is Not Visible

First, the examination should verify that this does not correspond to the normal cycle of filling and emptying of the fetal bladder.

If confirmed, the first suspicion should be bladder exstrophy, in which there is no normal bladder and instead a soft tissue mass is seen beneath the insertion of the umbilical cord. Also, no cystic structure is seen between the two umbilical arteries. Usually US is sufficient to reach this diagnosis [15].

One or Both Kidneys Are Not Visible

Bilateral renal agenesis is incompatible with postnatal life. The condition is associated with oligohydramnios and pulmonary hypoplasia.

In such conditions, no renal structure is visible within the lumbar areas. If necessary, fetal MR imaging can be performed in order to confirm the anomaly [14, 15]. MRI can also facilitate the diagnosis of ectopic kidneys.

Unilateral renal agenesis is common. There are usually no associated anomalies and the prognosis is good. Imaging should aim at determining whether a dysplastic kidney replaces the normal kidney or whether the kidney has developed in an ectopic position.

The Urinary Tract Is Dilated (Second and Third Trimester)

The diagnosis of a urinary tract dilatation is based upon an anterior-posterior diameter of the renal pelvis above 7 mm, a ureter above 3 mm, or a bladder above 5 cm.

The role of imaging is to determine the level of obstruction and the status of the remaining parenchyma. Assessment of associated anomalies, amniotic fluid volume and lung hypoplasia will help to determine the prognosis.

Fetal MR imaging may help in providing additional anatomical information for this evaluation [14, 15].

The Kidneys Are Hyperechoic (Second and Third Trimester)

As mentioned above, the echogenicity of the kidneys decreases with time and corticomedullary differentiation should be present by 17-18 weeks.

In some instances, the kidney parenchyma appears frankly hyperechoic and/or corticomedullary differentiation (CMD) is not present. The sonographic analysis should be as detailed as possible and should evaluate size, echogenicity, the presence of cysts, calcifications or other anomalies.

The main causes of hyperechoic kidneys are hereditary polycystic kidney diseases. Familial and genetic inquiries might help with diagnosis.

Other causes include syndromes, metabolic diseases, toxins, infections and vascular causes. A meticulous and systematic work-up will help to approach a correct diagnosis [16, 17]. To date, the role of MRI is limited for the analysis of the renal parenchyma, except for the detection of cysts.

There Are Cysts on the Kidneys (Second or Third Trimester)

As for the previous case, the approach should be meticulous, based on a systematic analysis of the kidneys.

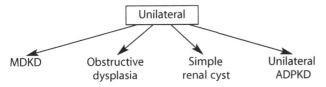

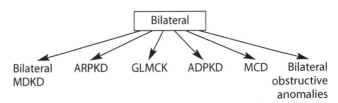

MDKD, Multicystic dysplastic kidney; ADPKD, Autosomal dominant polycystic kidney; ARPKD, Autosomal recessive polycystic kidney; GLMCK, Glomerulocyst kidney; MCP, Medullary cystic dysplasia

It is also important to look for associated anomalies corresponding to syndromes with renal cystic involvement [18].

There Are Intra-abdominal Calcifications

Intra-abdominal calcifications and echogenic masses are relatively common findings during fetal US. They may arise from any fetal part (e.g., liver, gallbladder, kidneys, spleen, adrenals).

Detection of such anomalies should prompt a detailed survey for additional findings, and a maternal history. In most cases, conservative management is sufficient. However, for some, a transfer to a tertiary care centre will be necessary.

In case of peritoneal calcifications, an important associated finding would be dilated intestinal loops, which would orient the diagnosis towards meconium peritonitis.

Another important finding would be an underlying fetal mass with calcifications (see below) [19-21].

There Is an Abdominal Mass (Second and Third Trimester)

In case of an abdominal mass, the role of imaging is to determine its anatomical origin, its content and the anatomic relation with the regional structures. The most common cystic tumor is an ovarian cyst.

The most common solid-type tumor is renal or adrenal in origin.

Cystic tumors	Solid-type tumors
- ovarian cyst	- mesoblastic nephroma
- mesenteric cyst	- neuroblastoma
- lymphangioma	- teratoma
- cystic teratoma	- hemangioma
- cystic neuroblastoma	- intra-abdominal sequestration
- urethral cyst	
- duplication cyst	

Follow-up is by US for neonatal management and eventual surgery [22].

In conclusion, a step-by-step analysis helps to define the anomalies affecting the fetal abdomen. For selected indications, US first and MR imaging thereafter, can be used to evaluate the malformation.

References

1. Filly RA, Feldstein VA (2000) US evaluation of normal fetal anatomy. In: Callen PW (ed) Ultrasonography in obstetrics and gynecology, 4 edn. WB Saunders, Philadelphia, pp 221-276

2. Avni FE, Rypens F, Donner C (2002) Routine obstetrical US examination in the second and 3rd trimester. In: Avni FE (ed) Perinatal imaging. Springer Verlag, Berlin, pp 1-12

3. Farhataziz N, Engels JE, Ramus RM et al (2005) Fetal MRI of urine and meconium by gestational age for the diagnosis of GU and GI abnormalities. AJR Am J Roentgenol 184:1891-1897

4. Trop I, Levine D (2001) Normal fetal anatomy as visualized with fast MRI. Top Magn Reson Imaging 12:3-17

5. Saguintaah M, Couture A, Veyrac C et al (2002) MRI of the fetal GI tract. Pediatr Radiol 32:395-404

6. Amin RS, Nikolaidis P, Kawashima A et al (1999) Normal anatomy of the fetus at MRI imaging. Radiographics 19:S201-S214

7. Yamashita Y, Namimoto T, Abe Y et al (1997) MR imaging of the fetus by a HASTE sequence. AJR Am J Roentgenol 168:513-519

8. Shinmoto H, Kashima K, Yuasa Y et al (2000) MR imaging of non CNS fetal abnormalities. Radiographics 20:1227-1243

9. Chaumoitre K, Amous Z, Bretelle F et al (2004) Diagnostic prénatal d'atrésie de l'œsophage par IRM. J Radiol (Paris) 85:2029-2031

10. Longer JC, Hussain H, Khan A et al (2005) Prenatal diagnosis of esophageal atresia using US and MRI. J Pediatr Surg 36:804-807

11. Veyrac C, Couture A, Saguintaah M, Baud C (2004) MRI of fetal GI tract abnormalities. Abdom Imaging 29:411-420

12. Cassart M, Lingier P, Massez A et al (2006) Sonographic prenatal diagnosis of malpositioned stomach. Pediatr Radiol (in press).

13. Hill BJ, Joe BN, Qayyum A et al (2005) Supplemental value of MRI in fetal abdominal disease detected in prenatal US. AJR Am J Roentgenol 184:993-998

14. Cassart M, Massez A, Metens T (2004) Complementary role of MRI after US in assessing bilateral urinary tract anomalies in the fetus. AJR Am J Roentgenol 182:689-695

15. Gearhart JP, Benchain J, Jeffs RD, Sanders RC (1995) Criteria for prenatal diagnosis of classical bladder exstrophy. Obstet Gynecol 185:961-964

16. Carr MR, Benaceraff BR, Estroff JA, Mandel J (1995) Prenatally diagnosed hyperechoic kidneys with normal amniotic fluid. J Urol 153:442-444

17. Nicolaides KH, Cheng HH, Abbas A et al (1992) Fetal renal defects: associated malformations and chromosomal defects. Fetal Diagn Ther 7:1-11

18. Avni FE, Garel L, Cassart M et al (2006) Perinatal assessment of hereditary cystic renal diseases. Pediatr Radiol (in press).

19. Mc Namara A, Levine D (2005) Intraabdominal fetal echogenic masses. Radiographics 25:633-645

20. Eckoldt F, Helling KS, Woderich R et al (2003) Meconium peritonitis and pseudo-cyst formation prenatal diagnosis and postnatal course. Prenat Diagn 23:904-908

21. Chan KL, Tang MHY, Tse HY et al (2005) Meconium peritonitis: prenatal diagnosis, postnatal management and outcome. Prenat Diagn 25:676-682

22. Kuroda T, Kitano Y, Honna T et al (2004) Prenatal diagnosis and management of abdominal diseases in pediatric surgery. J Pediatr Surg 39:1819-1822

Genitourinary Sonography in the Child

I. Gassner, T.E. Geley

Department of Pediatrics, University Hospital Innsbruck, Innsbruck, Austria

Introduction

Sonography is usually the first imaging modality applied and is a powerful tool for the evaluation of infants and children suspected of having genitourinary tract anomalies. The intention of this lecture is to provide a broad overview of common genitourinary anomalies and to highlight the strength of ultrasound for the evaluation of these conditions.

Anomalies of the Urinary Tract

Renal Agenesis

Renal agenesis may result from aplasia of the Wolffian duct or absence of the ureteral bud with consecutive lack of metanephrogenic tissue induction.

Unilateral renal agenesis is rather common, occurring in about 1 in 1,000 newborn infants [1]. There is a strong association of renal anomalies with Müllerian duct anomalies. Therefore, in females, the urinary tract and the reproductive system should always be evaluated as a unit.

Renal agenesis may also be mimicked by a multicystic dysplastic malformation of the kidney later in life since the multiple cysts seen in the affected infant disappear with time. In 10% of cases unilateral renal agenesis is associated with aplasia of the ipsilateral adrenal gland. In all other cases a characteristic elongated feature of the adrenal gland is found. Bilateral renal agenesis (Potter syndrome) is incompatible with life and most infants die shortly after birth.

Crossed Renal Ectopia

In crossed renal ectopia one kidney is displaced across the midline and lies on the opposite side of the ureteral insertion into the bladder. Four types of renal crossed ectopia are described (with fusion, without fusion, solitary, bilateral), with the crossed-fused ectopia being the most common.

Standard as well as colour Doppler ultrasound techniques document the location of ureteral orifices through the ureteral jet phenomenon.

Megaureter

The diameter of a normal ureter is rarely more than 5 mm and, therefore, the ureter is not visualised on pre- and postnatal ultrasound. Megaureter as a general term describes a dilated ureter with or without associated dilatation of the upper collecting system. Ureteral dilatation may be in response to anatomical or functional obstruction or vesicoureteral reflux, but may also occur in their absence.

Primary megaureter corresponds to an obstructive dilatation of the ureter above an adynamic segment at the ureterovesical junction. It is caused by hypoplasia and atrophy of muscle fibres in the distal segment of the ureter associated with an increase in collagen fibres in the pathologic segment and muscular hypertrophy of the proximal ureter.

Ultrasound demonstrates the dilated ureter and an increased peristalsis.

Secondary megaureter occurs as a result of reflux, urethral obstructions or bladder abnormalities such as posterior urethral valves or a neuropathic bladder.

Ureteral Duplication

Ureteral duplication (Fig. 1) is the most frequent renal anomaly. The duplications vary from partial to complete separation of the collecting system. Incomplete duplication is thought to result from early branching of a single ureteral bud, resulting in a common distal stem with two ureteral segments impinging on the metanephric blastema.

Complete ureteral duplication results from the formation of two ureteral buds on the same side. During absorption and migration of the distal portion of the mesonephric duct into the developing bladder, the orifices of the ureter draining the lower segment of the kidney migrates more cephalad and lateral than the orifice of the ureter draining the upper segment of the kidney.

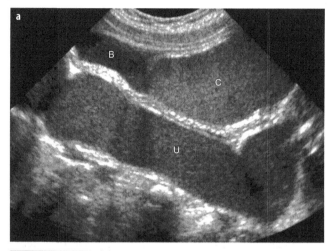

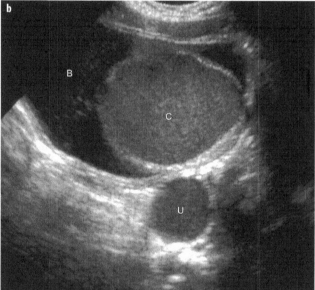

Fig. 1. Complete ureteropelvic duplication on the left with obstructive upper-pole ureterocele. Urinary tract infection in the upper pole collecting system in a 21-day-old male. **a** Longitudinal, **b** transverse pelvic scan. The dilated upper pole ureter (*U*) and the ectopic ureterocele (*C*) are full of debris (purulent exudate), *B*, bladder. (Reprinted with permission from [2])

This embryological relationship is known as the Weigert-Meyer-law.

When the area of the ureter to the lower segment buds is displaced closer to the urogenital sinus than normal, the orifice migrates more lateral and cephalad and the lower segment is more likely to be associated with vesicoureteral reflux.

When the area of the ureter to the upper segment, on the other hand, is displaced more proximally on the mesonephric duct than normal, the ureteral orifice will be ectopic in location and may open at the level of the bladder neck or even more distally into the urethra, vestibule or vagina.

Vesicoureteral reflux is the most common abnormality seen in association with complete ureteral duplication and commonly affects the lower segment due to the fact that the ureter to the lower segment has a more laterally placed orifice and a shortened submucosal tunnel. The ureter from the upper pole may function normally or may be obstructed, but reflux into the upper pole is rare.

Sonography clearly demonstrates malformations of the kidney, such as a dilated ureter due to either stenosis or reflux and ballooning of the submucosal segment of the upper ureter in the bladder (ureterocele). The ureteral jet sign locates the orthotopic as well as the ectopic ureteral orifice.

Ureteral Ectopia in Single and Duplex Collecting Systems

A ureter that opens anywhere but into the trigone of the bladder is considered ectopic (Fig. 2). About 20% of ectopic insertions of the ureter drain a kidney with a single collecting system. The remainder are associated with the affected ureter draining the upper pole of a duplex kidney.

In males, the ectopic ureter may empty into the lower bladder, posterior urethra, seminal vesicle, vas deferens or ejaculatory duct. In females it may insert into the lower bladder, urethra, vestibule, vagina, uterus or remnants of the Gartner's duct. Ureteral ectopia is more common in females and affected girls are frequently found to be incontinent due to the ectopic ureter terminating at a level distal to the continence mechanisms of the bladder neck and external sphincter. Ectopic ureters may show reflux, but obstruction is more common. When the collecting system is dilated the lack of an intravesical ureterocele suggests an insertion of the ectopic ureter on another side, such as the bladder neck or the proximal urethra. Ultrasound documents a dilated ureter on a lower and more medial level than expected and the exact location of the orifice may be documented via the ureteral jet sign.

Ureterocele in Single and Duplex Collecting Systems

Ureteroceles represent cystic dilatation of the intravesical segment of the ureter as a response to obstruction, and may be associated with single or duplex ureters (Fig. 1). They are called orthotopic or simple when found with a single collecting system, and ectopic when found with a duplicated collecting system. Ectopic ureteroceles are positioned beyond the confines of the trigone and frequently represent the distal portion of the upper pole ureter. On ultrasound the ureterocele appears as a cystic structure within the bladder. The ureteral jet sign documents the orifice of simple ureteroceles opposite the bladder wall. In ectopic ureteroceles the orifice is commonly located next to the bladder wall.

Posterior Urethral Valves (Case no. 1 on CD-ROM)

Posterior urethral valves are the commonest urethral abnormality occurring in boys. A thick membrane is found

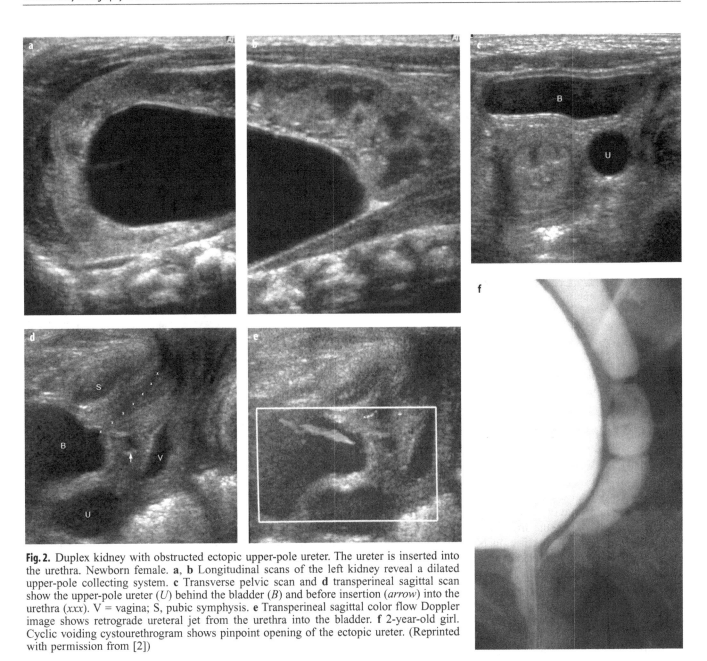

Fig. 2. Duplex kidney with obstructed ectopic upper-pole ureter. The ureter is inserted into the urethra. Newborn female. **a, b** Longitudinal scans of the left kidney reveal a dilated upper-pole collecting system. **c** Transverse pelvic scan and **d** transperineal sagittal scan show the upper-pole ureter (*U*) behind the bladder (*B*) and before insertion (*arrow*) into the urethra (*xxx*). V = vagina; S, pubic symphysis. **e** Transperineal sagittal color flow Doppler image shows retrograde ureteral jet from the urethra into the bladder. **f** 2-year-old girl. Cyclic voiding cystourethrogram shows pinpoint opening of the ectopic ureter. (Reprinted with permission from [2])

in the posterior urethra with a pinhole opening positioned posteriorly near the verumontanum. During voiding, the anterior portion of the membrane bulges. This urethral obstruction causes high intraluminal pressure during the early phases of foetal development, leading to abnormal bladder function and anatomy (trabeculation, bladder neck hypertophy), renal dysplasia, hydronephrosis, and vesicoureteral reflux. Vesicoureteral reflux often persists after relief of the obstruction. Prenatal and postnatal ultrasound document bilateral hydroureteronephrosis associated with parenchymal dysplasia and a thick-walled bladder. In cases of severe hydronephrosis, rupture of the intrarenal collecting system at the calyceal fornix leads to perirenal urinoma and urine ascites.

Anomalies of Renal Vessels (Fig. 3)

Each kidney is normally supplied by a single renal artery, although one or more accessory renal arteries are not uncommon. The renal artery originates from the abdominal aorta and runs behind the vena cava to reach the hilar region of the kidney.

In patients with interruption of the inferior vena cava with azygos continuation, the azygos vein increases in size and might be mistaken for the inferior vena cava. Cross-sectional imaging techniques document the course of the renal artery to be ventral to the azygos vein. Azygos continuation is frequently associated with cardiac and situs anomalies and awareness of the anatomic rela-

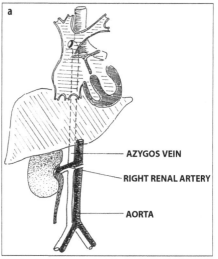

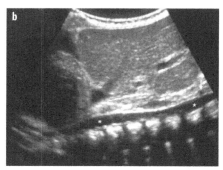

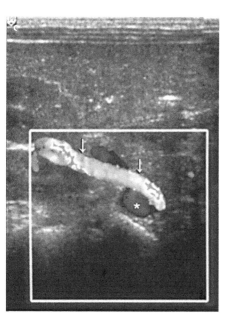

Fig. 3. Azygos continuation of inferior vena cava. **a** Drawing. **b** Longitudinal scan and **c** transverse color-coated duplex sonogram show right renal artery (*arrows*) ventral to azygos vein (*asterisks*)

tionship between the renal artery and the azygos vein can aid in diagnosis [3].

Anomalies of the Female Reproductive System

Embryology

The internal genital organs, as well as the lower urinary system, originate from two paired urogenital structures that develop in both sexes, the mesonephric ducts (Wolffian ducts) and the paramesonephric ducts (Müllerian ducts).

In female development the Müllerian ducts are divided into two segments. The distal segments move towards the midline and soon fuse into a single tube, the uterovaginal canal. The resulting septum that divides the uterovaginal canal disappears soon after. Failure of *lateral fusion* of the Müllerian ducts results in a wide variety of abnormalities of the uterus, cervix and vagina. The development of the vagina is induced by the fusion of the uterovaginal canal with the urogenital sinus (*transversal fusion*). Due to the close developmental relationship between the genital and the urinary tract, association of anomalies in both systems are common [4].

Normal Appearance and Ultrasound Techniques

During normal growth and development the uterus and ovaries undergo a series of changes in size and configuration.

Under the influence of maternal and placental hormones, the neonatal uterus is remarkably prominent with a thick myometrium and a definable endometrial lining [5].

At two to three month of age, the uterus regresses to its prepubertal size and tubular configuration. The endometrium is usually not visualised, making it rather difficult to evaluate uterine anomalies in infants and older children.

The post-pubertal uterus has the adult pear-shape appearance and the echogenicity and thickness of the endometrial lining varies according to the menstrual cycle [6].

High-resolution, real-time sonography has become the first-step imaging technique for the evaluation of the pelvis in infants, children and adolescents. Using the filled bladder as an acoustic window, the internal genital organs and the lower urinary tract are easily evaluated. In infants and young children who are not able to maintain a full bladder, filling of the bladder with sterile saline solution via a 5 to 8 French feeding tube might be necessary [7]. The same principle can also be used to outline the vagina (water vaginography), the rectum (water enema) or the urogenital sinus in complex congenital anomalies of the genitourinary tract. A transperineal sonographic approach should always be considered in cases of anomalies of the lower pelvis, since it allows an excellent documentation of the urethra, the periurethral soft tissue, the rectum and the distal genital tract.

Müllerian Duct Anomalies

Based upon the embryological development of the female genital system, uterovaginal malformations are classified as Müllerian agenesis in cases of a developmental defect of the caudal portion of the Müllerian ducts (Mayer-Rokitansky-Küster-Hauser syndrome), disorders of the lateral fusion resulting from failure of the two Müllerian ducts to fuse and disorders of the vertical fusion that are caused by faults in the union between the Müllerian tubercle and derivatives of the urogenital sinus (transverse vaginal septum, cervical agenesis, disorders of the hymen).

Mayer-Rokitansky-Küster-Hauser Syndrome

The Mayer-Rokitansky-Küster-Hauser syndrome is characterised by the absence of the entire or, more frequently, the proximal two thirds of the vagina, absence or abnormalities of the uterus and malformations of the upper urinary tract. The most frequently found subtype of the syndrome consists of two rudimentary uterine horns located on a higher level than expected and normal Fallopian tubes, ovaries and kidneys.

Sonographic evaluation aided by instillation of fluid into the bladder as well as the rectum may demonstrate the absence of vagina and uterus. MR imaging is frequently needed to clearly document the ovaries and the rudimentary uterus.

Uterus Didelphys (Fig. 4)

Disorders of the lateral fusion of the distal segments of the two Müllerian ducts include septate, bicornuate, didelphys and unicornuate uterus. In the absence of obstruction, these malformations are asymtomatic during

childhood or at puberty. A uterus didelphys or bicornuate uterus can readily be documented on sonographic evaluation of the newborn.

Imperforate Hymen (Fig. 5)

Although the hymen membrane is entirely of urogenital sinus origin, imperforate hymen is commonly listed together with defects of the vertical fusion of the Müllerian ducts. Imperforate hymen may either be symptomatic in the newborn period or after onset of puberty when development of hydrocolpos/hydrometrocolpos or hematocolpos/hematometrocolpos, respectively occurs. Sonographic evaluation shows the cystic dilatation of the vagina with the less distensible uterus attached to it. Internal echoes reflect cellular debris. Fluid may also be found in the peritoneal cavity due to spillage of genital secretion via the Fallopian tubes. Larger hydro- or haematocolpos may obstruct one or both ureters resulting in hydronephrosis.

Association of Lateral and Vertical Fusion Anomalies (Case no. 2 on CD-ROM)

The frequent association of vertical with lateral fusion anomalies means that it is useful to consider vaginal anomalies according to the presence or the absence of obstruction. Nonobstructive vaginal anomalies encompass bifid vagina, longitudinal vaginal septum and incomplete transverse septum. Among the obstructive vaginal anomalies are imperforate hymen, complete transverse vaginal septum, unilateral obstructive longitudinal vaginal septum, obstruction of a unilateral rudimentary horn and atresia of the uterine cervix or the vagina. Sometimes obstructive disorders already present at birth due to accumulated genital secretion. More commonly, however, the

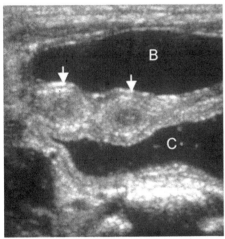

Fig. 4. Bicornuate uterus. 6-day-old newborn female newborn with congenital segmental dilatation of the colon (C). Transverse image through the pelvis shows two separate uterine horns (*arrows*), B = bladder. (Reprinted with permission from [4])

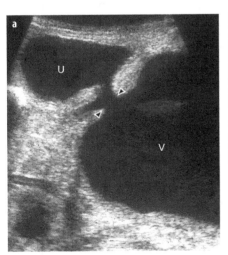
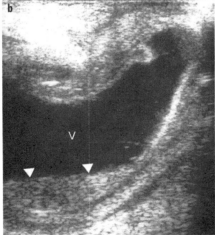
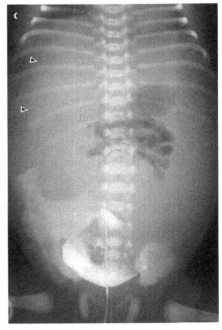

Fig. 5. Imperforate hymen with hydrometrocolpos and ascites due to spillage of genital secretions via the fallopian tubes into the peritoneal cavity. **a, b** Sagittal scans. The vagina (V) as well as the uterus (U) are dilated, with broad communication through the cervical ostium (*open arrowheads*). The vagina shows a fluid-debris level (*closed arrowheads*). **c** Distended, fluid-filled abdomen. The air-filled loops of bowel cluster in the center of the abdomen. The lateral edge of the liver (*arrowheads*) is visible. (Reprinted with permission from [4])

patient seeks medical advice at puberty with cyclic abdominal pain and a pelvic mass is found. The whole spectrum of Müllerian duct anomalies from the obstructed hemivagina in association with an uterus didelphys to the unicornuate uterus, which reflects the extreme end of the spectrum, are almost always associated with severe ipsilateral renal anomalies (renal agenesis, renal dysplasia, ectopia, ipsilateral ectopic ureter, and hydronephrosis).

This strong association should urge the physician to evaluate always both systems when a malformation is detected in one of them.

Urogenital Sinus Malformation

Urogenital sinus is suspected during physical examination of a newborn with a normally placed anus in association with either ambiguous genitalia or normal female external genitalia but only a single opening within the vestibulum. It is either found isolated or in association with chromosomal and hormonal abnormalities or as a cloacal variant.

Female Hypospadia

In female hypospadias the urethral meatus is positioned in the anterior wall of the vagina. Proximal hypospadias often show a narrowing of the urethra with signs of urinary outflow obstruction and are commonly associated with cloacal anomalies and female pseudohermaphroditism. Diagnostic evaluation will, therefore, be discussed below.

Distal hypospadia is more likely to have a urethra of normal diameter with no meatal stenosis and is frequently asymptomatic. In these girls the urethral meatus is on the roof of the vagina just inside the introitus and the urethra has to be catheterised blindly.

Congenital Adrenal Hyperplasia

In most instances, female pseudohermaphroditism results from the exposure of a female fetus to excessive androgens. The most common causes are congenital adrenal hyperplasia (an autosomal recessive disorder of adrenal steroidogenesis). The increased level of androgens within the foetal bloodstream causes virilisation of the external genitalia, which may vary from minimal phallic enlargement of the clitoris to almost complete masculinisation. At birth these patients present with marked clitoral enlargement, a variable degree of labioscrotal fold fusion and rugation. The opening of the urogenital sinus at the clitoral base may mimic penile hypospadia. Urinary tract anomalies are common and encompass renal agenesia, ectopia, and cystic dysplasia as well as uni- and bilateral hydronephrosis, vesicoureteral reflux and signs of urinary outflow obstruction.

The primary task of the radiologist is to demonstrate the level of communication between the vagina and the urethra, the anatomy of the internal genitalia, to rule out kidney anomalies and to document adrenal gland hyperplasia.

Sonographic evaluation of the patient is usually the first-step imaging technique, followed by conventional radiology using contrast material. Transabdominal ultrasound will demonstrate the internal genitalia, the kidneys and adrenal glands, and show any obstructions such as hydrocolpos and hydrometrocolpos [8]. Demonstration of enlarged adrenal glands with wavy limb configuration, however, is highly indicative of congenital adrenal hyperplasia [6].

Fluoroscopic studies with water-soluble contrast material are required to examine the exact anatomy of the malformation.

Cloacal Malformation

The cloacal malformation, the most complex type of imperforate anus, is a complex congenital malformation with a common outflow of the urinary, genital and intestinal tract into a urogenital sinus. Cloaca is exclusively seen in phenotypic females.

The diagnosis of cloacal malformation is made when, in addition to an absent anus, only one perineal orifice is found between the labia. *Every newborn girl with imperforate anus should be considered to have a cloacal malformation until proven otherwise.*

Associated anomalies include uterus didelphys [9], renal anomalies, ectopia of the ureter, bladder diverticula, lower spinal cord abnormalities, anomalies of the pelvic osseous structures such as sacral agenesis or hypoplasia, dysraphism and pubic diastasis.

Obstruction of the cloaca may occur at any level and determines whether the proximal distended urinary and/or genital system is filled solely with genital secretions or contains urine and/or meconium as well.

Ultrasound is the most efficient first-step imaging technique in the diagnostic work-up of these patients. Performed early after birth, no or only little intestinal gas will be present and a clearer documentation of the intrapelvic structures can be obtained. An abdominal mass in the neonate with cloacal malformation is almost always a distended vagina and/or uterus filled with urine and/or meconium because the path of least resistance for their egress was into the vagina instead of the cloaca. Obstruction of the common outlet can lead to retrograde flow via the fallopian tubes and accumulation of intraabdominal fluid. In cases where urine enters the rectum and colon, the meconium may calcify *in utero* and intraluminal calcification can be documented sonographically as well as radiologically. The distance between the blind end of the rectum and the perineum should be measured by transperineal ultrasound, and the kidneys should be evaluated, as well as the spinal cord [6].

Sonographic features of spinal anomalies, occurring with a frequency of nearly 50% in patients with cloacal malformations, are either a high lying plump conus or a tethered cord with a thickened filum terminale.

The next step in the imaging process are fluoroscopic studies using water-soluble contrast material to visualise the often unpredictable and erratic courses of the communication between the multiple structures, and to provide functional information about reflux and competence of the urinary sphincter.

MR imaging is gaining acceptance in imaging congenital abnormalities of the genital tract, but should be used in conjunction with other imaging modalities.

References

1. De Bruyn R (2005) The urinary tract. In: de Bruyn R (ed) Pediatric ultrasound. Elsevier Churchill Livingstone, pp 39-112
2. Gassner I (2005) Fetal genitourinary anomalies. Perinatal and postnatal management with imaging techniques. Radiologe 45:1067-1077
3. Geley TE, Unsinn KM, Auckenthaler TM et al (1999) Azygos continuation of the inferior vena cava: sonographic demonstration of the renal artery ventral to the azygos vein as a clue to diagnosis. AJR Am J Roentgenol 172:1659-1662
4. Gassner I, Geley TE (2004) Ultrasound of female genital anomalies. Eur Radiol 4:L107-L122
5. Nussbaum Balsk AR, Sanders RC, Gearhart JP (1991) Obstructed uterovaginal anomalies: demonstration with sonography, Part I: Neonates and infants. Radiology 179:79-83
6. Teele R, Share J (1992) Ultrasonography of the female pelvis in childhood and adolescence. Radiol Clin North Am 30:743-758
7. Kiechl-Kohlendorfer U, Geley TE, Unsinn KM, Gassner I (2001) Diagnosing neonatal female genital anomalies using saline-enhanced sonography. AJR Am J Roentgenol 177:1041-1044
8. Nussbaum Balsk AR, Sanders RC, Rock JA (1991) Obstructed uterovaginal anomalies: demonstration with sonography. Part II: Teenagers. Radiology 179:84-88
9. Jaramillo D, Lebowitz RL, Hendren WH (1990) The cloacal malformation: Radiologic findings and imaging recommendation. Radiology 177:441-448

Intussusception: An Approach to Management

A. Daneman

University of Toronto, and Division of General Radiology and Body Imaging, Department of Diagnostic Imaging, The Hospital for Sick Children, Toronto, Ontario, Canada

Intussusception is not an uncommon phenomenon in children and is one of the commoner causes of the acute abdomen between six months and five years of age. The vast majority of intussusceptions arise in the ileum and are either ileocolic or ileo-ileocolic. They are thought to occur because of hyperplasia of the lymphoid tissue in the ileum, possibly as a result of a viral infection [1, 2].

There are other types of intussusceptions that may relate to pathologic lead points [3], gastro-jejunostomy tubes or those intussusceptions that are seen in the postoperative period. These will be discussed separately at the end of this chapter.

The purpose of this chapter is to provide a summary of the diagnostic approaches and management of the various types of intussusception in children. For an in-depth review of the current literature on this subject the reader is referred to references 1-3.

Ileocolic and Ileo-Ileocolic Intussusception

A review of the history of the management of intussusception shows that there has been a continuing evolution of management techniques [4]. Changes in management of this condition over the last 20 years have evolved despite the lack of large, controlled, prospective, comparative studies. This has caused some controversy and some criticism in the literature [1-3, 5]. Indeed, successful management can be achieved in one of a number of different ways [1-3, 5-15]. In future years, the management of intussusception will probably continue to evolve.

Diagnosis

Children presenting with ileocolic or ileo-ileocolic intussusception commonly do not present with the classical clinical triad of abdominal pain, red currant jelly stool and a palpable abdominal mass. Presentation may, therefore, be nonspecific. For this reason, the clinician often has to rely on imaging procedures to promptly and accurately diagnose or exclude intussusception. The diagnosis can be made by either sonography, plain abdominal radiographs or by contrast studies of the colon [7-11].

Sonography

It has been shown in many series that sonography is 100% accurate in depicting the presence or absence of the common type of ileocolic or ileo-ileocolic intussusceptions in children [1, 7-9]. These lesions have a characteristic sonographic appearance and are usually found just under the abdominal wall, most commonly on the right side of the abdomen (Fig. 1, 2). Sonography is the modality of choice for the evaluation of patients suspected of having an intussus-

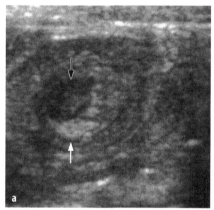
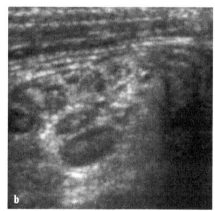

Fig. 1. Sonograms of a child with ileocolic intussusception. **a** Transverse scan through the intussusception shows the typical target sign that can be easily detected just below the abdominal wall anteriorly. The characteristic of this target sign that enables the diagnosis of intussusception to be made is the crescent of echogenicity (*white arrow*), which represents the fat in the mesentery that has been drawn into the intussusception between the layers of the intussusceptum. The black arrow indicates a hypoechoic area representing an enlarged lymph node within the mesentery. **b** Sonogram of the adjacent mesentery shows multiple nodes which have a normal echogenicity. The presence of the nodes in the mesentery reflects the lymphoid hyperplasia that is commonly found in these patients

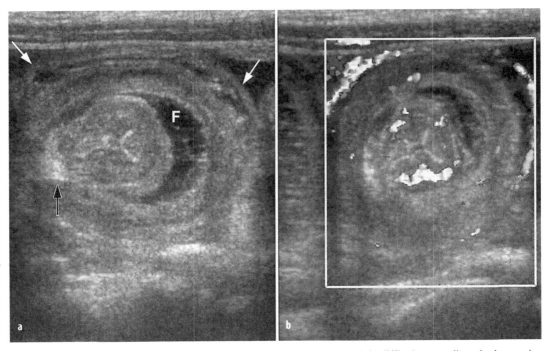

Fig. 2. Sonograms of child with ileocolic intussusception. **a** This intussusception shows a more complex target sign than shown in Figure 1. The echogenic fat in the mesentery is again noted (*black arrow*) between the layers of the intussusceptum. There is also fluid (*F*) trapped between the layers of the intussusceptum as a result of increased pressure and transudation of this fluid. The intussuscipiens is quite thinned (*white arrows*) and can be seen along the periphery of the intussusception also, separated from the outer layer of the intussusceptum by some fluid. **b** The color Doppler evaluation of the intussusception shows good flow to both the intussusceptum and the intussuscipiens along the periphery. It is difficult to predict whether an intussusception will reduce based on the ultrasound findings. The presence of fluid within the intussusception as shown in this patient suggests the intussusception may not reduce, whereas good blood flow to the intussusception suggests it will reduce easily. This intussusception was successfully reduced by pneumatic reduction

ception because it is a noninvasive, accurate procedure. An excellent review of the sonographic appearance of intussusception is provided in the article by del Pozo et al. [9].

Plain Abdominal Radiographs

There are some characteristic signs of an intussusception on a plain radiograph, including the meniscus sign, the target sign and, less commonly, a soft tissue mass [10, 11]

(Fig. 3, 4). Some institutions still rely on the plain radiograph for the diagnosis or exclusion of intussusception, but there is no study that has proven it to be as accurate as sonography [1, 10, 11]. In our institution we have relied on the plain radiograph only in those instances where there is a clinical consideration of peritonitis. In this clinical setting the plain radiograph is essential to exclude perforation, which is the major contraindication for attempted enema reduction.

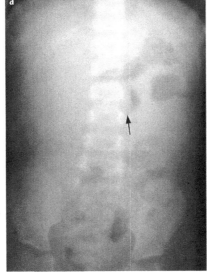
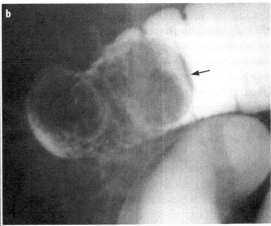

Fig. 3. Child with ileocolic intussusception, which extended into the transverse colon. **a** Abdominal radiograph shows a gasless right hemiabdomen due to the presence of the intussusception on the right. The black arrow indicates a soft tissue meniscus sign that represents the leading end of the intussusceptum in the transverse colon. **b** A hydrostatic contrast enema confirms the presence of the leading edge of the intussusceptum (*arrow*) in the transverse colon

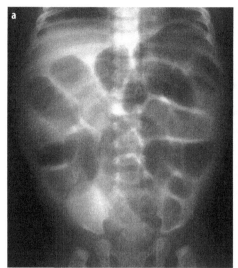
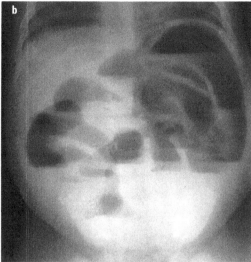

Fig. 4. Child with ileocolic intussusception causing marked small bowel obstruction. Supine (**a**) and upright (**b**) abdominal radiographs show marked distention of the small bowel with gas and air fluid levels indicating obstruction. The appearance is nonspecific. When this degree of small bowel distention occurs the other plain radiographic signs such as the gasless right hemi-abdomen, meniscus sign and target sign are usually not visible. Diagnosis of the exact etiology of the obstruction will then depend more on detailed clinical information

Contrast Enema

Despite the proven value of sonography, some institutions still consider the contrast enema as the quickest and most cost-effective method of excluding or confirming the presence of intussusception [1]. This, however, represents a more invasive diagnostic procedure and requires radiation. In some series using the contrast enema for diagnosis, 50% of the enemas may be negative for intussusception [1]. Using sonography as the diagnostic modality enables one to avoid performing unnecessary contrast enemas in those patients without intussusception [1, 6].

Reduction

There are many series in the recent literature that have shown a reduction rate of intussusception varying from 80% to as high as 95% [2, 12-15]. These series have used either fluoroscopic or sonographic guidance for reducing the intussusception and the series have used either hydrostatic [barium, water soluble contrast, saline] or pneumatic reduction (Fig. 5, 6). The fact that different techniques have been used with similar success rates suggests that it is not important which technique is used. There has been much controversy in the last 20 years regarding which technique is the best, but because the various techniques are probably equal in terms of success rates, the most important factors are to keep the safety of the child in mind and that individual radiologists use the technique with which they are most comfortable and experienced.

Nonoperative reduction of an intussusception should only be attempted after the surgical team has evaluated the patient and the patient is clinically stable, well hydrated, has no evidence of peritonitis and has an intravenous line in place [2]. The major contraindications to performing the enema are the clinical findings of peritonitis or shock or the signs of perforation on an abdominal radiograph [2].

We use pneumatic reduction because it is a simple, quick and clean technique [2]. The technique is also easy to learn. Furthermore, it has been shown clinically and experimentally that air enema is usually associated with smaller perforations and less fecal contamination of the peritoneum than hydrostatic enema [2, 16]. The advan-

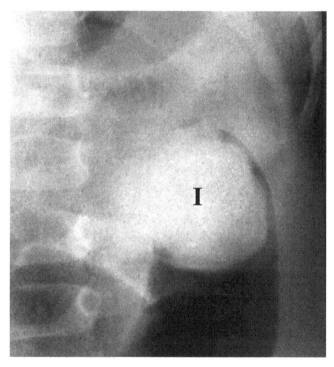

Fig. 5. Air enema in child with ileocolic intussusception that has reached the splenic flexure. The air enema easily outlines the leading edge of the intussusceptum (*I*) in the region of the splenic flexure

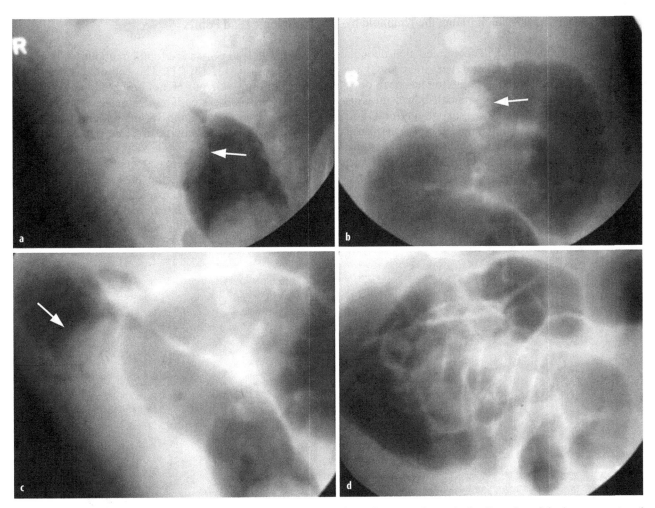

Fig. 6. Air enema reduction of ileocolic intussusception. **a** Initial image from air enema shows the leading edge of the intussusceptum (*arrow*) in the rectosigmoid region. **b** Later during the enema, the intussusceptum has been reduced into the transverse colon (*arrow*). Note the distended distal colon with air. **c** This shows the intussusceptum (*arrow*) reduced into the mid ascending colon. Note the air-distended sigmoid colon. **d** Complete reduction of the ileocolic intussusception is achieved and air fills not only the colon but multiple loops of small bowel, confirming complete reduction, as no residual intussusceptum can be identified

tage of sonography, however, is that it does not involve radiation. However, there is little information in the literature regarding the ease of recognition of perforation when using sonographic guidance. Even if one uses an air enema, sonography is an excellent modality to use for confirming reduction in those patients in whom it is difficult to determine whether reduction is complete on an air enema [2, 17]. Perforation rates should be under 1% [2, 16]. The surgical team must be available to intervene if complications occur during the enema.

In order to improve reduction rates, delayed, repeated reduction attempts can be used as long as the intussusception does move on the initial attempted reduction, and the child becomes asymptomatic and maintains stable vital signs [18]. It has been shown that this approach is a safe and effective technique with a good success rate [3, 18]. We have used this approach in approximately 15% of our patients with intussusception, achieving successful reduction in 50% of those intussusceptions not reduced on the first attempt [2, 18]. There does not appear to be a fixed

optimal timing between attempts, and the delayed second or third attempts can be made several hours after the first attempt [18]. However, it is essential to maintain strict clinical observation of the child between attempts. We have not experienced any perforations using this approach. There is not enough data in the literature to determine the optimal number of attempts that may be tried and this should be weighed against the risk of unnecessary added radiation in each patient if fluoroscopic guidance is used.

Recurrent intussusception occurs in approximately 10% of all children who have successful initial reduction [2, 19]. Two thirds of children having a recurrence will only have one recurrence and most will occur within the first few days (or even hours) after the initial reduction. The remaining third might have multiple (even ten or more) recurrences and these may occur as isolated episodes or randomly in clusters, sometimes over several years [2, 19]. Children who have recurrent intussusceptions usually have easy reductions. It has been suggested that intramuscular injection of steroids may decrease early recurrence by ameliorating the lymphoid hyperplasia [2].

Spontaneous reduction of ileocolic and ileo-ileocolic intussusceptions may occur. However, in recent years spontaneous reduction of intussusception has been documented more frequently in some small bowel intussusceptions depicted incidentally by sonography or CT [3, 20] (Fig. 7). These are usually small bowel intussusceptions with no recognizable pathologic lead point and may be seen in symptomatic or asymptomatic patients.

Pathologic Lead Points

Pathologic lead points are found in about 5-7% of all intussusceptions [3, 18, 21]. The commonest are Meckel diverticulum, polyps, Henoch-Schonlein purpura and cystic fibrosis. Less common causes are lymphoma, duplication cyst (Fig. 8) and various inflammatory lesions of the bowel. Management of these patients remains a challenge.

The contrast or air enema techniques are not always diagnostic in documenting the presence of a pathologic lead point. Sonography is extremely useful in this regard, as it has been shown that it may depict two thirds of pathologic lead points and may provide a specific diagnosis in one third of these [3, 18, 21] (Fig. 8). However,

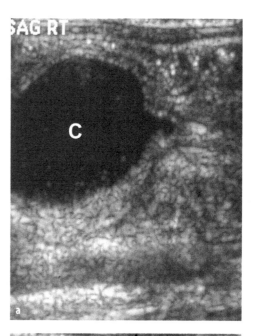

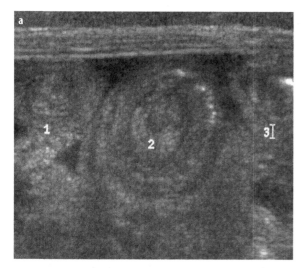

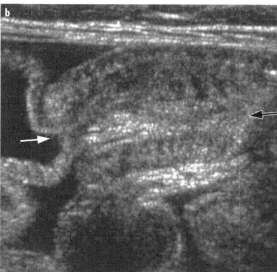

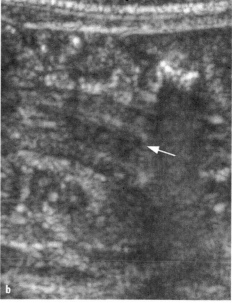

Fig. 7. Sonogram in a child with malabsorption shows three incidental small bowel intussusceptions (1, 2, 3). In this image, the sonogram depicts intussusception number two to best advantage. Note the crescent of mesentery between the layers of the intussusceptum. Also note more anteriorly the punctate areas of increased echogenicity that represent air trapped between the outer layer of the intussusceptum and the thinned intussuscipiens along the periphery. **b** Longitudinal scan through the intussusception number two (*arrows*) shows the so-called sandwich sign with some echogenic mesentery noted centrally. The intussusceptum enters the intussuscipiens from the region of the white arrow. At the time of evaluation this patient had a small amount of ascites

Fig. 8. Intussusception in a young child due to a duplication cyst (*C*). The sonogram has been obtained longitudinally through the intussusception (*arrow*). The duplication cyst is easily identified as a pathologic lead point

it remains a diagnostic challenge as to how to search for pathologic lead points in those patients in whom there is a high index of suspicion for such a lesion and in whom the sonogram is negative. In such cases, the choice of which other imaging modalities to use will depend on the clinical situation in each particular patient.

We recommend attempted enema reduction in all patients with a lead point if there is no contraindication to nonoperative reduction [3, 18].

Postoperative Intussusception

Intussusception may occur as a complication in less than 1% of laparotomies. The diagnosis is often not considered because it is so uncommon. Sonographic evaluation of any abdomen in the first few weeks following a laparotomy should include a search for a postoperative intussusception. These are usually more difficult to diagnose on sonography than the usual ileocolic intussusceptions, as they are small bowel intussusceptions and are usually surrounded by large, dilated loops of obstructed bowel. They usually require surgical reduction.

Gastrojejunostomy Tubes

Intussusceptions may complicate the presence of a gastrojejunostomy (GJ) tube [22] (Fig. 9). Most of the patients presenting with this complication are usually clinically stable and do not require urgent reduction of the intussusception. Most can be managed by replacing the tube with a standard or a shortened GJ tube or with a gastrostomy tube. However, manipulation of the GJ tube and flushing with air or saline may also be helpful. Surgery is rarely required for reduction.

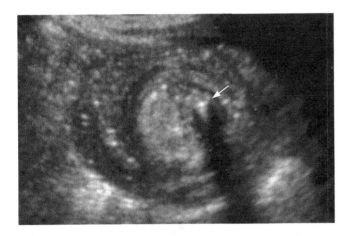

Fig. 9. Sonogram shows an intussusception due to a gastrojejunostomy tube (*arrow*). The tube is easily recognised in the centre of the intussusception as an echogenic focus with posterior acoustic shadowing

References

1. Daneman A, Navarro O (2003) Intussusception Part 1: A review of diagnostic approaches. Pediatr Radiol 33:79-85
2. Daneman A, Navarro O (2004) Intussusception Part 2: An update on the evolution of management. Pediatr Radiol 34:97-108
3. Navarro O, Daneman A (2004) Intussusception Part 3: Diagnosis and management of those with an identifiable or predisposing cause and those that reduce spontaneously. Pediatr Radiol 34:305-312
4. McDermott VGM (1994) Childhood intussusception and approaches to treatment: a historical review. Pediatr Radiol 24:153-155
5. Daneman A, Navarro O (2005) Intussusception: the debate endures. Pediatr Radiol 35:95-96
6. del-Pozo G, Albillos JC, Tejedor D et al (1999) Intussusception in children: current concepts in diagnosis and enema reduction. Radiographics 19:299-319
7. Pracros JP, Tran-Minh VA, Morin DE et al (1987) Acute intestinal intussusception in children: contribution of ultrasonography (145 cases). Ann Radiol 30:525-530
8. Verschelden P, Filiatraut D, Garel L et al (1992) Intussusception in children: reliability of US in diagnosis – a prospective study. Radiology 184:741-744
9. del-Pozo G, Abillos JC, Tejedor D (1996) Intussusception: US findings with pathologic correlation – the crescent-in-doughnut sign. Radiology 199:688-692
10. Eklof O, Thonell S (1984) Conventional abdominal radiography as a means to rule out ileocaecal intussusception. Acta Radiol Diagn 25:265-267
11. Sargent MA, Babyn P, Alton DJ (1994) Plain abdominal radiography in suspected intussusception: a reassessment. Pediatr Radiol 24:17-20
12. Gu L, Alton DJ, Daneman A et al (1988) Intussusception reduction in children by rectal insufflation of air. AJR Am J Roentgenol 150:1345-1348
13. Rohrschneider WK, Troger J (1995) Hydrostatic reduction of intussusception under US guidance. Pediatr Radiol 25:530-534
14. Todani T, Sato Y, Watanabe Y et al (1990) Air reduction for intussusception in infancy and childhood: ultrasonographic diagnosis and management without X-ray exposure. Z Kinderchir 45:222-226
15. Wang G, Liu S (1988) Enema reduction of intussusception by hydrostatic pressure under ultrasound guidance. A report of 377 cases. J Pediatr Surg 23:814-818
16. Daneman A, Alton DJ, Ein S et al (1995) Perforation during attempted intussusception reduction in children – a comparison of perforation with barium and air. Pediatr Radiol 25:81-88
17. Rohrschneider W, Troger J, Betsch B (1994) The post reduction donut sign. Pediatr Radiol 24:166-160
18. Navarro OM, Daneman A, Chae A (2004) Intussusception: the use of delayed, repeated reduction attempts and the management of intussusceptions due to pathologic lead points in pediatric patients. AJR Am J Roentgenol 182:1169-1176
19. Daneman A, Alton DJ, Lobo E et al (1998) Patterns of recurrence of intussusception in children: a 17 year review. Pediatr Radiol 28:913-919
20. Kornecki A, Daneman A, Navarro O et al (2000) Spontaneous reduction of intussusception: clinical spectrum, management and outcome. Pediatr Radiol 30:58-63
21. Navarro O, Dugougeat F, Kornecki A et al (2000) The impact of imaging in the management of intussusception owing to pathologic lead points in children. A review of 43 cases. Pediatr Radiol 30:594-603
22. Hughes UM, Connolly BL, Chait PG, Muraca S (2000) Further report of small-bowel intussusceptions related to gastrojejunostomy tubes. Pediatr Radiol 30:614-617

Imaging the Child with an Abdominal Mass

U.V. Willi

Department of Radiology, University of Zurich Children's Hospital, Zurich, Switzerland

General Considerations

The suspicion or diagnosis, even if it is nonspecific, of an abdominal mass in a child raises concern and anxiety. The pediatric radiologist may be the first person either to suspect or to diagnose a mass, quite commonly by ultrasonography (US). Therefore, adequate psychological interaction with the patient and the parent(s) is part of his or her professional competence. The findings should generally not be discussed while the examination is underway. Specific diagnostic statements should be avoided, even by the experienced examiner. Caution should be exercised before giving preliminary histological and prognostic hypotheses. The involved clinician, possibly the oncologist, should be informed promptly about the morphological findings and the information exchanged between the examiner and the patient and/or accompanying parent(s). This regards the situation of a suspicious mass that has been demonstrated and where a malignant process might exist or be likely. If the mass turns out to be a hydronephrosis or a similar obviously benign process, such concerns are less relevant.

Abdominal masses in children are often cystic and almost always benign, especially in the younger child (i.e., newborn and infants). In a majority of these cases, the mass originates from the urinary tract, typically due to some obstructive malformation and/or dysfunction (Fig. 1). Beside neoplasia and malformation, the underlying causes of such masses may be pathological conditions such as inflammation (usually due to infection), trauma (including iatrogenesis) or metabolic or other systemic diseases, including malignancy.

Proper imaging technique includes the correct choice of the imaging tool(s) and, if there is a need for more than one modality, their use in the appropriate order. This will shorten the time to diagnosis, and avoid uncertainty and unnecessary discussion, as well as help to limit costs. The role of the pediatric radiologist, therefore, is not only to make the diagnosis, but he or she also has a consulting duty toward the clinician who might think that, for example, all questions may be answered using magnetic resonance imaging (MRI). It is crucial that the examiner be aware of the strengths and limits of the method(s) used and those available for use.

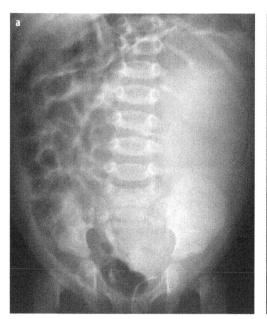
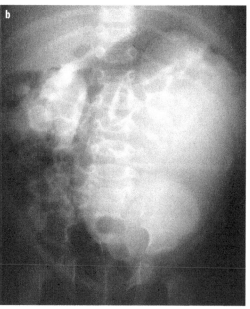

Fig. 1. Bilateral pyeloureteric junction obstruction in a 6-week-old boy. **a** Plain radiograph of abdomen shows large mass on the left displacing descending colon. Mass was clinically impressive. **b** Film three hours post-intravenous contrast injection shows excessive dilatation of left renal pelvis and calyces with relative high contrast intensity; moderate right hydronephrosis. Scintigraphic estimation of renal function was 69% on the left, 31% on the right. Bilateral hydronephrosis had been discovered by fetal ultrasonography

Clinical Aspects

When evaluating a child's abdominal mass, the patient's age, sex, history and clinical findings are the most important parameters to be included in the process of establishing a diagnosis. This renders pediatric radiology a distinct clinical specialty. Two different processes may look morphologically similar, yet have completely different pathogenesis and significance. With the necessary clinical information and professional experience, one should be able to make a reasonable or even distinct diagnosis in a given case (Fig. 2, 3). On the other hand, the abdominal mass may be an incidental observation by the child or the parent and there may be no additional symptoms. A child with *nephroblastoma*, unless traumatized, commonly presents with a large abdominal mass, without pain and apparently in good health. Parents may report that the mass appeared quite suddenly. Such a remark is not unusual, since nephroblastoma is known for its rapid growth. *Neuroblastoma*, on the other hand, may lead to symptoms such as pallor, fatigue and failure to thrive. Morphologically, each of these two retroperitoneal tumors has specific characteristics that render the diagnosis in the majority of instances. However, each may present a differential diagnostic challenge (Fig. 4, 5).

An *inflammatory mass* is commonly caused by an infectious process, such as appendicitis or infection of the urogenital tract. Therefore, the signs and symptoms, including laboratory data, are those of an infectious disease and are often associated with abdominal pain. Local or diffuse pain, although quite nonspecific,

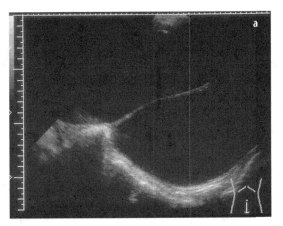

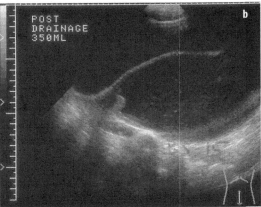

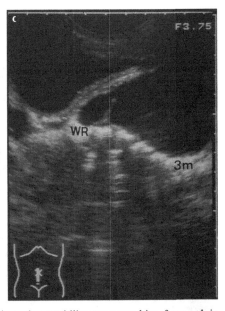

Fig. 3. Hematocolpos in a 15-year-old adolescent with acute urinary retention. Midsagittal ultrasonography through anterior lower abdomen shows two partially superimposed cystic structures similar to Fig. 2 (**a** before and **b** after spontaneous micturition). With a less filled bladder, numerous tiny echoes due to menstruation and uterine cervix are noticeable

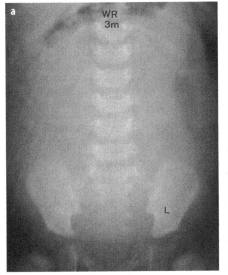

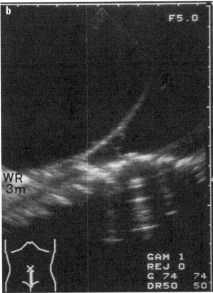

Fig. 2. Cystic teratoma in a 3-week-old girl with urinary retention. **a** Plain film of abdomen shows huge midline mass reaching from pelvic floor to displaced stomach. Midsagittal ultrasonographic scans through anterior lower abdomen show two partially superimposed cystic structures (**b** before, **c** after catheterization of bladder). Catherization helps in distinguishing antero-superior bladder with changing volume from infero-posterior cystic teratoma. Tiny linear structure in cranial aspect of teratoma is a hint for diagnosis

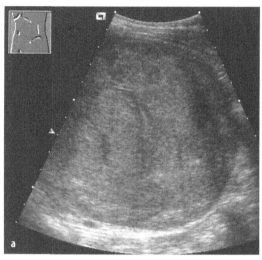

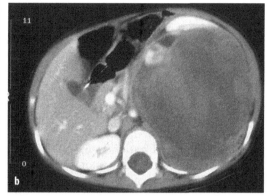

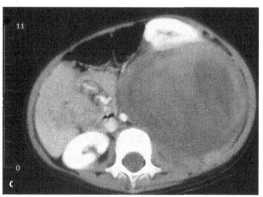

Fig. 4. Nephroblastoma in a 2-year-old boy with painless left abdominal mass. Left coronal ultrasonographic scan shows apparently solid tumor mass in left flank suspected to be a Wilms' tumor (**a**). Intravenously enhanced CT scans through mid part of well defined tumor (**b, c**) shows its dorsally exophytic growth; irregular contrast enhancement suggests partial tumor necrosis

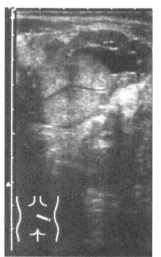

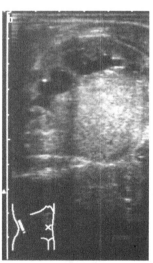

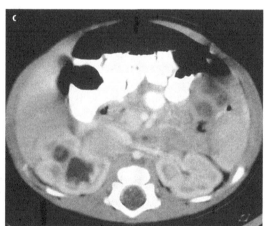

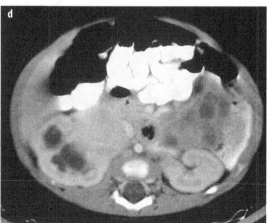

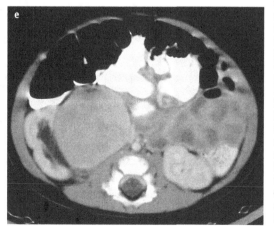

Fig. 5. Neuroblastoma in a 6-week-old boy causing ipsilateral urinary obstruction. Transverse ultrasonography with the child prone (**a**) and coronal scan (**b**) demonstrate solid echogenic mass next to right kidney; obstructive hydronephrosis from proximal extrinsic ureteral compression due to tumor. Renal artery is engulfed by mass (**a**); arterial Doppler signal not illustrated. Intravenously contrast-enhanced CT shows correlating features on three consecutive scans (**c, d, e**), including displacement and compression of inferior vena cava

is the most frequent symptom in abdominal disease, whether or not there is an appreciable anatomical correlate. Pain may also be a sequela of a noninflammatory mass that has been traumatized. Beside pain, functional abnormality of an organ system, fever, loss of weight and/or appetite, systemic disease, and even severe illness are all nonspecific in conjunction with an abdominal mass and do not, per se, indicate malignancy. Some may, however, be characteristic of a specific disease process such as *lymphoma, leukemia* or *metastatic disease.*

Urinary retention may be a serious symptom. Therefore, a pre- or rather, *retrorectal mass* causing the symptom must be excluded or differentiated (Fig. 1, 2). On the other hand, clinical uncertainty means that 'urinary retention' is a notoriously claimed symptom leading to imaging procedures recommended because of inadequate evaluation of the patient's history (e.g., no fluid intake for many hours with a subsequent lack of urine production and, thus, an empty bladder).

Approach to an Abdominal Mass

In attempting to diagnose and characterize an abdominal mass, the anatomical site of origin should be sought. Abdominal compartmentalization (as shown in Table 1) may help to localize a mass in one patient, but may be theoretical in another. Due to its large size, a mass may present as being intra-abdominal even though it may have originated in the retroperitoneum. It might be difficult to decide whether a mass is located in the abdomen or in the chest or whether it involves both compartments (such as in cases of neuroblastoma). Nephroblastoma and neuroblastoma are 'typical' retroperitoneal masses of childhood, and their renal or extrarenal origin may be readily recognizable, although an 'unusual case' may unpredictably present. As for a pelvic mass, it is useful to differentiate whether its origin is prerectal, rectal (i.e., stool) or retrorectal. A hepatic mass is usually recognizable as such and can mostly be differentiated from an anterior abdominal mass of another origin. The final imaging diagnosis or differential diagnosis will depend on the macroscopic tissue characterization of a mass (i.e., solid, cystic, mixed), its architecture and definition, whether it is solitary or multiple (possibly metastatic) and involving one specific or more than one organ system.

Table 1. Differential site of origin of an abdominal mass

Peritoneum versus retroperitoneum
Abdomen versus thorax versus both
Kidney versus extrarenal location
Pelvis versus upper anterior abdomen
Liver versus extrahepatic location

Imaging an Abdominal Mass

US is probably the most popular imaging method in children. Its use is becoming more widespread, also among pediatricians who may not place it in any further imaging context. However, a *plain radiography of the child's abdomen in recumbent position* is strongly recommended when there is suspicion of an abdominal mass and in view of further exploration of the abdomen by imaging means. An initial appreciation of the mass process with regard to its location, size, density (e.g., calcifications) and effect upon adjacent structures (including the skeleton) and its possible interference with the gastrointestinal and/or urinary tracts may be useful to guide the course of imaging evaluation. With this preliminary information, subsequent US is often more straightforward and rewarding, taking into account also the child's history, clinical findings and laboratory results. The finding from the initial abdominal radiography (or US) may prompt an additional radiography of the chest that may, in a positive or negative way, contribute to the diagnostic work-up.

US is the most versatile and effective method for taking a first thorough look at the child's abdominal content. It is generally important to use US to initially explore the child's abdomen systematically and carefully. In an abdominal mass, US is often sufficient to establish a reasonable diagnostic assumption based on the anatomical facts. Often, even a specific diagnosis becomes probable by US, so that a given hypothesis about a solid lesion then may need only biopsy for confirmation and possible initiation of treatment. For a nonspecific solid mass found by US, biopsy is the obvious next step (Fig. 6). The strength of US lies in its ability to allow the appreciation of anatomical structures; its limits are in the estimation of organ function, even if there are certain exceptions. On the other hand, Doppler US is used routinely for demonstrating the presence or absence of arterial and/or venous blood flow. It also helps, among the definition of numerous other anatomical structures, to distinguish the hepatic segments. US is the only imaging tool that can provide diagnostic information by making use of physiological organ movement from respiration. Free movement of the liver over a renal or suprarenal mass (due to nephroblastoma or neuroblastoma) indicates that the peritoneum is likely not to be involved by the retroperitoneal mass. Similarly, demonstration of some local change of relationship between an adrenal neuroblastoma and the ipsilateral kidney indicates likely anatomical separation between the two structures. In the follow-up evaluation of an abdominal mass by US, other criteria become useful parameters, such as persistence or change of size, shape, and echogenicity of a given mass. In the morphologically ambiguous situation of a hematoma, its echo characteristics typically change within days, while a solid tumor's do not, unless it has been traumatized.

The improved availability of 'high end' imaging equipment such as MRI and multislice computed to-

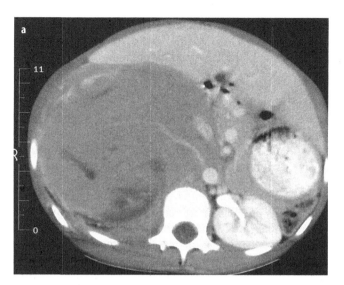

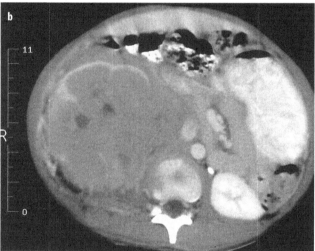

Fig. 6. B-non-Hodgkin lymphoma in a seven and a half year-old boy who had shown pallor and fatigue for a few weeks. CT with intravenous contrast enhancement shows mid portion of right flank mass (**a**, **b**). Mass appears mostly solid and seems to grow intra- and perirenally. Despite the unusual morphological aspect (and reduced health of the patient) the misdiagnosis of nephroblastoma was made, prompting suboptimal treatment and subsequent fatal outcome. Biopsy would have been indicated prior to therapy

mography (MSCT), leads to their more frequent use for evaluating abdominal masses in children. Given the professional effort to protect children from unnecessary radiation and following the 'ALARA' concept (as low as reasonably achievable), there is a tendency to make use of diagnostic MRI. On the other hand, MSCT allows fast and efficient imaging, which is quite attractive for use in children, as it renders complicated anesthesia unnecessary. In neuroblastoma, especially of the thoracic or thoraco-abdominal type that has a tendency to involve the spinal canal, if available, MRI is the modality of choice. One has to be aware of the fact that in spinal involvement by neuroblastoma, neurological abnormality or dysfunction is often rather mild or even absent. MRI is

recommended in a solid or cystic pelvic mass, especially if it is due to some gynecologic malformation (e.g., hydro- or hemato-metrocolpos) or neoplasia. The need for immobility means that the pelvis and retroperitoneum are better suited for evaluation by MRI than the anterior abdomen, which is more exposed to physiological motion from cardiac and respiratory dynamics. While the imaging technique is considerably improved through the use of cardiac and respiratory gating and rapid sequences, there are often difficulties in aiming for high diagnostic precision, especially in infants and young children. MRI is, nevertheless, recommended in tumorous abnormalities of the liver and biliary tract for morphological analysis of the mass, as well as the involved canalicular hepatic structures.

MSCT and CT are excellent at defining an abdominal mass, either benign or malignant. CT characterizes the mass by measuring its density, it localizes the mass and demonstrates its extension, both with high precision. In most instances it is possible to locate the organ or site of origin of a mass. In a malignancy, tumor spread may be accurately recognized, as well as enlarged or unenlarged lymph nodes, as possible metastatic manifestations. The degree of uptake of systemically introduced contrast material by a solid mass allows estimation of its perfusion (i.e., vitality) and, conversely, the lack of perfusion may point toward necrosis of the mass. The same applies to MRI. Perfusion criteria may be valuable when evaluating a potentially metastatic lesion using either method. MSCT and CT are most accurate and practical for diagnosing nephroblastoma, its spread and further complications within the regions of the abdomen, chest and skull. Two-dimensional and Doppler US for the evaluation of venous tumor spread up to the right atrium are the complementary examinations of choice. MSCT and CT are excellent for diagnosing and staging abdominal lymphoma and other infiltrative or complex abdominal masses (Fig. 7). However, MRI may be used with comparable accuracy.

In view of possible functional disturbance of the urogenital and/or gastrointestinal tract by the mass, scintigraphy and/or conventional digital radiographic/fluoroscopic contrast studies may be necessary in the diagnostic work-up. These will yield functional as well as additional or confirmatory anatomic information. Biliary scintigraphy may be considered for a cystic hepatic mass in order to demonstrate or exclude a direct or indirect relationship of the mass with the biliary system. Skeletal scintigraphy may be helpful for evaluating metastatic disease, i.e., in staging of neuroblastoma or other bone metastasizing abdominal malignancies. However, MRI may be used instead of scintigraphy in the diagnostic work-up of metastatic bone disease. Meta-iodobenzylguanidine (MIBG) scintigraphy is valid for demonstrating various forms of primary and/or metastatic neuroectodermal tumors.

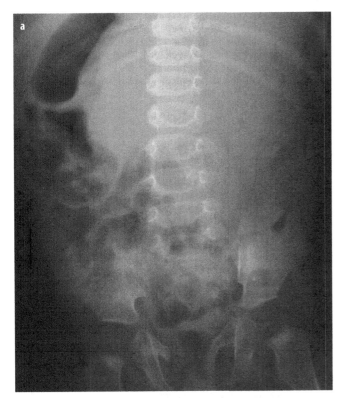

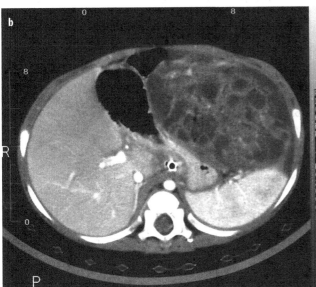

Fig. 7a, b. Gastric wall teratoma in a 7-month-old boy with painless abdominal mass. **a** Plain abdominal radiograph shows large mass in left upper abdomen displacing stomach and intestinal structures and containing calcifications. **b** Axial CT scan with intravenous contrast enhacement through upper abdominal area demonstrates large intra-abdominal, well-defined heterogeneous mass of generally low density in close relationship with thin left gastric wall and ventrally to pancreatic tail and spleen

Biopsy ·

In a potentially malignant mass, histological characterization or proof is required in almost all instances prior to deciding on specific therapy (immediate or secondary tu-

mor excision after initial chemotherapy). In lymphoma or leukemia, surgery is usually not indicated. Transcutaneous biopsy under direct vision by US or controlled by CT is a well established procedure in children, and should be performed under general anesthetic. CT is recommended as a safe alternative if direct guidance by US is difficult to achieve or is unsafe because of the small size or problematic location of the target lesion (e.g., a paravertebral process).

Malignant Abdominal Mass

The most common malignant abdominal masses are of embryological origin, i.e., neuroblastoma, nephroblastoma (Wilms' tumor), and hepatoblastoma followed by lymphoma, germ cell tumor and soft tissue sarcoma (Table 2). Although it is usually possible to locate the site of origin of a retroperitoneal tumor as renal or extrarenal, there may be occasional morphological difficulties in the differentiation between neuroblastoma and nephroblastoma. As stated before, the clinical condition may be helpful in distinguishing the two entities, although biopsy will yield the diagnostic basis for further management and therapeutic decisions. The differential diagnoses of nephroblastoma are listed in Table 3. Lymphoma and leukemia have to be considered as differential diagnostic alternatives in some unusual morphological presentations (Fig. 6). Both may also be considered in the differential diagnosis of rhabdomyosarcoma or a primitive neuroectodermal tumor (PNET). Depending on the differentiation, germ cell tumors are often benign. With regard to the ovary, the differential diagnoses of malignant germ cell tumors are listed in

Table 2. Common malignant abdominal tumors in the child

Nephroblastoma (Wilms' tumor)
Neuroblastoma, including hepatic metastases in stage IVs
Hepatoblastoma
Lymphoma
Germ cell tumor
Soft tissue sarcoma (rhabdomyosarcoma, PNET, Ewing)

Table 3. Differential diagnosis of nephroblastoma

Nephroblastoma (favorable and unfavorable histology)
Nephroblastomatosis (precursor of nephroblastoma, often bilateral, synchronous or not synchronous)
Clear cell sarcoma (formerly bone metastasizing tumor of kidney)*
Rhabdoid renal tumor (sarcoma)*
Renal cell carcinoma
Transitional cell carcinoma
Malignant renal lymphoma
Intrarenal growth of neuroblastoma
Congenital mesoblastic nephroma (benign)
Multilocular cystic nephroma (benign)

* high grade malignancy

Table 4. Tumor of the ovary

A) GERM CELL:
  Seminoma (i.e., dysgerminoma)
  'Mature' teratoma (20% malignant)
  'Immature' teratoma (100% malignant)
  Embryonal carcinoma
  Yolk sac tumor (usually high grade malignancy)
  Choriocarcinoma

B) SPECIALIZED GONADAL STROMA:
  Granulosa-theca cell tumor
  Sertoli cell tumor

C) OTHERS:
  Rhabdomyosarcoma
  Neuroectodermal tumor
  Lymphoma, leukemia

Table 4. The soft tissue sarcomas comprise the rhabdomyosarcoma, the primitive neuroectodermal tumor (PNET) and the Ewing sarcoma.

Conclusions

Prompt diagnosis and characterization of an abdominal mass in a child is an ever new challenge of diagnostic imaging. Awareness of the specific pediatric conditions (pathophysiology, changing anatomy of the growing organism, age-related and characteristic pathology) is a prerequisite with regard to a correct interpretation of the findings, as well as to the prompt and successful preceeding acquisition of imaging data. The experience and bias of the radiologist performing the evaluation, in terms of the choice of diagnostic instruments, will and should influence the choice of the technical procedure(s). However, there are procedural recommendations that have general validity. Professional expertise combined with state-of-the-art technology allows highly accurate diagnostic imaging, sometimes even by the simple means of US and X-ray. Technically more powerful and sophisticated equipment such as MRI and MSCT may be indispensable and the method(s) of choice in numerous cases. Yet, one should remember that there are always challenges to differential diagnosis and the very unexpected case may be waiting even for the skilled and experienced diagnostician.

Suggested Reading

Renal tumor, nephroblastoma
Agrons GA, Wagner BJ, Davidson AJ, Suarez ES (1995) Multilocular cystic renal tumor in children: radiologic-pathologic correlation. Radiographics 15:653-669
Broecker B (2000) Non-Wilms' renal tumor in children. Urol Clin North Am 27:463-469
El Kababri M, Khattab M, El Khorassani M et al (2004) Clear cell sarcoma of the kidney. A study of 13 cases. Arch Pediatr 11:794-799 (article in French)
Geller E, Smergel EM, Lowry PA (1997) Renal neoplasms of childhood. Radiol Clin North Am 35:1391-1413

Glick RD, Hicks MJ, Nuchtern JG et al (2004) Renal tumors in infants less than 6 months of age. J Pediatr Surg 39:522-525
Han TI, Kim MJ, Yoon HK et al (2001) Rhabdoid tumour of the kidney: imaging findings. Pediatr Radiol 31:233-237
Jenkner A, Camassei FD, Boldrini R et al (2001) 111 renal neoplasms of childhood: a clinicopathologic study. J Pediatr Surg 36:1522-1527
Lowe LH, Isuani BH, Heller RM et al (2000) Pediatric renal masses: Wilms tumor and beyond. Radiographics 20:1585-1603
Lonergan GJ, Martinez-Leon MI, Agrons GA et al (1998) Nephrogenic rests, nephroblastomatosis, and associated lesions of the kidney. Radiographics 18:447-468
Luo CC, Lin JN, Jaing TH et al (2002) Malignant rhabdoid tumour of the kidney occurring simultaneously with brain tumour: a report of two cases and review of the literature. Eur J Pediatr 161:340-342
McLorie GA (2001) Wilms' tumor (nephroblastoma). Curr Opin Urol 11:567-570
McNeil DE, Brown M, Ching A, deBaum MR (2001) Screening for Wilms tumor and hepatoblastoma in children with Beckwith-Wiedemann syndromes: a cost-effective model. Med Pediatr Oncol 37:349-356
Muir TE, Cheville JC, Lager DJ (2001) Metanephric adenoma, nephrogenic rests, and Wilms' tumor: a histologic and immunophenotypic comparison. Am J Surg Pathol 25:1290-1296
Shenk JP, Engelmann D, Ziegler B et al (2005) Radiologic differentiation of rhabdoid tumor from Wilms' tumor and mesoblastic nephroma. Urologe A 44:155-161 (article in German)
Scott DJ, Wallace WH, Hendry GM (1999) With advances in medical imaging can the radiologist reliably diagnose Wilms' tumours? Clin Radiol 54:321-327
Trobs RB, Hansel M, Friedrich T, Bennek J (2001) A 23-year experience with malignant renal tumors in infancy and childhood. Eur J Pediatr Surg 11:92-98
Vujanic GM, Sandstedt B, Harms D et al (2002) Revised international society of paediatric oncology (SIOP) working classification of renal tumors of childhood. Med Pediatr Oncol 38:79-82

Adrenal masses, neuroblastoma
Agrons GA, Lonergan GJ, Dickey GE, Perenz-Monte JE (1999) Adrenocortical neoplasms in children: radiologic-pathologic correlation. Radiographics 19:989-1008
Alexander F (2000) Neuroblastoma. Urol Clin North Am 27:383-392
Berdon WE, Stylianos S, Ruzal-Shapiro C et al (1999) Neuroblastoma arising from the organ of Zuckerkandl: an unusual site with a favorable biologic outcome. Pediatr Radiol 29:497-502
de Luca JL, Rousseau T, Durand C et al (2002) Diagnostic and therapeutic dilemma with large prenatally detected cystic adrenal masses. Fetal Diagn Ther 17:11-16
Hachitanda Y, Hata J (1996) Stage IVS neuroblastoma: a clinical, histological, and biological analysis of 45 cases. Hum Pathol 27:1135-1138
Hiorns MP, Owens CM (2001) Radiology of neuroblastoma in children. Eur Radiol 11:2071-2081
Ilias I, Pacak K (2005) Diagnosis and management of tumors of the adrenal medulla. Horm Metab Res 37:717-721
Kadah NM, Dessouky NM (2003) Functioning adrenal tumors in children: a report of 17 cases. Saudi Med J 24:S46-S47
Nadler EP, Barksdale EM (2000) Adrenal masses in the newborn. Semin Pediatr Surg 9:156-164
Rescorla FJ (2006) Malignant adrenal tumors. Semin Pediatr Surg 15:48-56

Hepatic mass
Donelly LF, Bisset GS 3rd (1998) Pediatric hepatic imaging. Radiol Clin North Am 36:413-427
Fabre M, Yilmaz F, Buendia MA (2004) Hepatic tumors in childhood: experience on 245 tumors and review of the literature. Ann Pathol 24:536-555 (article in French)

Iyer CP, Stanley P, Mahour GH (1996) Hepatic hemangiomas in infants and children: a review of 30 cases. Am Surg 62:356-360

Lack EE, Ornvold K (1986) Focal nodular hyperplasia and hepatic adenoma: a review of eight cases in the pediatric age group. J Surg Oncol 33:129-135

Meyers RL Scaife ER (2000) Benign liver and biliary tract masses in infants and toddlers. Semin Pediatr Surg 9:146-155

Reymond D, Plaschkes J, Luthy AR et al (1995) Focal nodular hyperplasia of the liver in children: review of follow-up and outcome. J Pediatr Surg 30:1590-1593

Reynolds M (1999) Pediatric liver tumors. Semin Surg Oncol 16:159-172

Senyuz OF, Celayir AC, Kilic N et al (1999) Hydatid disease of the liver in childhood. Pediatr Surg Int 15:217-220

von Schweinitz D, Gluer S, Mildenberger H (1995) Liver tumors in neonates and very young infants: diagnostic pitfalls and therapeutic problems. Eur J Pediatr Surg 5:72-76

Ovarian mass

1) Lee HJ, Woo SK, Kim JS, Suh SJ (2000) 'Daughter cyst' sign: a sonographic finding of ovarian cyst in neonates, infants and young children. AJR Am J Roentgenol 174:1013-1015

McCarville MB, Hill DA, Miller BE, Pratt CB (2001) Secondary ovarian neoplasms in children: imaging features with histopathologic correlation. Pediatr Radiol 31:358-364

Morowitz M, Huff D, von Allmen D (2003) Epithelial ovarian tumors in children: a retrospective analysis. J Pediatr Surg 38:331-335

Pomeranz AJ, Sabnis S (2004) Misdiagnoses of ovarian masses in children and adolescents. Pediatr Emerg Care 20:172-174

Schultz KA, Sencer SF, Messinger Y et al (2005) Pediatric ovarian tumors: a review of 67 cases. Pediatr Blood Cancer 44:167-173

Skiadas VT, Koutoulidis V, Eleytheriades M et al (2004) Ovarian masses in young adolescents: imaging findings with surgical confirmation. Eur J Gynaecol Oncol 25:201-206

Abdominal and pelvic mass

Defoor W, Minevich E, Sheldon C (2002) Unusual bladder masses in children. Urology 60:911

Haddad MC, Birjawi GA, Hemadeh MS et al (2001) The gamut of abdominal and pelvic cystic masses in children. Eur Radiol 11:148-166

Konen O, Rathaus V, Dlugy E et al (2002) Childhood abdominal cystic lymphangioma. Pediatr Radiol 32:88-92

Luo CC, Huang CS, Chao HC et al (2004) Intra-abdominal cystic lymphangioma in infancy and childhood. Chang Gung Med J 27:509-514

Luo CC, Huang CS, Chu SM et al (2005) Retroperitoneal teratomas in infancy and childhood. Pediatr Surg 21:536-540

McHugh K, Pritchard J (2001) Problems in the imaging of three common paediatric solid tumours. Eur J Radiol 37:72-80

Sebire NJ, Fowler D, Ramsay AD (2004) Sacrococcygeal tumors in infancy and childhood: a retrospective histopathological review of 85 cases. Fetal Pediatr Pathol 23:295-303

Wang JS, Lee HC, Sheu JC et al (1999) Pancreatic tumors in children: report of three cases. Acta Paediatr Taiwan 40:335-338

Wotton-Gorges SL, Thomas, KB, Harned RK et al (2005) Giant cystic abdominal masses in children. Pediatr Radiol 35:277-1288

Yang DM, Jung DH, Kim H et al (2004) Retroperitoneal cystic masses: CT, clinical, and pathologic findings and literature review. Radiographics 24:1353-1365

Imaging (MRI, Scintigraphy)

Angerpointner TA (2005) Abdominal tumours in children: 3-D visualisation and surgical planning. J Pediatr Surg 40:1219

Connolly LP, Drubach LA, Ted Treves S (2002) Applications of nuclear medicine in pediatric oncology. Clin Nucl Med 27:117-125

Goo HW, Choi SH, Ghim T et al (2005) Whole-body MRI of paediatric malignant tumours: comparison with conventional oncological imaging methods. Pediatr Radiol 35:766-773

Hoffer FA (2005) Magnetic resonance imaging of abdominal masses in the pediatric patient. Semin Ultrasound CT MR 26:212-223

Pfluger T, Leinsinger G, Sander A et al (1999) Magnetic resonance imaging of benign and premalignant tumors in childhood. Radiologe 39:685-694 (article in German)

Shun PI, McCowage G, Howman-Giles R (2002) Positron emission tomography in recurrent hepatoblastoma. Pediatr Sur Int 21:341-345

Biopsy

Drut R, Drut RM, Pollono D et al (2005) Fine-needle aspiration biopsy in pediatric oncology patients: a review of experience with 829 patients (899 biopsies). J Pediatr Hematol Oncol 27:370-376

Hussain HK, Kingston JE, Domizio P et al (2001) Imaging-guided core biopsy for the diagnosis of malignant tumors in pediatric patients. AJR Am J Roentgenol 176:43-47

Sklair-Levy M, Lebensart PD, Applbaum YH et al (2001) Percutaneous image-guided needle biopsy in children – summary of our experience with 57 children. Pediatr Radiol 31:732-736

Thiesse P, Hany MA, Combaret V et al (2000) Assessment of percutaneous fine needle aspiration cytology as a technique to provide diagostic and prognostic information in neuroblastoma. Eur J Cancer 36:1544-1551

Vujanic GM, Kelsey A, Mitchell C et al (2003) The role of biopsy in the diagnosis of renal tumor of childhood: results of the UKCCSG Wilms tumor study 3. Med Pediatr Oncol 40:18-22

Pediatric oncology

Gadner H, Gaedicke G, Niemeyer C, Ritter J (2006) Pädiatrische Hämatologie und Onkologie, (German) Springer, Berlin Heidelberg

Pizzo PA, Poplack DG (eds) (2002) Principles and practice of pediatric oncology, 4th edn. Lippincott, Philadelphia

Voute PA, Kalifa C, Barrett A (1998) Cancer in children, 4th edn. Oxford University Press, Oxford